Clinical Guide to Cardiology

The *Clinical Guides* Series

Series Editor: Christian Camm

The Clinical Guides are a brand new resource for junior doctors and medical students.

They provide practical and concise day-to-day information on common conditions, symptoms and problems faced in the clinical environment. They are easy to navigate and allow swift access to information as it is needed, with step-by-step guidance on decision making, investigations and interventions, and how to survive and thrive on clinical rotation and attachment.

This new title is also available as an e-book.
For more details, please see
www.wiley.com/buy/9781118755334
or scan this QR code:

Clinical Guide to Cardiology

Edited by

Christian F. Camm
John Radcliffe Hospital, Oxford, UK

A. John Camm
St. George's University of London, London, UK

WILEY Blackwell

This edition first published 2016 © 2016 by John Wiley & Sons, Ltd

Registered office: John Wiley & Sons, Ltd, The Atrium, Southern Gate, Chichester, West Sussex, PO19 8SQ, UK

Editorial offices: 9600 Garsington Road, Oxford, OX4 2DQ, UK
The Atrium, Southern Gate, Chichester, West Sussex, PO19 8SQ, UK
111 River Street, Hoboken, NJ 07030-5774, USA

For details of our global editorial offices, for customer services and for information about how to apply for permission to reuse the copyright material in this book please see our website at www.wiley.com/wiley-blackwell

Library of Congress Cataloging-in-Publication Data

Clinical guide to cardiology / edited by Christian F. Camm, A. John Camm.
     p. ; cm.
   Includes bibliographical references and index.
   ISBN 978-1-118-75533-4 (pbk.)
   I. Camm, Christian F. (Christian Fielder), editor.   II. Camm, A. John, editor.
   [DNLM: 1. Heart Diseases–diagnosis.   2. Heart Diseases–therapy.   WG 141]
   RC682
   616.1'2–dc23

                                        2015025343

A catalogue record for this book is available from the British Library.

Wiley also publishes its books in a variety of electronic formats. Some content that appears in print may not be available in electronic books.

Cover image: iStockphoto/© Nerthuz

Set in 8.5/10.5pt Frutiger Light by Aptara Inc., New Delhi, India

1   2016

Contents

Contributors

Laura Ah-Kye
King's College Hospital NHS Foundation Trust, London, UK

Kristopher Bennett
Whipps Cross Hospital, London, UK

Christian F. Camm
John Radcliffe Hospital, Oxford, UK

Lucy Carpenter
Barts Health NHS Trust, London, UK

Yang Chen
Imperial College Healthcare NHS Trust, London, UK

Ji-Jian Chow
Imperial College Healthcare NHS Trust, London, UK

James Cranley
Papworth Hospital NHS Foundation Trust, Cambridge, UK

George Davies
Oxford University Hospitals NHS Trust, Oxford, UK

Akshay Garg
King's College Hospital NHS Foundation Trust, London, UK

Harminder S. Gill
King's College Hospital NHS Foundation Trust, London, UK

Katie Glover
Guy's and St Thomas' NHS Foundation Trust, London, UK

Stephanie Hicks
King's College Hospital NHS Foundation Trust, London, UK

Fritz-Patrick Jahns
King's College Hospital NHS Foundation Trust, London, UK

Sophie Maxwell
Walsall Manor Hospital, Walsall, UK

Blair Merrick
Hammersmith Hospital, London, UK

Madeline Moore
King's College Hospital NHS Foundation Trust, London, UK

Sarah Morrow
Chelsea and Westminster Hospital, London, UK

Rahul K. Mukherjee
King's College Hospital NHS Foundation Trust, London, UK

Anna Robinson
King's College Hospital NHS Foundation Trust, London, UK

Arvind Singhal
Chelsea and Westminster Hospital NHS Foundation Trust, London, UK

Nicholas Sunderland
King's College Hospital NHS Foundation Trust, London, UK

Anneline te Riele
University Medical Centre, Utrecht, the Netherlands

Maria Tsakok
Hammersmith Hospital, London, UK

Robert A. Watson
Imperial College Healthcare NHS Trust, London, UK

Acronyms and Abbreviations

2D	two-dimensional
3D	three-dimensional
A2	aortic valve component of heart sound 2
AAA	abdominal aortic aneurysm
ABG	arterial blood gas
ABPM	ambulatory blood pressure monitoring
ACC	American College of Cardiology
ACE	angiotensin-converting enzyme
ACEi	angiotensin-converting enzyme inhibitor
ACR	albumin:creatinine ratio
ACS	acute coronary syndrome
ACTH	adrenocorticotropic hormone
ADP-P2Y	adenosine diphosphate-P2Y receptor
AF	atrial fibrillation
AHA	American Heart Association
AI	angiotensin I
AII	angiotensin II
AKI	acute kidney injury
ALD	alcoholic liver disease
ALP	alkaline phosphatase
ALS	advanced life support
AMA	American Medical Association
AMB	acute marginal branch
AMTS	Abbreviated Mental Test score
APS	antiphospholipid syndrome
aPTT	activated partial thromboplastin time
AR	aortic regurgitation
ARB	angiotensin-II receptor blocker
ARDS	acute respiratory distress syndrome
AS	aortic stenosis
ASD	atrial septal defect
AST	aspartate aminotransferase
ATP	adenosine triphosphate
AV	atrioventricular
AVN	atrioventricular node
AVNRT	AV-nodal re-entrant tachycardia
AVPU	alert/responsive to voice/responsive to pain/unresponsive
AVRT	atrioventricular re-entrant tachycardia
AVSD	atrioventricular septal defect
BAH	bilateral adrenocortical hyperplasia
BAV	balloon aortic valvuloplasty
BCS	British Cardiovascular Society
BD	twice a day
BE	base excess
beta-hCG	beta human chorionic gonadotrophin
BM	Boehringer-Mannheim – capillary glucose test
BMI	body mass index
BNP	brain natriuretic peptide

BP	blood pressure
BPH	benign prostatic hyperplasia
bpm	beats per minute
CABG	coronary artery bypass graft
CAC	coronary artery calcium
CAD	coronary artery disease
Cath Lab	(coronary) catheterization laboratory
CCB	calcium-channel blocker
CCF	congestive cardiac failure
CCP	cyclic citrullinated peptide
CCU	cardiac care unit
CK-MB	creatine kinase – MB isoform
CKD	chronic kidney disease
CMV	cytomegalovirus
CN	coagulase negative
CNS	central nervous system
CO	cardiac output
CoA	coarctation of the aorta
COPD	chronic obstructive pulmonary disease
COX	cyclo-oxygenase
CPAP	continuous positive airway pressure
CPR	cardiopulmonary resuscitation
CRP	C-reactive protein
CRT	cardiac resynchronization therapy
CRT-D	cardiac resynchronization therapy + cardiac defibrillator
CT	computed tomography
CTPA	computed tomography pulmonary angiogram
CTR	cardiothoracic ratio
CV(S)	cardiovascular (system)
CVA	cerebrovascular accident
CVD	cerebrovascular disease
CVP	central venous pressure
CXA	X-ray coronary angiography
CXR	chest X-ray
DAPT	dual anti-platelet therapy
DC	direct current
DCM	dilated cardiomyopathy
DH	drug history
DHP	dihydropyridine
DKA	diabetic ketoacidosis
DM	diabetes mellitus
DVLA	Driver and Vehicle Licensing Agency
DVT	deep vein thrombosis
EBV	Epstein–Barr virus
ECG	electrocardiogram
echo	echocardiogram
ED	emergency department
EDV	end-diastolic volume
EEG	electroencephalogram
EF	ejection fraction
EGDT	early goal-directed therapy
eGFR	estimated glomerular filtration rate
ELR	external loop recorder
EPS	electrophysiological study
ESC	European Society of Cardiology

ESM	ejection systolic murmur
ESR	erythrocyte sedimentation rate
ESV	end-systolic volume
EVAR	endovascular aneurysm repair
FAST	focused assessment with sonography for trauma
FBC	full blood count
FFP	fresh frozen plasma
FFR	fractional flow reserve
FH	family history
FY2	foundation year 2 doctor
G6PD	glucose-6-phosphate dehydrogenase
GCS	Glasgow coma scale
GFR	glomerular filtration rate
GI	gastrointestinal
GMP	guanosine monophosphate
GORD	gastro-oesophageal reflux disease
GP	general practitioner
GRA	glucorticoid-remediable aldosteronism
GRACE	Global Registry of Acute Coronary Events
GTN	glyceryl trinitrate
GZA	glycyrrhizic acid
HACEK	organisms associated with culture-negative infective endocarditis
Hb	haemoglobin
HbA1c	glycated haemoglobin
HBPM	home blood pressure monitoring
HCG	human chorionic gonadotrophin
HCM	hypertrophic cardiomyopathy
HDL	high density lipoprotein
HDU	high dependency unit
HF	heart failure
HF-PEF	heart failure with preserved ejection fraction
HF-REF	heart failure with reduced ejection fraction
HIT	heparin-induced thrombocytopenia
HIV	human immunodeficiency virus
HOCM	hypertrophic obstructive cardiomyopathy
HPC	history of the presenting complaint
HR	heart rate
HTN	hypertension
IABP	intra-aortic balloon pump
IC	intercostal
ICD	implantable cardioverting defibrillator
ICH	intracerebral haemorrhage
IE	infective endocarditis
IGG	immunoglobulin G
IHD	ischaemic heart disease
ILR	internal loop recorder
IM	intramuscular
INR	international normalized ratio.
ISMN	isosorbide mononitrate
ITU	intensive therapy unit
IV	intravenous
IVCD	intraventricular conduction delay
IVDU	intravenous drug user
IVUS	intravascular ultrasound
JVP	jugular venous pulse/pressure

LA	left atrium
Lac	lactate
LAD	left anterior descending coronary artery
LBBB	left bundle branch block
LCx	left circumflex artery
LDH	lactate dehydrogenase
LDL cholesterol	low density lipoprotein cholesterol
LFT	liver function test
LGV	large goods vehicle
LL	left leg
LMA	laryngeal mask airway
LMCA	left main coronary artery
LMWH	low molecular weight heparin
LQTS	long QT syndrome
LV	left ventricular/left ventricle
LVEDP	left ventricular end-diastolic pressure
LVEDV	left ventricular end-diastolic volume
LVEF	left ventricular ejection fraction
LVESD	left ventricular end-systolic diameter
LVH	left ventricular hypertrophy
LVOT	left ventricular outflow tract
LVOTO	left ventricular outflow tract obstruction
MAHA	microangiopathic haemolytic anaemia
MAOI	monoamine oxidase inhibitor
MAP	mean arterial pressure
MAU	medical assessment unit
MCA	middle cerebral artery
MCV	mean corpuscular volume
MDCT	multi-detector row computed tomography
MDM	multidisciplinary meeting
MDT	multidisciplinary team
MEN	multiple endocrine neoplasia
MI	myocardial infarction
MIBG	meta-iodobenzylguanidine
MR	mitral regurgitation
MRA	mineralocorticoid receptor antagonist
MRI	magnetic resonance imaging
MS	mitral stenosis
MVP	mitral valve prolapse
NAC	N-acetylcysteine
NBM	nil by mouth
NICE	National Institute for Health and Care Excellence
NOAC	novel oral anticoagulant
NPA	nasopharyngeal mask airway
NSAID	non-steroidal anti-inflammatory drug
NSTE ACS	non-ST-elevation acute coronary syndrome
NSTEMI	non-ST-elevation myocardial infarction
NYHA	New York Heart Association
OCT	optical coherence tomography
OD	once a day
OMB	obtuse marginal artery
OMT	optimal medical therapy
OR	odds ratio
OSCE	objective structured clinical examination
P2	pulmonary valve constituent of the second heart sound

PAD	peripheral arterial disease
P_aO_2	partial pressure of arterial oxygen
PCA	patient-controlled analgesia
PCC	prothrombin complex concentrate
PCI	percutaneous coronary intervention
PCR	protein:creatinine ratio
PCV	passenger-carrying vehicle
PDA	patent ductus arteriosus
PDE-5	phosphodiesterase-5
PE	pulmonary embolism
PEF	peak expiratory flow
PET	positron emission tomography
PFO	patent foramen ovale
PG	prostaglandin
PICC	peripherally inserted central catheter
PLV	posterior left ventricular branch
PMC	percutaneous mitral commisurotomy
PMH	past medical history
PND	paroxysmal nocturnal dyspnoea
PO	*per os* – taken orally
PP	pulse pressure
PPI	proton-pump inhibitor
PR	*per rectum*
PRN	*pro re nata* – as needed
PT	prothrombin time
PUO	pyrexia of unknown origin
PVI	pulmonary vein isolation
QDS	four times a day
QTc	corrected QT interval
RA	right atrium
RAA	renin–angiotensin–aldosterone
RBBB	right bundle branch block
RCA	right coronary artery
RCM	restrictive cardiomyopathy
RCT	randomized controlled trial
RF	risk factor
ROSC	return of spontaneous circulation
RR	respiratory rate
RRR	relative risk reduction
RV	right ventricular
RVOT	right ventricular outflow tract
RVST	right ventricular systolic pressure
S1	heart sound 1
S2	heart sound 2
S3	heart sound 3
S4	heart sound 4
SAN	sinoatrial node
S_aO_2	saturation of arterial oxygen
SAVR	surgical aortic valve replacement
SBAR	situation/background/assessment/recommendation
SC	subcutaneously
SG	specific gravity
SHO	senior house officer
SIRS	systemic inflammatory response syndrome
SLE	systemic lupus erythematosus

SOB	shortness of breath
SOBOE	shortness of breath on exertion
SPECT	single-photon emission computed tomography
SpO$_2$	oxygen saturation
SpR	specialist registrar
SSRI	selective serotonin reuptake inhibitor
STE ACS	ST-elevation acute coronary syndrome
STEMI	ST-elevation myocardial infarction
SV	stroke volume
SVC	superior vena cava
SVR	systemic vascular resistance
SVT	supraventricular tachycardia
T-LOC	transient loss of consciousness
TA	transapical
TAVI	transaortic valve implantation
TB	tuberculosis
TDS	three times a day
TF	transfemoral
TFT	thyroid function test
TGA	transposition of the great arteries
TIA	transient ischaemic attack
TIMI	Thrombolysis In Myocardial Infarction (study)
TOE	transoesophageal echocardiogram
TR	tricuspid regurgitation
TSH	thyroid-stimulating hormone
TTE	trans-thoracic echocardiogram
TXA2	thomboxane A2
U&E	urea and electrolytes
UA	unstable angina
UFH	unfractionated heparin
USS	ultrasound scan
UTI	urinary tract infection
VBG	venous blood gas
VF	ventricular fibrillation
VKA	vitamin K antagonist
VSD	ventricular septal defect
VT	ventricular tachycardia
VTE	venous thromboembolism
WCC	white cell count
WHO	World Health Organization
WPW	Wolff–Parkinson–White syndrome

About the Companion Website

This book is accompanied by a companion website:

www.wiley.com/go/camm/cardiology

The website includes:

- MCQs
- EMQs
- SAQs
- Clinical cases
- Audio
- Audio scripts

PART 1
Examination Techniques

1 Examination Techniques

Christian F. Camm

John Radcliffe Hospital, Oxford, UK

1.1 COMMON CONDITIONS TO BE LOOKED FOR ON THE EXAMINATION

1. Arrhythmias ■
2. Valvular pathology ■
3. Endocarditis ■
4. Heart failure ■
5. Ischaemic heart disease ■
6. Inherited cardiac conditions ■
7. Poor perfusion/shock ■
8. Anaemia ■

1.2 CLINICAL EXAMINATION – PERIPHERIES

Table 1.1 Elements to be undertaken prior to examining the patient

Item	Detail
1. Appropriate hand hygiene	Wash hands with soap and water or alcohol hand rub
2. Introduce yourself	Full name and job title
3. Confirm patient identity	Check full name and date of birth, verify against wrist band
4. Gain permission for the examination	Explain your role and what the examination will involve
5. Enquire about pain	Particularly chest and shoulder pain
6. Position the patient	45° on examination couch or bed
7. Expose the patient appropriately	Entire chest (women can leave bras on) Remember to cover patient when not examining the chest itself

---

1. Arrhythmias ■ 2. Valvular pathology ■ 3. Endocarditis ■ 4. Heart failure ■ 5. Ischaemic heart disease ■ 6. Inherited cardiac conditions ■ 7. Poor perfusion/shock ■ 8. Anaemia ■

Clinical Guide to Cardiology, First Edition. Edited by Christian F. Camm and A. John Camm.
© 2016 John Wiley & Sons, Ltd. Published 2016 by John Wiley & Sons, Ltd.
Companion website: www.wiley.com/go/camm/cardiology.

Table 1.2 Examination features from the end of the bed

Item	Detail
1. Does the patient look well?	• Sitting up and talking, or reduced consciousness? • Difficulty breathing? • Severe cyanosis? • Pallor? • Sweating?
2. Are there any obvious scars?	• Midline sternotomy • Lateral thoracotomy • Saphenous vein harvest scar • Pacemaker/ICD device or scar
3. Lines in and out of patient	• IV infusions • Catheters • Oxygen
4. Patient monitoring	• Continuous ECG • Pulse oximetry • Haemodynamic monitoring (e.g. blood pressure)
5. Any medications around the patient	• Glyceryl trinitrate (GTN) spray or inhalers • Drug infusions • Warfarin (or anticoagulation cards/booklets)

Table 1.3 Examination findings in the nails

Item	Conditions
1. Clubbing	■ / ■
2. Splinter haemorrhages	■
3. Capillary refill time >2 seconds	■
4. Peripheral cyanosis	■ / ■
5. Nicotine stains	▨

Box 1.1 Stages of clubbing

1. Fluctuation and softening of the nail bed
2. Loss of normal nail bed angle (Lovibond's angle)
3. Increased convexity of the nail fold
4. Thickening of the whole distal finger
5. Striations and increased shine on nails and surrounding skin

Table 1.4 Examination findings in the hand

Item	Conditions
1. Tendon xanthomata	■ / ▨
2. Osler nodes	■
3. Janeway lesions	■
4. Palmar crease pallor	■
5. Temperature	■
6. Bruising (anticoagulation or antiplatelet agents)	■

1. Arrhythmias ■ 2. Valvular pathology ■ 3. Endocarditis ■ 4. Heart failure ■ 5. Ischaemic heart disease ▨ 6. Inherited cardiac conditions ■
7. Poor perfusion/shock ■ 8. Anaemia ▨

Table 1.5 Examination findings in the wrist

Item	Conditions
1. Pulse rate	■ / ■
2. Pulse rhythm	■
3. Radio-radial delay	■
4. Radio-femoral delay	■
5. Collapsing pulse	■
6. Blood pressure	■ / ■ / ■ / ■

Table 1.6 Examination findings in the eyes

Item	Conditions
1. Corneal arcus	■/age
2. Conjunctival pallor	■
3. Petechial haemorrhages	■
4. Xanthelasma over eyelids	■
5. Roth spots	■
6. Lens dislocation	■

Table 1.7 Examination findings in the mouth

Item	Conditions
1. Hydration status	general
2. Dentition	■
3. Central cyanosis	■ / ■
4. High arched palate (Marfan's)	■

Table 1.8 Examination findings in the neck

Item	Conditions
1. Carotid pulse – character	■ / ■
2. JVP	■

Box 1.2 How to examine the JVP

1. Located between heads of sternocleidomastoid
2. JVP has double pulse (rather than single found in carotid)
3. JVP can be occluded
4. JVP may be made more visible by lowering angle of the bed
5. Hepato-jugular reflux
6. Height measured from the sternal angle (angle of Louis)

---

1. Arrhythmias ■ 2. Valvular pathology ■ 3. Endocarditis ■ 4. Heart failure ■ 5. Ischaemic heart disease ▨ 6. Inherited cardiac conditions ■
7. Poor perfusion/shock ■ 8. Anaemia ▨

Box 1.3   Central pulse character

1. **Slow rising:** aortic stenosis
2. **Small volume:** tachycardia, volume depletion, cardiogenic shock, aortic stenosis
3. **Bounding:** CO_2 retention, Paget's disease, aortic regurgitation
4. **Collapsing:** aortic regurgitation
5. **Pulsus bisferiens:** combined aortic stenosis and regurgitation

Table 1.9 Examination findings in the legs. This is often undertaken after examining the praecordium

Item	Conditions
Pitting oedema	■
Saphenous vein harvest scars	

1.3 CLINICAL EXAMINATION – THE PRAECORDIUM

Table 1.10 Inspection features of the praecordium

Item	Conditions
1. Scars	/■/■
2. Pacemaker/ICD	■/■
3. Visible apex beat	■/■

Table 1.11 Palpation features of the praecordium

Item	Conditions
1. Apex beat	■
2. Thrills	■ (aortic and pulmonary valve pathology)
3. Right ventricular heave	■/■

Box 1.4   The apex beat

1. Most lateral and inferior precordial cardiac pulsation
2. Normal position – fifth intercostal space, inside mid-clavicular line
3. Lateral and inferior displacement represents LV dilation
4. Diffuse apex beat represents LV dilation
5. Tapping of the apex beat is seen in mitral stenosis
6. Double impulse is a sign of hypertrophic obstructive cardiomyopathy

1. Arrhythmias ■ 2. Valvular pathology ■ 3. Endocarditis ■ 4. Heart failure ■ 5. Ischaemic heart disease ■ 6. Inherited cardiac conditions ■
7. Poor perfusion/shock ■ 8. Anaemia ■

Table 1.12 Auscultation of the praecordium

Location	Valve auscultated
1. Apex	Mitral valve
2. Fourth intercostal (IC) space, left sternal edge	Tricuspid valve + aortic (regurgitation)
3. Second IC space, left sternal edge	Pulmonary valve
4. Second IC space, right sternal edge	Aortic (stenosis)
5. Axilla	Mitral (reguritation)
6. Carotids	Aortic (stenosis) + carotid bruits

Box 1.5   Auscultatory elements

- To be successful at auscultation, it is important to actively listen (ask yourself what you can hear)
- The auscultatory elements that make up each cardiac cycle must be identified
- When identified, each component should then be characterized:
  1. **First heart sound:** mitral and tricuspid valve closure
  2. **Second heart sound:** aortic and pulmonary valve closure
  3. **Additional sounds:** S3, S4
  4. **Murmurs**
  5. **Non-valvular sounds:** e.g. pericardial rub
  6. **Mechanical heart valve sounds**

Box 1.6   Reinforcement manoeuvres

1. **Rolled to left side:** for mitral valve murmurs
2. **Hold breath in expiration:** left-sided murmurs
3. **Hold breath in inspiration:** right-sided murmurs
4. **Sit patient forward:** aortic regurgitation

Box 1.7   The first heart sound

- Caused by blood hitting the closed mitral and tricuspid valves
- Represents the start of ventricular systole
- Usually a single sound
- Heard best at the cardiac apex
  1. **Split sound:** bundle branch block
  2. **Soft S1:** first-degree AV block, aortic regurgitation
  3. **Loud S1:** mitral stenosis
  4. **Variable intensity:** ventricular arrhythmias, variable AV block

Box 1.8   The second heart sound

- Caused by blood hitting the closed aortic and pulmonary valves
- Represents the end of ventricular systole
- Heard well over the entire praecordium

1. Arrhythmias ■ 2. Valvular pathology ■ 3. Endocarditis ■ 4. Heart failure ■ 5. Ischaemic heart disease ▨ 6. Inherited cardiac conditions ■
7. Poor perfusion/shock ■ 8. Anaemia ▨

- Usually a split sound on inspiration
- Pulmonary component follows aortic
  1. **Widely split:** right bundle branch block
  2. **Fixed splitting:** atrial septal defects
  3. **Soft aortic component:** aortic stenosis

Table 1.13 Examination findings on the back

Item	Conditions
Lung bases	■
Sacral oedema	■

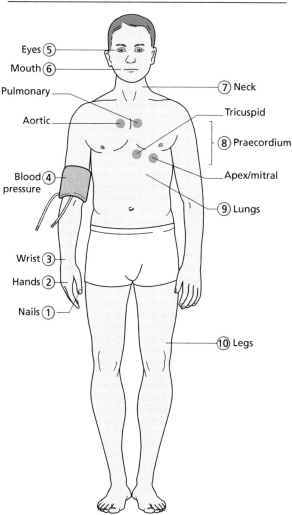

Figure 1.1 The examination circuit.

 (See Audio Podcast 1.1 at **www.wiley.com/go/camm/cardiology**)

1. Arrhythmias ■ 2. Valvular pathology ■ 3. Endocarditis ■ 4. Heart failure ■ 5. Ischaemic heart disease ▨ 6. Inherited cardiac conditions ■
7. Poor perfusion/shock ■ 8. Anaemia ▨

1.4 HOW TO PRESENT YOUR FINDINGS

Safety first approach
Details
- An approach that works well when not sure of your findings
- Useful for objective structured clinical examinations (OSCEs) to ensure that information is not missed
- Discuss the positive findings (and key negatives) in the order that you examined
- Give a potential diagnosis after presenting findings

Example

I examined this 52-year-old patient. He presented with shortness of breath and leg swelling. On inspection he was clearly dyspnoeic but otherwise appeared well. He was alert. There was a well healed midline sternotomy scar. His pulse was regular at 80 bpm. His blood pressure was 110/80 mmHg. The patient was well hydrated. The JVP was raised by 8 cm. There were no additional peripheral signs elucidated. On the praecordium he had no additional scars. His apex beat was not inappropriately located. On auscultation S1 and S2 were both heard. Additionally a third heart sound was heard across the praecordium. There were no additional sounds. There were inspiratory crackles at the lung bases and some sacral oedema. A clear scar along the course of the long saphenous vein was seen on the left leg, this was combined with bilateral pitting oedema reaching the mid-calf.

In conclusion, this patient presents with shortness of breath and signs suggestive of heart failure.

Ward-round based
Details
- An approach to be used when you are confident or pressed for time
- Give your suspected diagnosis first
- Discuss the examination findings that support the diagnosis and help to exclude others
- Discuss findings in the order of most supportive to least supportive of your diagnosis

Example

I examined this 52-year-old patient. He presented with shortness of breath and leg swelling. Examination revealed a patient with a clinical picture of congestive heart failure. This was supported by findings of inspiratory crackles at the lung bases, pitting oedema in the sacral region and bilaterally in the legs up to the mid-calf level. In addition, the JVP was raised to 8 cm above the angle of Louis. On auscultation S1 and S2 were clearly heard with the addition of a third heart sound. The patient has a history of coronary artery bypass surgery as supported by the midline sternotomy scar and long saphenous vein graft scar on the left leg. Given these findings, this suggests a history of heart failure potentially secondary to ischaemic heart disease.

1.5 EPONYMOUS SIGNS AND SYMPTOMS

Table 1.14 Eponymous signs in cardiology

Eponym	Details
Austin Flint murmur	Low-pitched rumbling murmur in mid-diastole due to aortic regurgitation causing mitral stenosis
Beck's triad	Three signs associated with cardiac tamponade: **i.** Low arterial blood pressure **ii.** Distended neck veins **iii.** Muffled heart sounds
Corrigan's pulse	A large-volume pulse which collapses away due to aortic regurgitation – observed at the carotid
De Musset's sign	Rhythmic nodding of the head due to increased pulse pressure in aortic regurgitation
Duroziez's sign	Compression of the femoral artery with the bell of the stethoscope leads to an audible diastolic murmur – aortic regurgitation
Ewart's sign	Collection of signs at the left lung base due to pericardial effusion: **i.** 'Woody' dullness to percussion **ii.** Increased vocal resonance **iii.** Bronchial breath sounds
Friedreich's sign	Significant drop in JVP during the diastolic phase due to constrictive pericarditis
Graham Steell murmur	Pulmonary regurgitant murmur heard in the left 2nd intercostal space
Janeway lesions	Non-tender, small erythematous nodular lesions on the palms/soles indicative of endocarditis
Kussmaul's sign	Paradoxical rise in JVP on inspiration, indicative of reduced right ventricular filling (e.g. right heart failure or constrictive pericarditis)
Mayne's sign	A drop >15 mmHg in diastolic blood pressure when the arm is raised – aortic regurgitation
Müller's sign	Bobbing of the uvula due to wide pulse pressure of aortic regurgitation
Oliver's sign	Downward tug of the trachea during systole – aneurysm of the aortic arch
Osler nodes	Painful, raised lesions on the hands/feet caused by immune complex deposition and suggestive of infective endocarditis
Osler's sign	Falsely elevated blood pressure due to calcification of the vessels
Quinke's pulse	Alternating blushing and blanching of the fingernails – aortic regurgitation
Roth spots	Retinal haemorrhages with a pale fibrin centre caused by immune complex deposition and suggestive of infective endocarditis
Still's murmur	Innocent flow murmur
Watson's waterhammer pulse	As with Corrigan's pulse, but observed over the radial artery

  For additional resources and to test your knowledge, visit the companion website at:

www.wiley.com/go/camm/cardiology

PART 2
Approach to Presenting Complaints

2 Chest Pain

Maria Tsakok
Hammersmith Hospital, London, UK

2.1 DEFINITION

Any pain or discomfort that is felt to originate in and around the thorax.

2.2 DIAGNOSTIC ALGORITHM

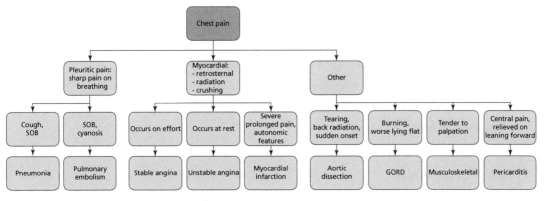

Figure 2.1 Algorithm for the diagnosis of chest pain.

2.3 DIFFERENTIALS LIST

Dangerous diagnoses
1. Acute coronary syndrome
2. Aortic dissection
3. Pulmonary embolism
4. Tension pneumothorax
5. Boerhaave's syndrome (oesophageal rupture)

Common diagnoses
1. Cardiac causes
   a. Stable angina
   b. Pericarditis
2. Pulmonary causes
   a. Pneumonia
   b. Pneumothorax
3. Gastrointestinal causes
   a. Gastro-oesophageal reflux disease
   b. Oesophageal spasm

Clinical Guide to Cardiology, First Edition. Edited by Christian F. Camm and A. John Camm.
© 2016 John Wiley & Sons, Ltd. Published 2016 by John Wiley & Sons, Ltd.
Companion website: www.wiley.com/go/camm/cardiology.

4. Musculoskeletal causes
   a. Rib contusions/fractures
   b. Intercostal muscle strains
   c. Costochondritis (including Tietze and Bornholm syndromes)

Diagnoses to consider
1. Psychiatric causes
2. Herpes zoster

2.4 KEY HISTORY FEATURES

(See Audio Podcast 2.1 at **www.wiley.com/go/camm/cardiology**)

Dangerous diagnosis 1
Diagnosis: Acute coronary syndrome

Questions
a. Is the pain crushing or heavy in nature?

These are the typical descriptions, but the pain may also be described as tight, gripping or pressing.

b. Does the pain radiate to the left arm or jaw?

These distinctive sites of radiation are highly suggestive of myocardial pain.

c. Are there associated autonomic symptoms?

Commonly nausea/vomiting and sweating.

d. Are there any cardiac risk factors?

See Box 2.1.

Box 2.1   Cardiac risk factors

Non-modifiable:

1. Increasing age
2. Male gender
3. Family history
4. Previous cardiovascular events
5. Diabetes

Modifiable:

1. Smoking
2. Hypertension
3. Obesity
4. Low physical activity

Dangerous diagnosis 2
Diagnosis: Aortic dissection

Questions
a. Is the pain tearing, central and extremely severe?

Interscapular when involving the descending aorta, anterior when involving the ascending aorta.

b. Does the pain radiate through to the back?

The pain may also radiate to the abdomen; these sites help distinguish dissection from ACS.

c. Sudden onset?

The pain occurs very suddenly, as the layers of the aorta are rapidly forced apart.

d. Was there associated collapse?

This implies large rupture and subsequent haemodynamic instability.

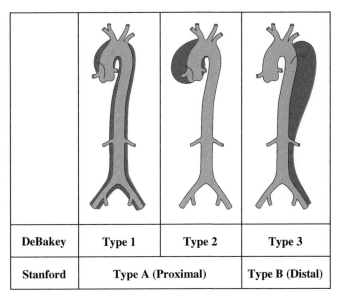

DeBakey	Type 1	Type 2	Type 3
Stanford	Type A (Proximal)		Type B (Distal)

Figure 2.2 Stanford classification.

Dangerous diagnosis 3
Diagnosis: Pulmonary embolism

Questions:
a. Does the pain worsen with inspiration, and is it 'sharp' or 'catching' in nature?

This is known as 'pleuritic' pain, and is usually localized to one side of the chest.

b. Was there acute-onset breathlessness or haemoptysis?

SOB is non-specific but if accompanied by haemoptysis, dizziness/syncope, may represent a significant PE.

c. Has the patient got any risk factors or features of deep venous thrombosis?

See Boxes 4.5 and 4.6 for risk factors for DVT and PE.

Dangerous diagnosis 4
Diagnosis: Tension pneumothorax

Questions
Note: Patients often present in acute respiratory distress and history is unobtainable – diagnosis is made on examination findings.
a. Any history of breathing difficulties or lung disease?

A pneumothorax occurring with pre-existing lung disease (COPD, asthma, TB etc.) is more likely to tension.

b. Has there been traumatic injury to the thorax?

Laceration of the lung may allow air to enter the pleural space but not to return, creating a 'one-way valve'.

Dangerous diagnosis 5
Diagnosis: Oesophageal rupture (Boerhaave's)

Questions

a. Did severe retching and vomiting precede the pain?

Retrosternal pain is usually felt suddenly – increased intra-oesophageal pressure due to vomiting is combined with negative intrathoracic pressure leading to oesophageal wall rupture.

b. Is there pain on swallowing, rapid and painful breathing or fever?

Patients with Boerhaave's rapidly develop odynophagia, tachypnoea/dyspnoea, fever and shock.

c. Is the patient an alcoholic or do they have a past medical history of gastric ulcers?

A history of alcoholism or gastric/duodenal ulcers increases the clinical suspicion of oesophageal rupture.

d. Has there been recent ablation to treat an arrhythmia?

Oesophageal thermal injury can occur during radiofrequency/cryoablation resulting in oesophageal rupture in the days to weeks post procedure.

Common diagnosis 1
Diagnosis: Stable angina

Questions

a. Is the pain a 'heavy' discomfort felt retrosternally?

The pain of angina is similar to that felt during ACS. It may also radiate to the left arm or jaw.

b. Is there a relationship between the onset of the pain and exercise?

Anginal pain is usually brought on by effort (exercise, stress, etc.) and relieved by <5 minutes' rest.

c. Are there any cardiac risk factors?

See Box 2.1.

d. Is the pain relieved by glyceryl trinitrate (GTN) spray/sublingual nitrate tablets?

GTN increases blood concentrations of nitric oxide, resulting in systemic vasodilation decreasing strain on the heart.

Common diagnosis 2
Diagnosis: Pericarditis

Questions

a. Is the pain relieved by sitting up and leaning forward, and exacerbated by inspiration, lying flat and coughing?

Pericardial pain differs from pleuritic pain by being both central and positional (worse lying down and better leaning forward).

b. Has there been a viral prodrome (cough, chills and weakness)?

Viral infection is the most common cause of pericarditis.

c. Does the medical history include a connective tissue disorder, severe renal disease, TB or malignancy?

These chronic conditions may result in inflammation of the pericardium.

d. Is the pain central and retrosternal, radiating to the arms and shoulders?

These are the typical characteristics of the pain.

Common diagnosis 3
Diagnosis: Pneumonia

Questions

a. Is the pain pleuritic in nature?

See Chapter 3 for description.

b. Are fever, rigors or new-onset confusion present?

These associated symptoms suggest an infective cause for the chest pain such as pneumonia.

c. Is there cough, productive of sputum?

A productive cough is typical of pneumonia. Sputum may be rusty coloured (as in pneumococcal infection) or purulent.

Common diagnosis 4
Diagnosis: Gastro-oesophageal reflux disease

Questions
a. Is the pain 'burning' in nature and related to meals?

The burning sensation is caused by the acidic contents of the stomach irritating the oesophageal squamous epithelium. It is felt retrosternally and is worse on lying down.

b. Are there any risk factors for GORD?

Hiatus hernia, obesity, overeating, smoking, alcohol and pregnancy all increase the risk of GORD.

c. Is the pain relieved by antacids?

Pain relief upon ingestion of antacids reliably indicates the chest pain is cause by reflux oesophagitis.

d. Is there belching, acid brash (acid/bile regurgitation), water brash (excessive swallowing) or pain on swallowing?

These symptoms constitute the oesophageal symptoms of GORD. Extra-oesophageal symptoms include nocturnal asthma, chronic cough, laryngitis and sinusitis.

Common diagnosis 5
Diagnosis: Oesophageal spasm

Questions
a. Is the pain retrosternal and does it involve the throat or epigastrium?

The characteristics of this pain vary (e.g. gripping, tight or stabbing) and can be difficult to differentiate from angina. It may radiate to the back, neck and arm.

b. Is there difficulty in swallowing?

Episodes of intermittent dysphagia and reflux-related symptoms (as above) can develop during spasm.

c. What precipitates the pain?

Hot or cold drinks may trigger an episode; pain is not exercise related.

Common diagnosis 6
Diagnosis: Musculoskeletal cause

Questions
a. Is there pain on movement of the chest?

This is typical of a musculoskeletal cause and decreases the likelihood of cardiac/pulmonary causes.

b. Is there a history of injury?

Intercostal muscle strain or rib contusion/fracture resulting from an injury are common causes.

Diagnosis to consider 1
Diagnosis: Psychiatric cause

Questions
a. Is there a history of anxiety or panic disorder?

Patients with a panic attack often complain of chest tightness and a sensation of impending doom. Useful screening questions are:

- In the past 6 months, have you suddenly felt anxious, frightened or very uneasy?
- In the past 6 months, has your heart suddenly began to race, have you felt faint, or couldn't you catch your breath for no apparent reason?

Diagnosis to consider 2
Diagnosis: Herpes zoster

Questions
a. Is the pain superficial and burning?

The pain may also be associated with hyperaesthesia/paraesthesia.

b. Is the pain confined to a particular area?

The pain is located in a unilateral, dermatomal distribution.

2.5 KEY EXAMINATION FEATURES

Dangerous diagnosis 1
Diagnosis: Acute coronary syndrome

Examination findings
a. Pallor, sweatiness, anxiety, distress

The ACS patient has a characteristic cold, clammy, grey appearance.

b. Blood pressure

Blood pressure may be high or low. Low blood pressure suggests haemodynamic shock.

c. Signs of acute complications

See Box 2.2.

Box 2.2 Signs of acute myocardial infarction complications

1. **Acute heart failure:** raised JVP, third heart sound, basal crepitations
2. **Papillary muscle rupture:** new pansystolic murmur
3. **Ventricular septal rupture:** new pansystolic murmur
4. **Ventricular free wall rupture:** signs of cardiac tamponade or shock

---

Dangerous diagnosis 2
Diagnosis: Aortic dissection

Examination findings
Note: Patients often present in shock with haemodynamic compromise so aggressive resuscitation and stabilization are required prior to formal examination.
a. Radio-radial delay

See Box 2.3.

b. Difference in BP (>20–25 mmHg systolic) between arms

This is an important sign and blood pressure should be checked in both arms in any patient presenting with severe chest pain.

c. Signs of cardiac tamponade

Beck's triad: low arterial blood pressure, muffled heart sounds and distended neck veins.

Box 2.3   Causes of radio-radial delay

1. Aortic dissection
2. Coarctation of the aorta
3. Cervical rib

Dangerous diagnosis 3
Diagnosis: Pulmonary embolus

Examination findings
a. Respiratory rate and heart rate

These are likely to be raised in a case of pulmonary embolism.

b. Signs of DVT

Oedema, erythema, tenderness or a palpable cord in the calf or thigh.

c. Signs of right heart strain

These include raised JVP, loud P2 (pulmonary valve constituent of the second heart sound) and a right ventricular heave. There is an increased work load on the right ventricle caused by increased pulmonary vascular resistance.

Dangerous diagnosis 4
Diagnosis: Tension pneumothorax

Examination findings
a. Hyper-resonance

Percussion reveals hyper-resonance on the affected side with reduced breath sounds on auscultation.

b. Shock

Hypotension, respiratory distress and tachycardia are seen as a result of reduced venous return to the heart.

c. Tracheal deviation

The mediastinum and trachea are pushed away from the side of tension pneumothorax.

d. Distended neck veins

This indicates impaired venous return in a tension pneumothorax.

Dangerous diagnosis 5
Diagnosis: Oesophageal rupture (Boerhaave's)

Examination findings
Note: Physical examination is not usually helpful, particularly early in the course.
a. Subcutaneous emphysema

An important diagnostic finding but has poor sensitivity in Boerhaave's rupture.

> **Box 2.4** Common causes of subcutaneous emphysema
>
> **1.** Pneumothorax
> **2.** Pneumomediastinum
> **3.** Trauma
> **4.** Infection (e.g. gas gangrene)
> **5.** Chest tube dysfunction

Common diagnosis 1
Diagnosis: Stable angina

Examination findings
Note: There are few clinical signs of stable angina.
a. Sweatiness, pallor, nausea, anxiety

This may be evident following any activity that increases myocardial oxygen demand.

Common diagnosis 2
Diagnosis: Pericarditis

Examination findings
a. Pericardial friction rub

The inflamed pericardial layers rubbing against each other cause a scratching/grating sound that may occupy all of systole and diastole. It is loudest in expiration and when leaning forward.

b. Pyrexia

Usually low-grade.

c. Ewart sign

Dullness and bronchial breathing between the tip of the left scapula and the vertebral column (may occur if there is an associated pericardial effusion) due to lower lobe compression of the left lung.

Common diagnosis 3
Diagnosis: Pneumonia

Examination findings
a. Signs of consolidation

Dull percussion note, reduced expansion, increased vocal resonance, bronchial breathing and potentially a pleural rub.

b. Pyrexia

Given the infective nature of pneumonia, patients usually present with a raised temperature.

c. Confusion

This may be the only sign in the elderly.

d. Tachypnoea and tachycardia

The extent of increase in respiratory rate is indicative of severity, justifying its inclusion in the CURB-65 score.

> **Box 2.5** CURB-65 Score: increasing score increases risk of mortality with community-acquired pneumonia
>
> - C – Confusion (Abbreviated Mental Test score (AMTS) ≤8)
> - U – Urea (>7 mmol/L)
> - R – Respiratory rate (≥30 per minute)
> - B – Blood pressure (<90 mmHg systolic)
> - 65 – Age (>65 years)

Common diagnosis 4
Diagnosis: Gastro-oesophageal reflux disease

Examination findings
No specific findings for this condition.

Common diagnosis 5
Diagnosis: Oesophageal spasm

Examination findings
No specific findings for this condition.

Common diagnosis 6
Diagnosis: Musculoskeletal cause

Examination findings
a. Pain reproduced on palpation

This is highly suggestive of the chest pain being derived from a precise location on the chest wall.

b. No signs of systemic involvement

This decreases the likelihood of a cardiac/pulmonary cause.

Diagnosis to consider 1
Diagnosis: Psychiatric cause

Examination findings
There are no specific examination findings although a mental state examination may be helpful. Diagnosis relies primarily on the history.

Diagnosis to consider 2
Diagnosis: Herpes zoster

Examination findings
a. Vesicular rash

The characteristic appearance is of small blisters on red, swollen skin distributed within a dermatome. However, the rash usually occurs after the onset of pain, making the diagnosis of herpes zoster initially more difficult.

(See Audio Podcast 2.2 and 2.3 at **www.wiley.com/go/camm/cardiology**)

2.6 KEY INVESTIGATIONS

Bedside

Table 2.1 Bedside tests of use in patients presenting with chest pain

Test	Justification	Expected result
Oxygen saturations	Important in any unwell/breathless patient, can help determine clinical severity	PE: decreased Pneumonia: decreased Pneumothorax: decreased
ECGs	Vital in any patient with chest pain. Serial ECGs are important in determining dynamic change.	See Box 2.6
Arterial blood gas (ABG)	Painful, only performed if patient is critically ill-and deteriorating	Respiratory failure (any cause): respiratory acidosis
Capillary glucose	Cardiovascular risk factor identification	Diabetes: high

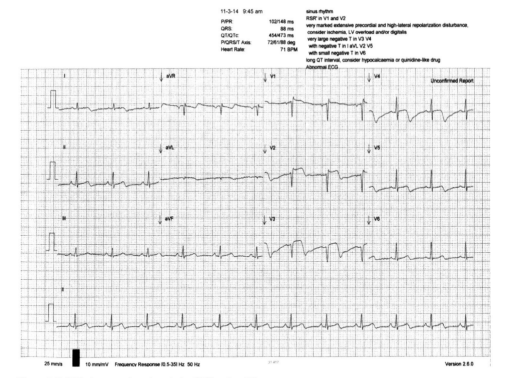

Figure 2.3 ECG changes of acute anterior ST-Elevation MI.

Box 2.6   Possible ECG findings in chest pain

1. STEMI: hyperacute T waves, ST elevation, new left bundle branch block
2. NSTEMI: ST depression, T wave inversion or normal
3. PE: right ventricle strain pattern (inverted T in V1 to V4, right bundle branch block, right axis deviation, peak P waves, S1Q3T3 (deep S waves in lead I, Q waves and inverted T waves in lead III)), sinus tachycardia, atrial fibrillation or normal
4. Pericarditis: saddle-shaped ST segment elevation across multiple leads, not associated with an arterial distribution

Box 2.7   Diagnosing MI

Diagnosis of MI requires two out of three of:

- History of ischaemia
- Serial ECG changes
- Raised cardiac enzymes

If troponin is normal ≥6 hours after onset of pain, and ECG is normal, risk of missing MI is extremely small

Blood tests

Table 2.2 Blood tests of use in patients presenting with chest pain

Test	Justification	Expected result
Serial troponin	Vital in the diagnosis of MI (see Box 2.7) Can be taken at time of chest pain but key test is >6 hours after chest pain	Myocardial infarction: raised *NB: PE, myocarditis and heart failure can also raise troponin levels*
Full blood count	Raised white cell count suggests an infective/inflammatory process is occurring	Pneumonia: white cell count is raised
Renal function tests	Required prior to angiogram to check baseline renal function – contrast medium is nephrotoxic. Dissection involving the renal arteries will also cause acute kidney injury	Aortic dissection involving renal arteries: raised urea and creatinine
Lipids	Important cardiovascular risk factor	Myocardial infarction: often raised, may represent a predisposing genetic condition (e.g. familial hypercholesterolaemia)
D-dimer	Used to rule out PE (see Box 2.8) Should only be used if genuine suspicion of PE	Unlikely to be PE: low D-dimer
Amylase	Used to rule out acute pancreatitis, a rare cause of chest pain (more commonly presents with epigastric pain)	Pancreatitis: raised
CRP/ESR	Useful to suggest an infective/inflammatory process is occurring	Pneumonia: raised Pericarditis: raised

Box 2.8 Sensitivity and specificity of D-dimer

A positive result is sensitive but not specific (i.e. all PEs should raise D-dimer, but there are other causes)
A negative result effectively rules out the presence of PE

(See Audio Podcast 2.4 at **www.wiley.com/go/camm/cardiology**)

Imaging

Table 2.3 Imaging modalities of use in patients presenting with chest pain

Test	Justification	Expected result
Chest X-ray	There may be the typical appearance of a particular pathology	See Box 2.9
Echocardiography	Look for structural heart disease or cardiac failure (may not be performed in the acute setting)	Heart failure: poor LV function MI: Poorly contracting wall segments Dissection: visualized (TOE only). Trans-thoracic echocardiogram (TTE) will only show a complication of dissection such as aortic regurgitation
Chest CT	Chest CT: imaging modality of choice for dissection and Boerhaave's CT pulmonary angiography: A sensitive and specific test to determine if emboli are in pulmonary arteries. However, has a large radiation dose so should only be used if there is a strong possibility of PE	Dissection: aortic intramural haematoma visualized and/or intimal flap Boerhaave's syndrome: oesophageal wall oedema and thickening, or extra-oesophageal air PE: emboli visualized in the pulmonary tree
Cardiac CT angiography	Contrast-enhanced CT angiography is increasingly being used as a sensitive and specific alternative to standard evaluation in acute chest pain	Myocardial infarction: narrowed or blocked coronary arteries

Box 2.9 Potential CXR findings in patients presenting with chest pain

1. **Aortic dissection:** widened mediastinum
2. **PE:** often normal, but may see wedge-shaped infarct
3. **Pneumothorax:** a peripheral area devoid of lung markings
4. **Pneumonia:** consolidation/opacification of the affected lung
5. **Boerhaave's:** mediastinal emphysema, pleural effusion

Special

Table 2.4 Special tests to be considered in patients presenting with chest pain

Test	Justification	Expected result
Exercise ECG (no longer recommended as a routine investigation)	Can confirm cardiac ischaemia Poor sensitivity and specificity	Angina: look for planar or down-sloping ST segments on the ECG of greater than 1 mm
Myocardial perfusion scan	Can confirm and further characterize the area and severity of ischaemia	Angina: a perfusion defect is seen during stress but not at rest Old myocardial infarct: defect is present at rest and during exercise
Upper gastrointestinal endoscopy	Can identify a GI cause of chest pain when other causes have been ruled out	Oesophagitis: may see inflamed raw endothelium Ulcers: may visualize oesophageal or peptic ulcers Oesophageal rupture: may visualize the rupture
Cardiac angiography	This is combined with percutaneous intervention during acute STEMI to reperfuse ischaemic myocardium	Myocardial infarction: narrowed or blocked coronary arteries

2.7 WHEN TO CALL A SENIOR

Situations
In the context of chest pain there are several situations in which a senior needs to be called:

- The pain is felt to be cardiac in origin
- The patient is haemodynamically compromised
- The patient is hypoxic

The three scenarios described here illustrate each situation:
A) The patient presents with crushing chest pain occurring at rest. The patient has significant cardiac risk factors. ACS is the likely diagnosis
B) The patient presents with tearing chest pain and a gradually dropping blood pressure. Aortic dissection is the likely diagnosis
C) The patient presents with pleuritic chest pain and haemoptysis. Saturations are 86% on room air. Significant pulmonary embolism is the likely diagnosis
Please note that there is considerable overlap between these scenarios. ACS may cause all of the above, whilst also leading to other pathology, such as an aortic dissection or cardiac tamponade. Similarly, a significant pulmonary embolism will cause haemodynamic compromise and hypoxia. All the above scenarios require urgent senior review as quickly as possible.

What should be completed by the time the senior arrives
Common to all scenarios
- Brief history and examination (including BP in both arms)
- Blood tests – full set including FBC, renal function tests, clotting, troponin, lipids, glucose and group and save
- 12-lead ECG
- Chest X-ray (portable if required)
- The patient has been put on cardiac monitoring
- The patient has been put on oxygen
- IV access has been obtained (for scenario B large-bore access is key)

Scenario A
- ACS protocol has been initiated (see Chapter 9)

Scenario B
- Cross-match blood

Scenario C
- Perform an ABG

What should be arranged by the time the senior arrives
Common to all scenarios
- Regular observations
- Appropriate analgesia
- Echo request (cardiology SpR usually will do a bedside echo upon assessment of the patient but formal echocardiogram will be required at an available opportunity)

Scenario A
- Serial ECGs
- Serial troponin

Scenario B
- CT chest-abdo-pelvis request
- Contact ITU so they are aware of patient

Scenario C
- CT pulmonary angiogram request

KEY CLINICAL TRIALS

Key trial 2.1
Trial name: Framingham Heart Study.
Participants: 5209 healthy men and women, aged 30–62.
Study design: Observational study examining factors associated with the development of cardiovascular heart disease.
Findings: Cigarette smoking, increased cholesterol, high blood pressure, diabetes, physical inactivity, and obesity are independent risk factors for cardiovascular disease.
Reason for inclusion: Seminal study that first identified the major cardiac risk factors.
Reference: http://www.framinghamheartstudy.org/about-fhs/index.php

Key trial 2.2
Trial name: ISIS-2
Participants: 17 187 patients presenting within 24 hours after onset of suspected acute MI.
Intervention: Streptokinase or aspirin or both.
Control: Placebo.
Outcome: Streptokinase alone and aspirin alone give significant reduction in 5-week vascular mortality.
Reason for inclusion: Provided early evidence for aspirin and thrombolysis.
Reference: ISIS-2 (Second International Study of Infarct Survival) Collaborative Group. Randomised trial of intravenous streptokinase, oral aspirin, both, or neither among 17,187 cases of suspected acute myocardial infarction: ISIS-2. Lancet. 1988;2(8607):349-360.

Key trial 2.3
Trial name: FAME-2 Trial.
Participants: 1220 stable patients with suspected coronary artery disease.
Intervention: Fractional-flow reverse-guided percutaneous coronary intervention (PCI).
Control: Best medical therapy.
Outcome: Reduced composite of death/MI with PCI.

Reason for inclusion: PCI with drug-eluting stents significantly reduced revascularization compared to medical therapy.

Reference: De Bruyne B, et al. Fractional flow reserve-guided pci versus medical therapy in stable coronary disease. N Engl J Med. 2012;367(11):991-1001.

Key trial 2.4
Trial name: 4S Trial.
Participants: 4444 patients with angina or previous MI and serum cholesterol 5.5–8.0 mmol/L.
Intervention: Simvastatin.
Control: Placebo.
Outcome: Reduced all-cause mortality, fatal coronary events and myocardial revascularization procedures.
Reason for inclusion: Strong evidence for use of simvastatin as secondary cardioprotection following MI.
Reference: Randomised trial of cholesterol lowering in 4444 patients with coronary heart disease: the Scandinavian Simvastatin Survival Study (4S). Lancet. 1994;344(8934):1383-1389.

GUIDELINES

National Institute for Health and Clinical Excellence (NICE). Chest pain of recent onset (CG95). March 2010. http://guidance.nice.org.uk/CG95

European Society of Cardiology. Chest Pain (Management of). 2002. http://www.escardio.org/guidelines-surveys/esc-guidelines/Pages/chest-pain.aspx

FURTHER READING

Ringstrom E, Freedman J. Approach to undifferentiated chest pain in the emergency department: a review of recent medical literature and published practice guidelines. *Mt Sinai J Med.* 2006;73(2):499–505.
Provides a comprehensive and sensible approach to the diagnosis of chest pain in the emergency setting.
Spodick DH. Acute cardiac tamponade. *N Engl J Med.* 2003; 349:684–690.
A detailed review article on cardiac tamponade and its management. Clear explanation of the interesting physiology at play.
Wertli MM, Ruchti KB, Steurer J, Held U. Diagnostic indicators of non-cardiovascular chest pain: a systematic review and meta-analysis. *BMC Med.* 2013;11(1):239.
A good discussion of the importance of different signs and symptoms suggestive of non-cardiac chest pain.

 For additional resources and to test your knowledge, visit the companion website at:

www.wiley.com/go/camm/cardiology

3 Shortness of Breath

Sarah Morrow

Chelsea and Westminster Hospital, London, UK

3.1 DEFINITION

Subjective sensation of increased, uncomfortable, awareness of breathing.

Box 3.1   MRC dyspnoea scale. (For breathlessness in heart failure, see NYHA scale: Table 11.2)

1. Not troubled by breathlessness except on strenuous exercise
2. Short of breath when hurrying or walking up a slight hill
3. Walks slower than contemporaries on level ground because of breathlessness
4. Stops for breath after walking 100 m on level ground
5. Too breathless to leave house, or breathless while dressing

---

3.2 DIAGNOSTIC ALGORITHM

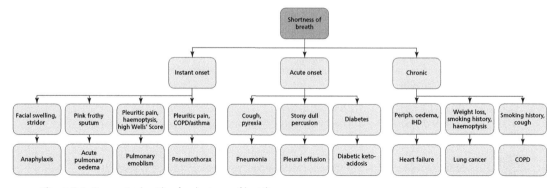

Figure 3.1 Diagnostic algorithm for shortness of breath.

3.3 DIFFERENTIALS LIST

Dangerous diagnoses
1. Acute pulmonary oedema
2. Pulmonary embolism (PE)
3. Pneumothorax
4. Acute asthma attack
5. Anaphylaxis

Common diagnoses
1. Chronic congestive cardiac failure
2. Pneumonia/infective exacerbation of COPD

Clinical Guide to Cardiology, First Edition. Edited by Christian F. Camm and A. John Camm.
© 2016 John Wiley & Sons, Ltd. Published 2016 by John Wiley & Sons, Ltd.
Companion website: www.wiley.com/go/camm/cardiology.

3. Pleural effusion
4. COPD

Diagnoses to consider
1. Diabetic ketoacidosis
2. Lung cancer
3. Pulmonary fibrosis

3.4 KEY HISTORY FEATURES

(See Audio Podcast 3.1 at **www.wiley.com/go/camm/cardiology**)

Dangerous diagnosis 1
Diagnosis: Acute pulmonary oedema

Questions
a. Recent central, crushing chest pain?

Myocardial infarction can result in rupture of the papillary muscles and cause acute mitral regurgitation and catastrophic pulmonary oedema.

b. Productive cough?

In pulmonary oedema, pink frothy sputum is classically coughed up. Differentiate from infective causes where sputum is green/yellow.

c. Associated congestive symptoms?

In particular, bilateral leg oedema, paroxysmal nocturnal dyspnoea and orthopnoea suggest cardiac failure.

d. Risk factors for IHD?

See Chapter 10.

Dangerous diagnosis 2
Diagnosis: Pulmonary embolism

Questions
a. Recent immobilization?
  i. *Long-distance travel – should ask about flights and long-distance coach/car journeys*
  ii. *Recent surgery/major surgery (<12 weeks ago)/prolonged bed rest (>3 days in the last 4 weeks)*

b. Haemoptysis?

PEs can cause infarction of pulmonary tissue resulting in coughing up of blood.

c. Swelling or pain in the calves?

Unilateral suggests deep vein thrombosis, bilateral swelling is more likely to be peripheral oedema.

d. Pleuritic chest pain?

Infarction of the lung can cause inflammation of the pleura, pain will be classically sharp and worst upon inspiration.

e. Past history of DVT or PE?

History of previous clotting is a major predictive factor for the development of further thrombosis.

Dangerous diagnosis 3
Diagnosis: Pneumothorax

Questions
a. Pre-existing lung disease?

COPD and asthma can generate lung bullae which may rupture to cause a pneumothorax. Infective lung pathology can also be causative.

b. Recent trauma to the chest?

Blunt/penetrating injuries can result in pneumothoraces.

c. Smoking history?

This is a major risk factor for pneumothorax. In addition to development of COPD, it is also an independent risk factor. Healthy smoking males have a lifetime pneumothorax risk of 12% (c.f. 0.1% in non-smokers).

d. Recent medical procedure

Iatrogenic interventions into the chest cavity (e.g. subclavian central line) can result in air entering the pleural space.

Dangerous diagnosis 4
Diagnosis: Acute asthma attack

Questions
a. Past history of asthma?

If a person is known to suffer from asthma, it is more likely to be an exacerbation of this which brings them into hospital with shortness of breath.

b. Character of the shortness of breath?

Classically described as being difficult to physically exhale.

c. Any trigger for the exacerbation?

Cold, emotion and allergic reactions such as to pets/dust can all trigger exacerbations.

Dangerous diagnosis 5
Diagnosis: Anaphylaxis

Questions
Note: Anaphylaxis is a clinical diagnosis and prompt treatment is vital. Time should not be wasted taking a full history first. However, key questions include:

a. Any swelling (particularly of the face, lips and throat)?

Swelling in subcutaneous and submucosal layers of the skin is referred to as angioedema and is particularly worrying in the throat because it can close off the airway.

b. Any rash?

The release of histamine from mast cells in the epidermis causes fluid release from superficial blood vessels, creating the 'wheal and flare' rash of urticaria.

c. Preceding 'feeling of impending doom'?

The systemic release of inflammatory cytokines often gives patients this classic sensation.

d. Previous allergic reactions/conditions such as asthma/eczema?

A known allergic condition increases likelihood of anaphylaxis. Furthermore, patients with asthma are more likely to have respiratory problems during episodes of anaphylaxis.

Common diagnosis 1
Diagnosis: Heart failure

Questions

a. Any symptoms of orthopnoea or paroxysmal nocturnal dyspnoea?

Suggestive of pulmonary oedema, in which dyspnoea is classically worse on lying down. Ask about the number of pillows which they need in order to sleep at night.

b. Exercise tolerance?

How far the patient is able to walk before becoming short of breath assesses their functional capability; also helpful for monitoring treatment progress (see NHYA scale, Table 11.2).

c. Past history of heart disease (IHD, cardiomyopathy, valvular etc.)?

Heart failure is a syndrome; therefore it must have a cause. Any pathological process which affects the heart can eventually lead to heart failure. Common pathologies include: ischaemic heart disease, cardiomyopathies and valvular heart disease.

Common diagnosis 2
Diagnosis: Pneumonia/ Infective exacerbation of COPD

Questions

a. Productive cough?

Yellow/green/'rusty' sputum is classically produced. Rusty sputum results from Streptococcus pneumoniae infections. In smokers, should determine any change in cough.

Box 3.2   Common causative organisms of community-acquired pneumonia

1. *Streptococcus pneumoniae*
2. *Haemophilus influenzae*
3. *Mycoplasma pneumoniae*
4. *Staphylococcus aureus* (especially after influenza infection)
5. *Legionella* species
6. *Chlamydia pneumoniae*

---

b. Fevers or rigors?

Signs of systemic infection.

c. Pleuritic chest pain?

The infection may cause inflammation of the pleura. Pain will be classically sharp and worse on inspiration.

Common diagnosis 3
Diagnosis: Pleural effusion

Questions

a. Recent respiratory illness?

Exudative pleural effusions are formed by fluid entering the pleural space through blood vessels with increased permeability. This can occur with bacterial pneumonia and carcinoma.

b. Other chronic illnesses?

Transudates are caused by filtration of fluid out of blood vessels, without increased permeability. Causes of this include increased venous pressure (e.g. cardiac failure) and those with decreased oncotic pressure (e.g. nephrotic syndrome, hepatic cirrhosis and malabsorption).

c. Pleuritic chest pain?

The fluid may cause inflammation of the pleura, classically sharp pain worse on inspiration; suggestive of pulmonary rather than cardiac cause.

Common diagnosis 4
Diagnosis: COPD

Questions
Note: Commonly, COPD is diagnosed following admission to hospital with other illnesses; during admission breathlessness is further investigated.

a. Smoking history?

Smoking is by far the most important risk factor for COPD; therefore determine the patient's 'pack year history'. Smoking cessation can improve symptoms and prognosis.

b. Speed of onset?

Chronic onset (over months/years) is one of the key differentiating factors of COPD.

c. Family or personal history of alpha-1 antitrypsin deficiency?

Alpha-1 antitrypsin is a molecule which is produced in the liver. One of its functions is to protect the lung tissue from neutrophil elastase, an enzyme which can break down connective tissue. Deficiency in alpha-1 antitrypsin predisposes to early development of COPD, especially in those exposed to cigarette smoke. The history is more acute than with classic COPD and affects a younger patient.

Diagnosis to consider 1
Diagnosis: Diabetic ketoacidosis (DKA)

Questions
a. Existing diagnosis of insulin-dependent diabetes?

Normally only type 1 diabetics may have episodes of DKA as even small amounts of insulin will prevent ketogenesis.

b. Symptoms of thirst, polydipsia and polyuria?

DKA is often the first presentation of diabetes. Therefore, general diabetes symptoms are often present.

c. Recent illness?

DKA is commonly triggered by an episode of illness, commonly infective such as a chest/urinary tract infection or diarrhoea and vomiting.

 (See Audio Podcast 3.2 at **www.wiley.com/go/camm/cardiology**)

Diagnosis to consider 2
Diagnosis: Lung cancer

Questions
a. Haemoptysis?

Coughing up blood on the background of a chronic cough is common with lung malignancy due to the cancer invading small blood vessels within the lung fields.

b. Systemic symptoms of malignancy?

In particular loss of weight or night sweats.

c. Smoking history?

The most common significant risk factor.

Diagnosis to consider 3
Diagnosis: Pulmonary fibrosis

Questions
a. Speed of onset?

Pulmonary fibrosis progresses gradually over time. Patients will therefore complain of a worsening shortness of breath over months to years.

b. Does the patient have any risk factors due to their work or their home environment?

Occupational or environmental exposure to inhaling dusts or chemicals may predispose to pulmonary fibrosis. In particular asbestosis, which results from asbestos exposure. 'Hypersensitivity pneumonitis' is an allergic form of pulmonary fibrosis, including 'farmer's lung' (exposure to mouldy hay).

c. Careful drug history?

Several medications, when taken chronically, can significantly increase a patient's risk of developing pulmonary fibrosis. In particular amiodarone, methotrexate and nitrofurantoin are all implicated. Radiotherapy to the thorax commonly damages and scars the lungs.

d. Any ongoing joint pain?

Any pathology which affects connective tissue may affect the lungs. In particular, rheumatoid arthritis often involves the lungs. SLE, scleroderma and ankylosing spondylitis also frequently cause pulmonary fibrosis.

3.5 KEY EXAMINATION FEATURES

Dangerous diagnosis 1
Diagnosis: Acute pulmonary oedema

Examination findings
a. Bi-basal crackles/crepitations

Classically fine and inspiratory. The bilateral nature suggests a systemic cause. In contrast, a local pathology would often only affect one side.

b. Third heart sound/gallop rhythm

Created by rapid ventricular filling (e.g. due to mitral regurgitation) or hypo- or akinesia of the ventricular wall (e.g. post-MI). Best heard with the bell of the stethoscope over the apex.

c. Associated congestive features

Other signs of heart failure include peripheral oedema and raised JVP.

d. Heart murmurs

Mitral regurgitation resulting from the rupture of the papillary muscles in a myocardial infarction can lead to acute and devastating pulmonary oedema (see Chapter 9).

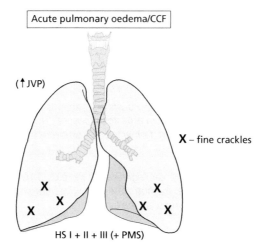

Figure 3.2 Examination findings in acute pulmonary oedema.

Dangerous diagnosis 2
Diagnosis: Pulmonary embolism

Examination findings
Note: Examination is often completely normal
a. Tachycardia

Although very non-specific, should increase suspicion of this diagnosis.

b. Raised JVP

Results from right-sided heart strain. May be associated with a loud P2 and parasternal heave.

c. Pleural friction rub

This describes an auscultatory finding caused by inflammation of the pleural layers, disrupting their lubrication and thus the ability of the layers to slide over one another when the chest wall moves. It is heard on both inspiration and expiration.

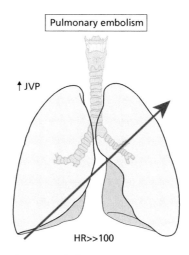

Figure 3.3 Examination findings in pulmonary embolism.

Dangerous diagnosis 3

Diagnosis: Pneumothorax

Examination findings

a. Tracheal deviation

Vitally important to exclude tension pneumothorax in any patient with acute shortness of breath. The trachea will deviate away from the affected side although this is notoriously difficult to pick up clinically.

b. Reduced chest expansion

Air in the pleural space will decrease available lung air space and thus expansion on the affected side.

c. Hyper-resonant percussion

The air trapped within the pleura produces a higher-pitched and more resonant percussion note than in an unaffected lung where normal lung tissue reaches closer to the chest wall.

d. Subcutaneous emphysema

Inspect for facial/neck swelling and palpate for characteristic 'fresh snow' feeling.

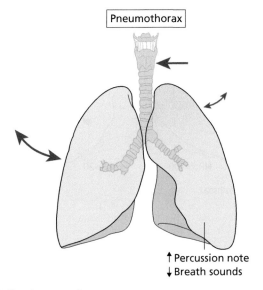

Figure 3.4 Examination findings in pneumothorax.

Dangerous diagnosis 4

Diagnosis: Acute asthma attack

Examination findings

Note: always do a peak flow (PEF) reading to help assess the asthmatic patient. Readings are compared to the 'best or predicted' PEF for that patient.

a. Wheeze

An expiratory wheeze is usually heard; however, in severe attacks the chest may be 'silent'.

Table 3.1 Features of asthma exacerbation (adapted from British Thoracic Guidelines 2012)

Moderate exacerbation	Severe exacerbation	Life-threatening exacerbation
PEF 50–75%	PEF 33–50%	PEF <33%
No features of severe	RR ≥25/min	Altered conscious level
	HR ≥110/min	Arrhythmia
	Inability to complete sentences	Hypotension
		Cyanosis
		Silent chest/poor respiratory effort

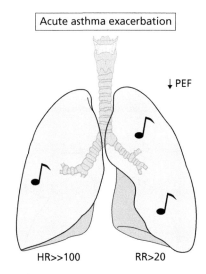

Figure 3.5 Examination findings in asthma.

Dangerous diagnosis 5
Diagnosis: Anaphylaxis

Examination findings
a. Widespread rash

The rash is classically urticarial ('wheal and flare'), due to release of inflammatory mediators (e.g. histamine).

b. Swelling

Facial (especially of the lips and tongue) and neck swelling is particularly common.

c. Stridor

Stridor results from partial obstruction of the upper airway due to soft tissue swelling. It is a loud, harsh sound heard on inspiration (in contrast to expiratory wheeze).

d. Signs of systemic shock

Extensive peripheral vasodilatation in anaphylaxis results in systemic shock. Signs include tachycardia and hypotension; check the observations early on. This is a worrying presentation and indicates the need for urgent management.

Common diagnosis 1
Diagnosis: Heart failure

Examination findings

a. Signs of left-sided heart failure:

As for acute pulmonary oedema (Dangerous diagnosis 1).

b. Signs of right-sided heart failure:

Peripheral (dependant) oedema, raised JVP and ascites.

(See Audio Podcast 3.3 at **www.wiley.com/go/camm/cardiology**)

Common diagnosis 2
Diagnosis: Pneumonia

Examination findings

a. Fever

Sign of systemic infection.

b. Reduced chest expansion

Infection in the lung parenchyma decreases available air space for expansion on the affected side.

c. Dull percussion note

The pus from the infection reduces the amount of air within the respiratory tree and therefore deadens the percussion note.

d. Bronchial breathing

Bronchial breathing is the sound of turbulent air flow in the upper airways; normally not conducted to the chest wall. However, consolidated lungs conduct sound more effectively thus transmitting these upper airway sounds.

e. Increased vocal resonance/fremitus

Similar explanation to that for bronchial breathing.

Box 3.3   Whispered pectoriloquy

- Patients is asked to whisper
- Normally, whispered tones are not audible when lung fields are auscultated
- Consolidation increases transmission of sounds through lung parenchyma making whispered tones audible
- This test uses the same mechanism as vocal resonance

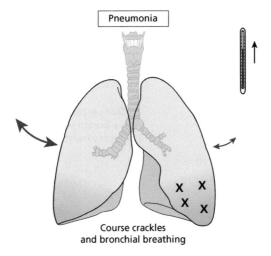

Pneumonia

Course crackles
and bronchial breathing

Figure 3.6 Examination findings in pneumonia.

Box 3.4   CURB-65 scoring system – predictive of mortality in community-acquired pneumonia

C – Confusion (AMTS <9)
U – Urea (>7 mmol/L)
R – Respiratory rate (>30/min)
B – Blood pressure (systolic pressure <90 mmHg)
65 – Age >65 years

Common diagnosis 3
Diagnosis: Pleural effusion

Examination findings
a. Reduced chest expansion

Fluid in the pleural space will decrease available lung air space for expansion on the affected side.

b. Stony dull percussion note

The density of the fluid within the pleural cavity, so close to the chest wall, produces a percussion note which is more dull than that of a consolidated lung.

c. Reduced breath sounds on auscultation

Due to the fluid within the pleural cavity preventing transmission of breath sounds to the chest wall.

d. Reduced vocal resonance/fremitus

Explanation as for reduced breath sounds.

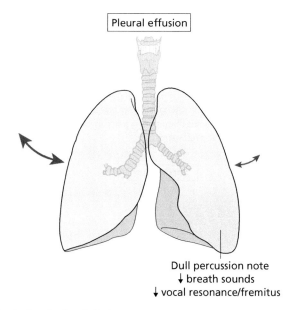

Figure 3.7 Examination findings in pleural effusion.

Common diagnosis 4
Diagnosis: COPD

Examination findings

a. Reduced crico-sternal angle

A patient with COPD will develop hyper-inflation of the lungs. This produces the characteristic 'barrel-shaped chest' and also reduces the crico-sternal distance to <3 cm.

b. CO_2 retention flap

Occurs in carbon dioxide retention; seen in type 2 respiratory failure (10% of COPD sufferers). If this is the case then they may also have a bounding pulse and be confused.

c. Hyper-resonance on percussion

This is similarly produced by hyper-inflation of the lungs leading to decreased parenchyma density.

d. Signs of right heart failure

COPD patients may develop signs of right heart failure over time due to increased pulmonary pressure. Check for raised JVP, loud P2, right ventricular heave and peripheral oedema.

Diagnosis to consider 1
Diagnosis: Diabetic ketoacidosis

Examination findings

a. Confusion

This is multifactorial and related to dehydration, acidosis and underlying infection. This can also be seen in other infections (e.g. pneumonia).

b. Kussmaul breathing

Deep, sighing breathing which produces respiratory compensation for the metabolic acidosis in DKA.

c. Smell of ketones on patient's breath

Ketones have the characteristic smell of pear-drop sweets.

d. Clinical signs of dehydration:

Sunken eyes, dry mucous membranes, reduced skin turgor, prolonged capillary refill time.

Diagnosis to consider 2
Diagnosis: Lung cancer

Examination findings

a. Cachexia and muscle-wasting

Due to the high metabolic demand of cancer.

b. Signs of super-imposed respiratory disease

In particular pleural effusion or respiratory infection may commonly complicate lung malignancy.

Diagnosis to consider 3
Diagnosis: Pulmonary fibrosis

Examination findings

a. Fine, inspiratory crackles on auscultation

'Late inspiratory fine' crackles are heard in pulmonary fibrosis (compared with the 'early/middle inspiratory' crackles found in pulmonary oedema). Furthermore, asking the patient to cough will reduce crackles relating to heart failure but have no effect on fibrotic crackles. Crackle location may also help determine the aetiology.

Box 3.5 Instructing a patient on how to perform a peak flow measurement

1. Hold peak flow meter on either side so fingers do not obstruct the moving part
2. Take a deep breath in
3. Place the mouthpiece into mouth and form a tight seal with lips
4. Exhale as forcefully as possible into the meter
5. Best reading of three should be documented

b. Finger clubbing

One of the main respiratory causes of clubbing is pulmonary fibrosis, differentials are bronchiectasis and lung cancer.

Table 3.2 Respiratory findings in shortness of breath diagnoses. With all of these conditions, the affected side will demonstrate reduced expansion. In conditions such as asthma where both lungs are affected, both sides expand less than normal.

Pathological process	Mediastinal displacement	Percussion note	Breath sounds	Vocal resonance	Added sounds
Consolidation	None	Dull	Bronchial	Increased	Coarse crackles
Pleural effusion	Away from lesion (if large)	Stony dull	Reduced or absent	Reduced or absent	None
Pneumothorax	Away from lesion (if tension)	Hyper-resonant	Reduced or absent	Reduced or absent	None
Asthma	None	Normal	Vesicular with prolonged expiration	Normal	Expiratory polyphonic wheeze

3.6 KEY INVESTIGATIONS

Bedside

Table 3.3 Bedside tests in patients with shortness of breath

Test	Justification	Potential result
Pulse oximetry	Important to check the effects of the condition upon the patient's oxygen saturations To monitor the effect of therapeutic oxygen	Often low with respiratory conditions
Peak flow	For patients with an asthma exacerbation: • Indicates episode severity • Monitors progress	Reduced peak flow reading suggests increased severity of asthma exacerbation
ABG	Indicates respiratory failure and type	See Box 3.8
Capillary glucose measurement	For diagnosis of DKA	Significantly raised in DKA: >11 mmol/L
ECG	Changes often found with conditions causing SOB	• Sinus tachycardia associated with PE • Signs of ischaemia precipitating acute pulmonary oedema See Box 2.6 for ECG changes with PE

Box 3.6 Crackle locations and suggested aetiology

Apical:

- Silicosis
- Sarcoidosis

Basal:

- Asbestosis
- Iatrogenic fibrosis secondary to drugs (e.g. methotrexate and amiodarone)

Box 3.7 How to take an arterial blood gas sample

1. Perform an 'Allen's test' to ensure the patency of the ulnar artery
2. Palpate the radial artery at the wrist
3. Clean the area thoroughly
4. Use a heparinized needle to insert at 45°
5. Adjust the position of the needle until flash-back is achieved
6. If this is arterial blood, the syringe will self-fill

Box 3.8 Reading the ABG

1. PaO_2: determines whether the patient is hypoxic (PaO_2 <8 kPa)
2. pH: >7.45 indicates an alkalosis; <7.35 indicates an acidosis
3. $PaCO_2$:
   a. If hypoxic and normo-/hypo-capnic – type 1 respiratory failure
   b. If hypoxic and hypercapnic – type 2 respiratory failure
   c. If acidotic, raised $PaCO_2$ indicates respiratory cause. If an alkalosis exists secondary to a respiratory cause, expect to see a low $PaCO_2$. If these do not apply, the cause is metabolic

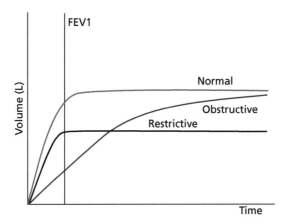

Figure 3.8 Graphical representation of restrictive and obstructive pulmonary function test results.

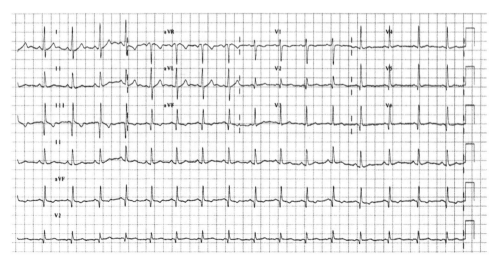

Figure 3.9 ECG of a patient with a pulmonary embolism showing the classic S1,Q3,T3 pattern.

Blood tests

Table 3.4 Blood tests in patients with shortness of breath

Test	Justification	Potential result	
FBC	High or low white cell count is a marker of infection	Raised WCC: pneumonia, infective exacerbation of COPD, or an infection precipitating DKA	
CRP and ESR	Inflammatory markers, to help diagnose infections and to track their course	These will be raised in infections. Note that the CRP 'lags' behind the changes in WCC	
Urea and electrolytes	Assess for acute kidney injury precipitated by dehydration in DKA Assess for kidney disease which might limit the use of diuretics in heart failure/pulmonary oedema	Raised creatinine suggests kidney disease. Look at any previous results to see whether this is part of an acute or chronic picture	
Serum glucose	To confirm capillary glucose reading	Raised in DKA	
Serum LDH and protein	To determine whether a pleural effusion is a transudate or an exudate using Light's criteria (by comparison with the concentrations of these in the pleural fluid)	Transudate: pleural/serum (P/S) protein ratio <0.5 P/S LDH ratio <0.6	Exudate: P/S protein ratio >0.5 P/S LDH ratio >0.6
D-dimer	To help exclude a PE	Of little use clinically if raised as this is very non-specific. However if negative can virtually exclude a PE	

(See Audio Podcast 3.4 at **www.wiley.com/go/camm/cardiology**)

Imaging

Table 3.5 Imaging modalities of use in patients with shortness of breath

Test	Justification	Potential result
Chest X-ray	Sufficient imaging to diagnose a number of respiratory pathologies	Variable dependent on pathology
Computed tomography pulmonary angiogram (CTPA)	If suspicious of a PE (high Well's score), this is the best investigation for diagnosis	PE: thrombus located in the pulmonary arterial system
CT chest	If the chest X-ray shows a potential malignancy this will help to characterize such a lesion	May also show nodes if metastasis of cancerous cells
Echocardiogram	For all patients in whom heart failure is suspected	Ventricular function and ejection fraction may both be reduced in patients with heart failure

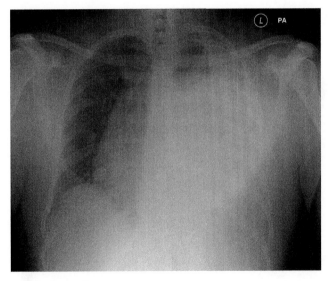

Figure 3.10 CXR showing a pleural effusion.

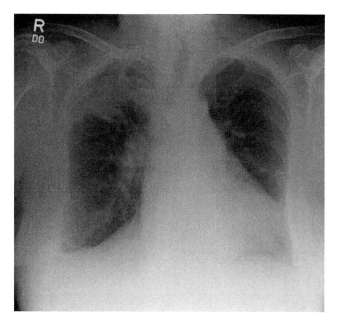

Figure 3.11 CXR showing a right upper-lobe pneumonia.

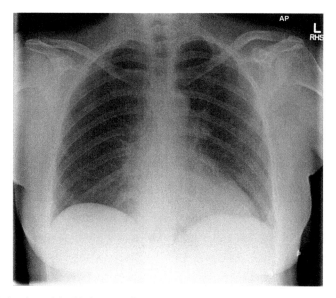

Figure 3.12 CXR showing a right sided pneumothorax.

Special tests

Table 3.6 Special tests of use in patients with shortness of breath

Test	Justification	Expected result
Pleural tap	To determine whether this is a transudate or an exudate by looking at the protein and LDH content of the fluid	In a transudate protein content is <30 g/L and LDH is <200 U/L. Exudate would contain more protein and LDH
Pleural/lung biopsy	May provide further information when pulmonary fibrosis is suspected	Most common fibrosis histology is 'usual interstitial pneumonia' which is found in 'idiopathic pulmonary fibrosis'

3.7 WHEN TO CALL A SENIOR

Situations
Divide these into the ABC assessment:

1. Airway: any situation where you believe that the airway is compromised – in particular from the examples shown above, tingling of the lips or swelling of the tongue with anaphylaxis should trigger an immediate senior referral

2. Breathing: hypoxia or hypercapnia not responding to initial management. These patients are likely to be candidates for non-invasive ventilation and this is an area where senior support is very valuable

3. Circulation:
    a. If you suspect a pulmonary embolism – particularly in a situation where the patient is tachycardic, hypoxic on their blood gases and has a high Well's score
    b. If there are signs that the patient has gone into acute heart failure and pulmonary oedema – especially if they may have had an acute cardiac event
    c. If there are any signs that the patient is in septic shock secondary to a pneumonia or hypovolaemic shock such as in DKA

What should be arranged by the time the senior arrives
Radiology
- Chest X-ray – does not necessarily have to be completed, however the senior will expect this to have been ordered by the time that they approach the bedside
- CTPA – if the initial assessment is suggestive of a PE

Other appropriate referrals
- For example – cardiology review would be very important in a situation where an acute cardiac event causing pulmonary oedema is suspected

What should be completed by the time the senior arrives
Bedside investigations
1. Observations
2. Arterial blood gas – an absolute must before calling the senior regarding a breathless patient
3. Capillary glucose measurement
4. Peak flow if indicated – for example in a known asthmatic

Management
1. Patient to be on oxygen therapy as appropriate – usually with saturations titrated to 94–98% (remember hypoxia will kill faster than hypercapnia so if in doubt always titrate to 94–98% even in a patient with COPD)
2. Patient to be given fluid resuscitation as appropriate – especially for the DKA patient or a septic patient

3. Initial therapeutic steps: such as salbutamol nebulizers in asthma exacerbations, furosemide in pulmonary oedema, antibiotics in a septic patient, insulin for DKA

GUIDELINES

British Thoracic Society. British guideline on the management of asthma. 2012. http://www.brit-thoracic.org.uk/Portals/0/Guidelines/AsthmaGuidelines/sign101%20Jan%202012.pdf

European Society of Cardiology. ESC guidelines for the diagnosis and treatment of acute and chronic heart failure. 2012. http://www.escardio.org/guidelines-surveys/esc-guidelines/GuidelinesDocuments/Guidelines-Acute%20and%20Chronic-HF-FT.pdf

FURTHER READING

Bense L, Eklund G, Odont D, et al. Smoking and the increased risk of contracting pneumothorax. Chest. 1987;92:1009-1012.

Demonstrates the learning point that smoking is a strong, statistically significant risk factor for pneumothorax.

Manning H, Schwartzstein RM. Pathophysiology of dyspnea. N Engl J Med. 1995;333:1547-1553. http://www.nejm.org/doi/full/10.1056/NEJM199512073332307

An interesting review discussing the pathophysiology of dyspnoea, including the mechanisms underlying why patients feel short of breath.

Lansing RW, Gracely RH, Banzett RB. The multiple dimensions of dyspnoea: review and hypotheses. Respir Physiol Neurobiol. 2009;167(1):53-60. http://www.ncbi.nlm.nih.gov/pmc/articles/PMC2763422/

A thorough discussion of the neurophysiology of dyspnoea including several models underlining the psychology of dyspnoea.

Thomas JR, von Gunten CF. Management of dyspnoea. J Support Oncol. 2003;1(1):23-32. http://www.ncbi.nlm.nih.gov/pubmed/15352640

A discussion of the management of oncology based dyspnoea.

  For additional resources and to test your knowledge, visit the companion website at:

www.wiley.com/go/camm/cardiology

4 Loss of Consciousness

Robert A. Watson
Imperial College Healthcare NHS Trust, London, UK

4.1 DEFINITION

Syncope is a transient loss of consciousness due cerebral hypoperfusion.

There are numerous causes of transient loss of consciousness (T-LOC), many of which are syncopal (i.e. due to cerebral hypoperfusion); other causes of T-LOC – such as epilepsy – are not syncopal events. However, for completeness this chapter will deal with T-LOC in general.

4.2 CLASSIFICATION

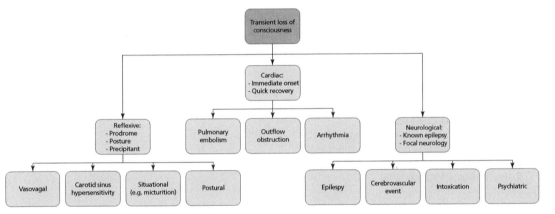

Figure 4.1 Classification of T-LOC aetiology

4.3 DIFFERENTIALS LIST

Dangerous diagnoses

1. Cardiovascular disorder (23%)
   a. Arrhythmia
   b. Outflow obstruction
   c. Pulmonary embolus
2. Neurological disorder (1%)
   a. Epileptic seizure
   b. Cerebrovascular event
3. Hypoglycaemia

Clinical Guide to Cardiology, First Edition. Edited by Christian F. Camm and A. John Camm.
© 2016 John Wiley & Sons, Ltd. Published 2016 by John Wiley & Sons, Ltd.
Companion website: www.wiley.com/go/camm/cardiology.

Box 4.1   Major causes of cardiac outflow obstruction

1. Aortic stenosis
2. Hypertrophic cardiomyopathy
3. Congenital structural disease (e.g. Fallot's tetralogy)
4. Prosthetic valve dysfunction

Box 4.2   Arrhythmic causes of collapse

1. Monomorphic ventricular tachycardia
2. Polymorphic ventricular tachycardia (torsades de pointes)
3. Supraventricular tachycardia with rapid ventricular response
4. Complete (third-degree) heart block
5. Sinus node arrest

Common diagnoses

1. Reflex syncope (58%)
   a. 'Vasovagal' syncope
   b. Carotid sinus hypersensitivity (vasovagal mechanism)
   c. Micturition syncope (vasovagal mechanism)
2. Postural (orthostatic) hypotension
   a. Dehydration
   b. Drugs

Diagnoses to consider

1. Intoxication (alcohol or other drugs)
2. Mechanical fall (may not result in/from T-LOC)
3. Intracardiac mass (atrial myxoma or thrombus)
4. Psychological syncope (1%)

Box 4.3   Drugs that can commonly cause T-LOC

1. Opiates
2. Barbiturates
3. Benzodiazepines
4. Beta blockers (due to bradycardia)
5. Diuretics (leading to postural hypotension)

4.4 KEY HISTORY FEATURES

(See Audio Podcast 4.1 at **www.wiley.com/go/camm/cardiology**)

General points

Key elements to any T-LOC history include:

- **Before the event:** what was the patient doing? Where were they? Was there any prodrome or precipitants?
- **During the event:** (reports from witnesses may be necessary for this) Did the patient spasm? Did they go blue? Was there loss of continence? Did they injure themselves?
- **After the event:** did they recover quickly or slowly? Did they feel flushed and hot? Did they have palpitations or chest pain?

The other sections of the history are also very important – past medical history (PMH), drug history (DH) and family history (FH) may all give clues to the underlying diagnosis.
(See Audio Podcast 4.2 at **www.wiley.com/go/camm/cardiology**)

Dangerous diagnosis 1
Diagnosis: Cardiac arrhythmia

Questions
a. Was there warning of syncope?

There is usually no warning of syncope caused by a cardiac arrhythmia, although it may be associated with preceding palpitations.

b. Were injuries sustained?

The lack of warning prevents patients breaking their fall, often resulting in serious injuries, commonly to the face.

c. How quick was the recovery?

A quick recovery (seconds–minutes) where the patient's pallor is replaced by flushing is usual. However, the patient may be psychologically shocked and can appear confused and dazed.

d. Known cardiac disease?

Patients with a history of structural heart disease are more prone to arrhythmias.

Box 4.4   Stokes Adams attacks

- Abrupt T-LOC due to a sudden fall in cardiac output caused by a cardiac arrhythmia
- Specific characteristics are initial pallor during T-LOC replaced by facial flushing during a rapid recovery

---

Dangerous diagnosis 2
Diagnosis: Outflow obstruction

Questions
a. Was the syncope associated with exercise?

Sudden-onset syncope during exercise is a red flag for outflow obstruction or other cardiovascular disease.

b. Episodes of chest pain?

Outflow obstruction is often associated with angina.

c. Aortic or mitral valve replacement?

Although uncommon, prosthetic valve dysfunction should be ruled out in this population.

Dangerous diagnosis 3
Diagnosis: Pulmonary embolus

Questions
a. Was the syncope associated with breathlessness?

Pulmonary embolism is likely to present with breathlessness but is a non-specific sign and may be associated with cardiac disease.

b. Any risk factors for venous thrombo-embolism?

See Boxes 4.5 and 4.6 for risk factors for DVT and PE.

c. Recent pain or swelling in the leg?

Unilateral swelling is suggestive of a DVT, however, other causes include cellulitis and a ruptured baker's cyst.

d. Any tachycardia, chest pain or haemoptysis?

Pulmonary embolism is often associated with these clinical features – pleuritic pain due to infarction of the lung and pleural inflammation, a sinus tachycardia and haemoptysis (secondary to infarction).

Box 4.5   Wells' score for DVT (Adapted from Wells et al. JAMA 2006;295(2):199-207)

1. Active cancer (treatment ongoing/in last 6 months)	1
2. Paralysis, paresis or recent plaster immobilization of the leg(s)	1
3. Recent bed rest for >2 days or major surgery in last 12 weeks	1
4. Localized tenderness along distribution of deep venous system	1
5. Leg swelling (whole leg)	1
6. Calf swelling >3 cm compared to other leg (10 cm below tibial tuberosity)	1
7. Pitting oedema only on symptomatic side	1
8. Non-varicose collateral superficial veins	1
9. Previous DVT	1
10. Alternative diagnosis as likely as DVT	−2

0 = low pretest probability, 1 or 2 = moderate pretest probability, 3 or more = high pretest probability

---

Box 4.6   Wells' score for PE (Adapted from Wells et al. JAMA 2006;295(2):199-207)

1. Clinical signs and symptoms consistent with DVT	3
2. PE the most likely diagnosis	3
3. Surgery or bed bound for >3 days in last 4 weeks	1.5
4. Previous DVT or PE	1.5
5. Pulse >100 bpm	1.5
6. Haemoptysis	1
7. Active cancer	1

4 or less = low pretest probability, 4.5–6 = moderate pretest probability, greater than 6 = high pretest probability

Dangerous diagnosis 4
Diagnosis: Epileptic seizure

Questions
a. Was there tonic–clonic jerking, tongue biting, or loss of continence?

Jerking may be suggestive of an epileptic seizure (can be confused with hypoxic jerks seen in other forms of syncope). Incontinence is also common in epilepsy but non-specific. Tongue biting (side of tongue), however, is virtually pathognomonic of a seizure.

b. Has this happened before and was the event similar?

A history of numerous stereotyped events may be suggestive of epilepsy.

c. How fast was the recovery?

Epileptic seizures are followed by a long (often several hours) post-ictal period of confusion.

Dangerous diagnosis 5

Diagnosis: Cerebrovascular event

Note: T-LOC is not a common presentation for a stroke; however, a posterior infarct may result in collapse.

Questions

a. Complaint of weakness, loss of sensation, or difficulty with speaking?

If the patient/witness reports a focal neurological deficit, this is suggestive of stroke.

b. Any 'funny turns' recently?

Cerebrovascular accidents are commonly preceded by TIAs where there are transient focal neurological deficits.

c. Does the patient have risk factors for stroke?

These are similar to those for cardiovascular disease (see Box 2.1) and are relatively non-specific.

Dangerous diagnosis 6

Diagnosis: Hypoglycaemia

Questions

a. Does the patient have diabetes?

Hypoglycaemia is most likely in patients with diagnosed and treated diabetes. The following questions are only necessary if the patient has diabetes.

b. What medication do they take?

Hypoglycaemia is almost always due to over-medication with insulin or oral hypoglycaemic agents (e.g. sulphonylureas). If the patient does not take these medications then hypoglycaemia is unlikely to be the cause.

c. Timing of last meal?

Hypoglycaemia commonly occurs when patient has not eaten for some time.

Common diagnosis 1

Diagnosis: Vasovagal syncope

Questions

a. Posture at time of collapse?

Most often occurs when standing, but may occur when sitting. This is very unlikely to occur if the patient was lying flat.

b. Was there a prodrome?

Is often preceded by a brief period of feeling dizzy, or 'faint' (pre-syncope). In addition, autonomic features (e.g. nausea and sweating) are common.

c. Was there a precipitant?

Vasovagal syncope usually has a clear precipitant – e.g. standing on a bus on a hot day, seeing blood or receiving bad news.

Box 4.7   Differentiating vasovagal syncope from more sinister causes – the 3 Ps

If all three are present, it is very likely to be a vasovagal mechanism:

- Prodrome
- Posture
- Precipitant

Common diagnosis 2
Diagnosis: Carotid sinus hypersensitivity

Questions
a. What was the patient doing/wearing at the time?

Occurs following sinus stimulation – e.g. turning of the head/wearing a tight collar.

b. What drugs is the patient taking?

Certain drugs (e.g. digoxin) increase the sensitivity of the carotid sinuses.

Common diagnosis 3
Diagnosis: Micturition syncope

Questions
a. What was the patient doing at the time?

If there is a history of raised intra-abdominal pressure – such as urinating, coughing or straining on the toilet – this is suggestive of this diagnosis.

Common diagnosis 4
Diagnosis: Postural hypotension

Questions
a. Was there an change in posture from sitting/lying to standing?

A drop in blood pressure on standing (postural drop) is the precipitating cause. This drop can be delayed and the patient may have walked a distance before fainting.

b. What drugs is the patient taking?

A number of drugs – anti-hypertensives and diuretics – can predispose to postural hypotension, particularly in combination.

c. Any predisposing conditions?

- Age: more likely in older patients
- CVA: through damage to sympathetic tracts
- Diabetes: due to autonomic neuropathy
- Multi-system atrophy (a Parkinson-plus syndrome): autonomic degeneration

Diagnosis to consider 1
Diagnosis: Intoxication (alcohol or other drugs)

Questions
a. Has the patient taken any drugs/alcohol recently?

A thorough drug history (particularly alcohol, opiates and sedatives) is vital to this diagnosis.

Diagnosis to consider 2
Diagnosis: Mechanical (trips and slips)

Questions
a. Was there an obvious mechanism for the fall/collapse?

This should be a diagnosis of exclusion. In elderly patients, even if there is an obvious mechanism for a fall, pathological causes should be excluded. Other factors may have contributed to a fall – such as poor eyesight or an unsafe home environment.

Diagnosis to consider 3
Diagnosis: Intracardiac mass (atrial myxoma or thrombus)

Questions
a. Is there a history of atrial fibrillation/flutter, or stroke/TIA?

These arrhythmias predispose to intracardiac thrombus formation, whilst a history of stroke or TIA indicates that the patient is high risk for thrombosis.

b. Are there any symptoms of heart failure or constitutional symptoms?

Atrial myxoma is the commonest form of cardiac neoplasia and can have a variety of clinical presentations. Dizziness and syncope is experienced by around 20% of patients (usually due to mitral valve obstruction – which is positional). The commonest symptoms are those of left heart failure (75% experience exertional dyspnoea).

Diagnosis to consider 4
Diagnosis: Psychological syncope

Questions
a. Is there a history of pseudo-seizures?

Patients prone to pseudo-seizure may well be frequent attenders or known to psychiatric services. However, patients with a mental health diagnosis may still have an organic cause for syncope so this should be excluded.

b. Has the patient recently experienced any psychological trauma?

Somatoform, dissociative and post-traumatic stress disorder can manifest as pseudo-seizures.

4.5 KEY EXAMINATION FEATURES

Dangerous diagnosis 1
Diagnosis: Cardiac arrhythmia

Key examination findings
a. Pulse rate and rhythm

This could be tachy- or bradycardic or irregular, suggesting an underlying rhythm disturbance. Rhythm is often normal at time of examination.

b. JVP

Cannon waves suggest the presence of third-degree heart block or ventricular tachycardia.

c. External injuries

It is important to check for these. Their presence implies a sudden onset of syncope.

(See Audio Podcast 4.3 at **www.wiley.com/go/camm/cardiology**)

Dangerous diagnosis 2
Diagnosis: Outflow obstruction

Key examination findings
a. Heart murmur

An ejection systolic murmur (+/- associated thrill and carotid radiation) is present with outflow obstruction (see Chapter 6). Normal mechanical heart sounds exclude serious prosthetic valve obstruction.

b. Apex beat

A double apex beat and systolic thrill at the sternal edge may be felt in HOCM.

Dangerous diagnosis 3
Diagnosis: Pulmonary embolus

Key examination findings
a. Respiratory and heart rate

These are likely to be raised in a case of pulmonary embolism.

b. Haemoptysis

Recent-onset haemoptysis in a young patient is suggestive of a PE.

c. Leg swelling

Suggests DVT.

Dangerous diagnosis 4
Diagnosis: Epileptic seizure

Key examination findings
a. Ongoing seizure activity

Status epilepticus should be ruled out, if present it is a medical emergency.

b. Tongue biting

The tongue should be actively checked. The presence of tongue biting is almost pathognomonic of an epileptic seizure (if on the side of the tongue – injuries to the tongue tip can occur as a result of a fall).

c. Mental state of patient

A drowsy, confused patient may well be post-ictal.

Dangerous diagnosis 5
Diagnosis: Cerebrovascular event

Key examination findings
a. Focal neurological deficit

The presentation of stroke is extremely varied depending on the vascular territory involved. However, unilateral weakness, dysphasia or hemianopia are common presenting signs.

b. Carotid bruit

Carotid artery atherosclerosis is a risk factor for stroke.

c. Irregularly irregular pulse

Suggestive of atrial fibrillation which is a factor in approximately 15% of strokes.

Dangerous diagnosis 6
Diagnosis: Hypoglycaemia

Key examination findings
a. Level of consciousness

Hypoglycaemia can cause a reduced Glasgow coma score (GCS) and hypoglycaemic coma. It can also lead to seizure activity.

b. Behaviour

Hypoglycaemic patients often display altered behaviour and can become irritable and aggressive.

c. Sweating

In an attempt to raise blood sugar levels there is a physiological adrenergic response provoking sympathetic symptoms such as sweating and tachycardia.

Common diagnosis 1
Diagnosis: Vasovagal syncope

Key examination findings
a. Absence of injury

The diagnosis of vasovagal syncope relies heavily on the history. However, the absence of external injuries suggests that the patient had warning and could fall safely.

Common diagnosis 2
Diagnosis: Carotid sinus hypersensitivity

Key examination findings
a. Injury

As with vasovagal syncope, the diagnosis of this condition relies on the history and a positive result on carotid sinus massage (see Section 4.6 Key investigations). However, in this type of syncope, patients often are unable to protect themselves as they fall and may have injuries associated with this.

Common diagnosis 3
Diagnosis: Micturition syncope

Key examination findings
There are no specific examination findings – diagnosis relies on the history.

Common diagnosis 4
Diagnosis: Postural hypotension

Key examination findings
a. Lying and standing blood pressure

A significant drop in blood pressure (>20 mmHg systolic) makes orthostatic hypotension a likely cause of syncope.

b. Hydration status

A full hydration status assessment should be performed to determine if the patient is hypovolaemic. Dehydration increases the risk of postural hypotension.

Diagnosis to consider 1
Diagnosis: Intoxication (alcohol or other drugs)

Key examination findings
a. Cerebellar examination

The patient may have dysarthria and ataxia associated with alcohol intoxication. However, formal examination is unlikely to be necessary.

b. Pupils

Pinpoint pupils suggest opiate intoxication.

c. Respiratory rate

A low rate is a non-specific sign of sedative use. If there is strong suspicion of opiate use, the patient should be monitored closely.

Diagnosis to consider 2
Diagnosis: Mechanical (trips and slips)

Key examination findings
a. Sequelae of fall

It is important to look for any injuries resulting from the fall – for example fractures or haematomas.

b. Neurological status

Do they have a neurological condition (e.g. peripheral neuropathy, Parkinson's disease etc.) which may predispose them to falling?

c. Mechanical factors

For example poor vision or poor footwear; these are easy to correct and may prevent future admissions.

Diagnosis to consider 3

Diagnosis: Intracardiac mass (atrial myxoma or thrombus)

Key examination findings

a. JVP

The JVP is classically raised with a prominent A wave.

b. Auscultation

A loud S1 may be heard (delayed closure of the mitral valve), or a delayed P2. An early diastolic sound may be heard in cases of atrial myxoma. Known as a tumour plop, this represents the tumour impacting against the ventricular wall. Other sounds of heart failure (such as S3 or S4) may be present.

Diagnosis to consider 4

Diagnosis: Psychological syncope

Key examination findings

There are no specific examination findings although a mental state examination may be helpful. Diagnosis relies primarily on the history.

4.6 KEY INVESTIGATIONS

Bedside tests

Table 4.1 Bedside tests undertaken when patient presents with syncope

Test	Justification	Potential result
Oxygen saturations	Simple non-invasive test	Low if PE
Capillary blood glucose ('BM')	Should be checked in ALL patients presenting with reduced level of consciousness	Low if hypoglycaemic
ECG	A good way to check for rhythm abnormalities	Usually normal May show ongoing arrhythmia/heart block

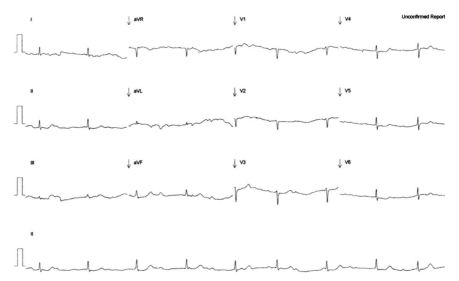

Figure 4.2 An ECG showing complete dissociation of atrial and ventricular systole. This is consistent with third-degree (complete) heart block. These patients often present with syncope – so-called Stokes Adam's attacks.

Blood tests

Table 4.2 Bedside tests undertaken when patient presents with syncope

Test	Justification	Potential result
Full blood count	Anaemia may exacerbate cerebral hypoperfusion, making syncope more likely	Low haemoglobin
Renal function tests and electrolytes	Electrolyte disturbance may cause a seizure or arrhythmias or may signify hypovolaemia	Electrolyte disturbances and/or raised urea and creatinine (dehydration)
C-reactive protein	Especially in the elderly, hypovolaemia secondary to sepsis can present as syncope	May be raised
D-dimer	Can consider to rule out PE	A normal result would effectively rule out a PE if pre-test probability is low
Cardiac enzymes (e.g. troponin I)	Myocardial ischaemia can precipitate, or be the result of a cardiac arrhythmia	May be raised. The timing of chest pain in relation to syncope may give a clue as to whether an MI was a cause or effect of syncope

Imaging

Table 4.3 Imaging modalities of use when patient presents with syncope

Test	Justification	Expected result
Chest X-ray	May show evidence of cardiac disease	Signs of heart failure or calcified valves
Echocardiography	Look for structural heart disease	May reveal structural defects such as hypertrophic obstructive cardiomyopathy or valve disease. It would be diagnostic to detect an endocardial mass although a TOE may be required
CT head	If CVA (stroke/TIA) is suspected this is vital, particularly if the patient has presented within a thrombolysis window	May show an area of infarction or haemorrhage
CTPA	If high pre-test probability of PE or D-dimer is raised this is the imaging modality of choice to show PE	Obstruction of one or more arteries in the pulmonary system

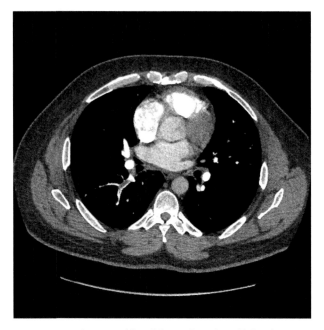

Figure 4.3 CT pulmonary angiogram showing a filling defect in the right and left pulmonary arteries consistent with bilateral pulmonary emboli.

Special

Table 4.4 Special tests to consider when a patient presents with syncope

Test	Justification	Potential result
Ambulatory/continuous ECG	Needed to identify rhythm disturbances that could cause syncope, although this is only likely if there is a high event rate	May capture dysrhythmias or conduction defects
EEG (electroencephalogram)	May provide evidence of epileptic seizure or prove a pseudoseizure	Spike and slow wave discharge in epilepsy. Normality in the presence of an on-going 'seizure' is suggestive of pseudo-seizure
Carotid sinus massage	Can be used to demonstrate carotid sinus hypersensitivity Do not perform if recent cerebral ischaemia or if a carotid bruit is present	A reduction in blood pressure and heart rate
Exercise test	For exercise-related syncope, this may be a way of provoking a dysrhythmia which can be captured on ECG	Evidence of ECG changes or dysrhythmia during exercise
Tilt table test	If postural hypotension/autonomic dysfunction is suspected	Patient is strapped to a horizontal table and then moved to vertical. Blood pressure and ECG monitoring takes place An onset of symptoms (lightheadedness), a drop in blood pressure or pulse, or syncope itself give a positive result

Box 4.8 How to perform a carotid massage

1. Assess for the presence of a carotid bruit – do not undertake if bruit present
2. Attach patient to a 12-lead ECG
3. Lie the patient flat
4. Locate the carotid sinus at the top third of the anterior border of the sternocleidomastoid muscle
5. Rub this area and assess for any T-LOC and cardiac pauses

4.7 WHEN TO CALL A SENIOR

Situations
In the context of syncope, there are two circumstances where a senior needs to be called:
A) If the patient has a cardiac or neurological cause for their syncope which is ongoing
B) If the patient might need specialist follow up
The two scenarios below illustrate each situation:

1. Patient presents with syncope due to third-degree heart block which is ongoing
2. A young patient with suspected SVT (now in sinus rhythm) that may require cardiology referral

What should be arranged by the time the senior arrives
Scenario 1
This is a high-risk situation as third-degree heart block can progress to asystole. Additionally the immediate management – atropine and external pacing – are best supervised by a more senior doctor (external pacing will require anaesthetic input). N.B. if the patient is showing 'adverse signs', such as respiratory distress or shock, this is a peri-arrest situation and may warrant a crash-call. Outside of this situation, the following should be arranged by the time the senior arrives:

- Cardiac monitoring
- 12-lead ECG
- Blood tests, including full blood count, renal function, clotting (as the patient will be considered for pacemaker insertion) and troponin (in case the heart block was precipitated by, or resulted from, a myocardial infarction)
- Chest X-ray – probably portable (the patient may have signs of heart failure requiring management)
- Echocardiogram – your senior may bring an echo machine with them (especially if they are the cardiology SpR), but if this is likely to take time to arrange, it can be helpful to request this in advance

Scenario 2
In this scenario the patient is stable but will almost certainly need specialist input and possible follow up and intervention. As above, a 12-lead ECG, basic blood tests and a chest X-ray are indicated and should be requested in a timely manner, however the senior will especially be interested in:

- A thorough history – especially the history of the presenting complaint (HPC) and PMH
- Information from the social history – this will determine location and possible nature of follow up
- Any information from previous admissions – previous discharge summaries or information from the GP will be useful in this scenario

What should be completed by the time the senior arrives
Scenario 1
In this scenario the senior would expect the following to be completed:

- Cardiac monitoring – the patient should be on continuous monitoring
- 12-lead ECG
- A full ABCDE assessment, including results of a quick clinical examination and measurement of bedside glucose

Scenario 2
The senior would expect:

- Thorough history
- 12-lead ECG and any previous ECGs

KEY CLINICAL TRIALS

Key trial 4.1
Trial name: Prevention of Syncope Trail (POST).
Participants: Inclusion criteria: positive tilt test and three preceding syncopal episodes.
Intervention: Metoprolol at highest tolerated dose (25–200 mg).
Control: Placebo.
Outcome: No significant difference between intervention and control.
Reason for inclusion: Beta blockers have poor evidence base for management of vasovagal syncope.
Reference: http://www.ncbi.nlm.nih.gov/pubmed/16505178.

Key trial 4.2
Trial name: Second Vasovagal Pacemaker Study (VPS II).
Participants: Outpatients with a mean of four syncope episodes.
Intervention: Dual-chamber pacemaker with rate drop response pacing.
Control: Dual-chamber pacemaker with sensing but no response.
Outcome: Syncope at six months – 42% with sensing but no pacing, 33% in the paced group. This was not statistically significant.
Reason for inclusion: Disproved earlier evidence demonstrating a benefit of placing pacemakers in this group.
Reference: http://www.ncbi.nlm.nih.gov/pubmed/12734133.

GUIDELINES

NICE. Transient loss of consciousness ('blackouts') management in adults and young people. NICE clinical guideline 109. August 2010. http://www.nice.org.uk/nicemedia/live/13111/50452/50452.pdf
European Society of Cardiology. Guidelines for the diagnosis and management of syncope. 2009. http://eurheartj.oxfordjournals.org/content/30/21/2631.full.pdf

FURTHER READING

Cannom DS. History of syncope in the cardiac literature. Prog Cardiovasc Dis. 2013;55(4):334–338. http://www.ncbi.nlm.nih.gov/pubmed/23472768.
Provides good general overview of syncope in the literature.
Thijs RD, Bloem BR, van Dijk JG. Falls, faints, fits and funny turns. J Neurol. 2009;256(2):155–167. http://www.ncbi.nlm.nih.gov/pubmed/19271109.
A recent, easy to read overview of syncope from a well respected journal.
O'Rourke RA. Clinical cardiology: The Stokes-Adams syndrome – definition and etiology; mechanisms and treatment. Calif Med. 1972; 117(1): 96–99. http://www.ncbi.nlm.nih.gov/pmc/articles/PMC1518479/?page=1.
Definition and aetiology of Stokes Adams attacks. A more focused reference
Bowman ES, Markand ON. Psychodynamics and psychiatric diagnoses of pseudoseizure subjects. Am J Psychiatry. 1996;153(1):57–63. http://www.ncbi.nlm.nih.gov/pubmed/8540592.
Association of pseudoseizures to psychiatric disease. A more focused reference.

For additional resources and to test your knowledge, visit the companion website at:

www.wiley.com/go/camm/cardiology

5 Palpitations

Harminder S. Gill

King's College Hospital NHS Foundation Trust, London, UK

5.1 DEFINITION

The sensation of a rapid, strong or irregular heartbeat caused by either an arrhythmia or experienced during normal sinus rhythm. It can be either physiological or pathological.

5.2 DIAGNOSTIC ALGORITHM

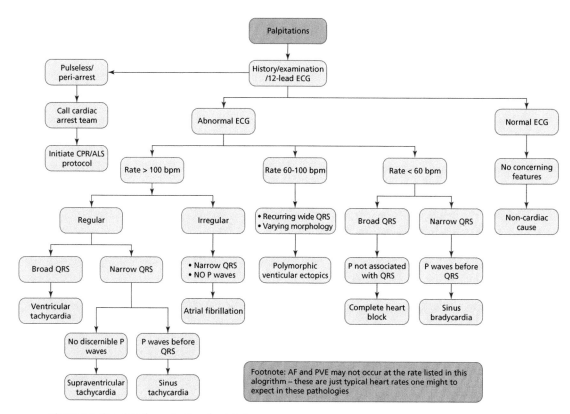

Figure 5.1 Flow chart for evaluation of palpitations.

5.3 DIFFERENTIALS LIST

Tachyarrhythmias
1. Supraventricular tachycardia
2. Ventricular tachycardia

Clinical Guide to Cardiology, First Edition. Edited by Christian F. Camm and A. John Camm.
© 2016 John Wiley & Sons, Ltd. Published 2016 by John Wiley & Sons, Ltd.
Companion website: www.wiley.com/go/camm/cardiology.

Bradyarrhythmias
1. Sinus bradycardia
2. Complete heart block

Extrasystoles
1. Ventricular ectopics
2. Atrial ectopics

Atrial fibrillation
1. With slow or fast ventricular rate

Sinus rhythm/tachycardia
1. Sinus rhythm
2. Sinus tachycardia

Box 5.1   Medical conditions associated with palpitations

1. Thyrotoxicosis: insomnia, heat intolerance, tremor, anxiety, fatigue, weight loss
2. Phaeochromocytoma: sweating, headache, weight loss, night sweats, fevers, FH of endocrine conditions
3. Hypoglycaemia: confusion, tremor, sweating, dizziness, DH of insulin
4. Hypercapnia: bounding pulse, flow murmur, asterixis, confusion/reduced conscious level, PMH of COPD
5. Pregnancy: various symptoms/signs depending on stage of pregnancy
6. Anaemia: reduced exercise tolerance, lethargy, pallor

Box 5.2   Exogenous substances associated with palpitations

1. Caffeine
2. Alcohol
3. Illicit drugs (e.g. cocaine)
4. Nicotine
5. Antihistamines (via muscarinic antagonism)

Box 5.3   Ventricular fibrillation

- Ventricular fibrillation has not been included in our differential list for palpitations
- This is because VF is not compatible with a cardiac output and thus life
- As such, the patient is unlikely to present with palpitations

---

5.4 KEY HISTORY FEATURES

Tachyarrhythmia 1
Diagnosis: Supraventricular tachycardia

Questions
a. Is there dizziness or chest discomfort/tightness associated?

A rapid rhythm can compromise coronary perfusion due to shorter diastolic filling times; this is experienced as tightness or discomfort in the chest.

b. Is there a warm/flushing sensation across the body?

This can occur due to the raised heart rate.

c. Has there been any polyuria after the episode?

Rapid atrial contraction results in release of atrial natriuretic peptide which results in polyuria.

d. Any past history of any SVT?

Patients who have previously been diagnosed are more likely to have a re-presentation with the same problem.

Tachyarrhythmia 2
Diagnosis: Ventricular tachycardia

Questions
a. Is there associated syncope/light-headedness/chest pain?

Ventricular tachycardia at faster rates will compromise cardiac output and reduced coronary/cerebral perfusion will be experienced.

b. Is there a sensation of 'fullness in the neck'?

Resulting from jugular venous distension.

c. Drug history including drugs associated with electrolyte depletion, e.g. diuretics and hypokalaemia?

Ventricular tachycardia can be precipitated by various electrolyte imbalances and which disturb the homeostasis of the myocytes.

d. Any past medical history of IHD/structural heart disease/cardiomyopathy?

Infarction and structural abnormalities may give rise to fibrosis which in turn acts as an ectopic focus.

e. Any family history of sudden cardiac death?

There are inherited syndromes which may predispose to VT (e.g. long QT channelopathies).

Bradyarrhythmia 1
Diagnosis: Sinus bradycardia

Questions
a. Are the palpitations slow, heavy and thudding in nature?

In bradycardia, there is no fluttering in the chest, the palpitations occur at a much lower rate

b. Is there dizziness?

Cerebral perfusion is compromised due to a reduced cardiac output and this can result in dizziness.

c. Is there lethargy and fatigue?

The reduced heart rate results in globally reduced perfusion which can be perceived as tiredness and generalized malaise.

Bradyarrhythmia 2
Diagnosis: Complete heart block

Questions
a. Is there any associated dizziness/weakness/fatigue/impaired exercise tolerance?

This is a product of the reduced cardiac output due to the greatly reduced ventricular rate; there is no rise in heart rate on exertion resulting in reduced exercise tolerance.

b. Is there any chest pain?

Complete heart block can occur in the acute setting of myocardial infarction, particularly inferior infarcts where blood supply to the AV node is also compromised.

c. Is there any past history of conduction defects (e.g. second-degree heart block)?

Any previous documentation of a conduction defect such as second-degree heart block, or tri-fascicular block gives a higher chance of development of complete conduction failure.

d. Drug history specifically for beta-blockers, calcium-channel antagonists, digoxin that can precipitate episodes?

Various rate-controlling agents have specific action to inhibit the AV node; in some cases this can be enough to precipitate complete heart block.

Extrasystoles 1
Diagnosis: Ventricular ectopics

Questions
a. Do the 'palpitations' come on while going to sleep?

This is typical for ventricular ectopics which are associated with an increased vagal tone related to parasympathetic drive before sleeping.

b. Are the symptoms positional, for instance while lying down on the left side?

Feeling a forceful ventricular contraction when the apex is lying in close apposition to the chest wall, suggests that this is a ventricular ectopic beat.

c. Do they correlate with episodes of emotion or exercise?

During these episodes ventricular ectopics occur more frequently than normally.

d. Is there any stimulant use, e.g. caffeine, amphetamine, methamphetamine and derivatives?

Stimulants alter the normal myocyte physiology, making the cells more excitable, which can result in premature ventricular contraction.

e. Is there history of structural heart disease?

Structural abnormalities of the myocardium can result in aberrant myocytes which can become foci for ventricular ectopics.

Extrasystoles 2
Diagnosis: Atrial ectopics

Questions:
a. Does the patient describe the palpitations as a 'skipped' or 'missed beat'?

Often the atrial ectopic itself is not 'felt' but the short refractory pause after is experienced as a missed beat.

b. Is there history of mitral valve disease?

Mitral valve disease often affects the atria by means of dilatation and this can predispose to atrial ectopics.

c. Is there history of cardiac failure?

In heart failure bi-atrial dilatation can give rise to atrial ectopics in the first instance, and then frequently will progress to atrial fibrillation.

d. Has the patient had any extended periods of a fast, irregular heart beat (atrial fibrillation)?

Regular atrial ectopics can become recurrent, turning into runs of atrial fibrillation.

Atrial fibrillation
Diagnosis: Atrial fibrillation

Questions
a. Any past medical history of AF?

Atrial fibrillation is one of the most common arrhythmias and frequently occurs in situations of stress or altered physiology, i.e. sepsis or post surgery. Therefore if there have been episodes of AF in these situations this more likely to become persistent in the future.

b. Is there associated dyspnoea/weakness?

AF increases the risk of thrombosis which can embolize and cause a cerebral infarct.

c. Is the patient able to tap out the beat? Is this regular or irregular?

This will give a clear indication of the rate and nature of the palpitations; in atrial fibrillation this beat will be irregularly irregular.

d. Is there a long-standing history of hypertension/IHD?

Ischaemic heart disease results in gradual damage to myocytes, which in turn can result in aberrant discharging of atrial myocytes.

Sinus rhythm/tachycardia
Diagnosis: Sinus rhythm/tachycardia

Questions
a. Any history of anxiety or functional disorders?

Sinus rhythm is usually asymptomatic, anxiety can result in 'awareness' of the heartbeat.

b. Does the patient have any cough/cold/lower urinary tract symptoms/diarrhoea and vomiting?

During infection cytokines and other vascular mediators exert effects on the myocardium and central mechanisms to raise the heart rate, which usually manifests as a sinus tachycardia.

c. Is there any recent blood loss?

A sudden loss in circulating volume results in an increase in sympathetic drive. This in turn can cause vasoconstriction and a sinus tachycardia, although this is usually only evident after a significant degree of blood loss.

d. Is there any history of fatigue/lethargy and reduced exercise tolerance?

Anaemia reduces the oxygen-carrying capacity and this is compensated by raising the heart rate to increase the rate at which blood is oxygenated and delivered to the tissues.

5.5 KEY EXAMINATION FEATURES

Tachyarrhythmia 1
Diagnosis: Supraventricular tachycardia

Key examination findings
a. Pulse

The rhythm is regular and typically at a rate of 140–200 bpm.

b. Blood pressure

This depends on the rate of tachycardia, at faster rate there is not adequate time or diastolic filling and cardiac output is greatly reduced, manifesting as hypotension.

Tachyarrhythmia 2
Diagnosis: Ventricular tachycardia

Key examination findings
a. Blood pressure

Ventricular tachycardia usually runs at rate of 150–300 bpm; as the rate increases, ventricular filling falls and cardiac output drops, resulting in hypotension.

b. JVP

Jugular venous distension occurs due to the reduced cardiac output; cannon ball 'a' waves may be seen due to atrial contraction on closed AV valves, resulting in a back-surge of blood up the jugular veins.

c. Heart sounds

These tend to be variable due to atrioventricular asynchrony.

Bradyarrhythmia 1
Diagnosis: Sinus bradycardia

Key examination findings
a. Pulse

The rhythm is regular and by definition at a rate of <60 bpm, although a mild sinus bradycardia (heart rate of 50–60 bpm) is a frequent finding in physically active individuals.

Bradyarrhythmia 2
Diagnosis: Complete heart block

Key examination findings
a. Hypotension

Frequently the cardiac output is diminished at lower rates.

b. Regular rhythm <60 bpm (usually 30–40 bpm)

The slow rate of complete heart block is the intrinsic rate of the escape rhythm; the electrocardiographic morphology of this will vary depending on the level of origin.

c. Inspiratory respiratory crackles

Sarcoidosis should be considered in patients presenting with complete heart block.

Extrasystoles 1
Diagnosis: Ventricular ectopics

Key examination findings
a. Pulse

There is usually an underlying regular rhythm, with odd misplaced beats with an increased volume and forceful character. Do not confuse this for AF; by palpating the pulse for a longer period the underlying sinus rhythm can be detected.

b. Murmur

Patients with structural heart disease are prone to ectopic beats from areas of scar, a murmur may be indicative of valvular disease/myocardial disease which leaves patients prone to ectopics.

Extrasystoles 2
Diagnosis: Atrial ectopics

Key examination findings
a. Pulse

Regular pulse will be palpated with extra beats which feel normal in volume and character (as it is a normal ventricular depolarization following premature atrial contraction). There will be pause after the premature atrial contraction which can usually be sensed.

b. Murmur

Mitral valve lesions are most frequently associated with atrial ectopics; a pansystolic murmur of mitral regurgitation or mid-diastolic murmur in mitral stenosis may be auscultated.

Atrial fibrillation
Diagnosis: Atrial fibrillation

Key examination findings
a. Pulse

The pulse will feel variable both in rhythm and rate ('irregularly irregular'), but also in in terms of volume and character.

b. Heart sounds

Ventricular filling varies from beat to beat and therefore the first heart sound changes with each beat.

Sinus rhythm/tachycardia
Diagnosis: Sinus rhythm

Key examination findings
a. Pulse

In sinus rhythm, the rate should lie between 60 and 100 bpm and be normal in rhythm and character. In sinus tachycardia the rate will be >100 bpm and thready on palpation.

b. Heart sounds

With a sinus tachycardia there is a hyper-dynamic state; this may include a third heart sound due to rapid ventricular filling. A fourth heart sound and systolic flow murmur may also be encountered.

c. Temperature and general examination

In sepsis there may be pyrexia which is often associated with a sinus tachycardia. In addition a general examination may reveal the patient to be peripherally shut down, or show specific signs localizing the infection.

(See Audio Podcast 5.1 and 5.2 at **www.wiley.com/go/camm/cardiology**)

5.6 KEY INVESTIGATIONS

Bedside

Table 5.1 Bedside tests of use in patients with palpitations

Test	Justification	Potential result
Blood pressure	Simple, fast	Haemodynamic instability
ECG	Diagnostically vital	Multiple, fundamental to management, may show abnormal rhythm

Blood tests

Table 5.2 Blood tests of use in patients with palpitations

Test	Justification	Potential result
Urea and electrolytes	Potassium influences myocardial stability	Hyperkalaemia, hypokalaemia, renal dysfunction
Magnesium	Influences myocardial stability	Hypomagnesaemia
Calcium	Influences the QT interval – predisposing to ventricular tachycardia	Hypocalcaemia
Thyroid function test	Abnormalities can predispose to both Brady- and tachy-arrhythmias	Hypothyroidism – low T4 Hyperthyroidism – high T4
Full blood count	Anaemia can cause sinus tachycardia/exacerbate other arrhythmias	Anaemia
	Neutrophilia may indicate infection	Neutrophilia
CRP	Inflammatory marker which suggests infection or inflammation	Infection – raised
Cardiac troponins	Use if there is concurrent chest pain – suggests ischaemia, which can underlie abnormal rhythms and palpitations	Raised in the setting of acute coronary syndromes

Imaging

Table 5.3 Imaging modalities of use in patients with palpitations

Test	Justification	Potential result
Echocardiogram	Structural and functional information	Structurally abnormal hearts are predisposed to palpitations due to aberrant conduction

Special tests

Table 5.4 Specialist tests of use in patients with palpitations

Test	Justification	Potential result
IV adenosine	In tachycardias where the rate makes the ECG difficult to interpret; adenosine can act as AV-nodal blocking agent to reveal the underlying rhythm. Short-acting bolus is administered and a 12-lead ECG/rhythm strip performed immediately	Useful for differentiating narrow-complex tachycardias; at rates >180 bpm it can be difficult to differentiate between sinus tachycardia, supraventricular tachycardia and atrial fibrillation or flutter
Cardiac magnetic resonance	Structural and functional information	This may show scar or fibrosis which can act as an ectopic focus for arrhythmias
24-hour ECG (Holter monitor)	Gives a greater sample for diagnosis of palpitations. Patients can press an event button when symptomatic for correlation with cardiac rhythm	May give an electrocardiographic diagnosis for the palpitations
Electrophysiological study	Invasive test to map conduction pathways and locate aberrant electrical activity	Can identify the source of an arrhythmia – can identify targets for ablation and thus also has elements of management
Implantable loop recorder (e.g. REVEAL device)	Where diagnosis uncertain and palpitations remain troublesome. Can remain *in situ* for months–years if needed	May give an electrocardiographic diagnosis for the palpitations

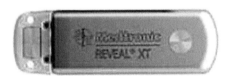

Figure 5.2 A REVEAL™ device – used for palpitations/syncope of unknown origin.
Source: courtesy of Medtronic.

(See Audio Podcast 5.3 at **www.wiley.com/go/camm/cardiology**)

5.7 WHEN TO CALL A SENIOR

Situations

Two major situations warrant senior input:
A) Any patient with evidence of haemodynamic instability where further, more advanced management, such as cardioversion, needs to be offered
B) If initial, simple management methods are unsuccessful in correcting the problem and the patient remains symptomatic, or is developing complications

An example of a situation which demonstrates each of these is:

1. A patient with palpitations who has VT on their monitoring and has become haemodynamically unstable with hypotension and evidence of end-organ dysfunction (e.g. confusion or reduced conscious level)

2. A patient with AF (with fast ventricular response) who is complaining of palpitations and dyspnoea despite beta-blocker treatment and is starting to develop signs of complications with decompensated heart failure, such as raised respiratory rate, desaturation and agitation

What should be arranged by the time the senior arrives
Scenario 1
This is a peri-arrest scenario and a crash call should be put out. While awaiting a crash team the patient should be managed using an ABCDE approach. In particular the following things should be prepared:

- **Chest X-ray:** often useful, to identify any pericardial effusion, pulmonary oedema or pneumonia
- **Anaesthetics liaison:** patient may require DC cardioversion, which is best done under sedation (although this should not delay cardioversion if the patient is *in extremis*)

Scenario 2
This patient is not at risk of immediate harm in this situation, however is likely to deteriorate if the underlying problem is not corrected. The initial management methods have not been successful and therefore more senior input will be required for more complex management methods. The following would be appropriate:

- **Chest X-ray:** to assess for the degree of complications, or show any pericardial effusion that could be precipitating the AF
- **Echocardiogram:** may be useful in identifying structural abnormalities

What should be completed by the time the senior arrives
Scenario 1
A rigorous approach to resuscitation in these patients is vital. Focusing on the basic aspects of treatment. This includes:

- **ABCDE:** this assessment approach should be used
- **Establishing IV access:** this is a situation where this HAS to be large bore (at least a green cannula) into a large vein. This may be for IV fluids, but also for amiodarone, adenosine or other medications
- **Blood tests:** FBC/urea and electrolytes (U&E)/Mg^{2+}/Ca^{2+}/CRP/LFTs/TFTs
- **Applying defibrillator pads and cardiac monitoring:** the patient may require DC cardioversion
- **Patients notes:** an approximate summary of the case

Scenario 2
The senior would expect:

- Full history and examination of the patient
- Full set of observations
- IV access
- Correction of hypotension/hypoxia with simple measures, e.g. oxygen and IV fluids where appropriate
- Cardiac monitoring for the patient

GUIDELINES

American College of Cardiology, American Heart Association, and the European Society of Cardiology. Supraventricular arrhythmias (ACC/AHA/ESC Guidelines for the Management of Patients with). 2003. http://www.escardio.org/guidelines-surveys/esc-guidelines/Pages/supraventricular-arrhythmias.aspx

American College of Cardiology, American Heart Association, and the European Society of Cardiology. Ventricular Arrhythmias and the Prevention of Sudden Cardiac Death (ACC/AHA/ESC 2006 Guidelines for Management of Patients With). 2006. http://www.escardio.org/guidelines-surveys/esc-guidelines/Pages/ventricular-arrhythmias-and-prevention-sudden-cardiac-death.aspx

European Society of Cardiology. Atrial fibrillation (Management of) 2010 and Focused Update (2012). 2010, 2012. http://www.escardio.org/guidelines-surveys/esc-guidelines/Pages/atrial-fibrillation.aspx

FURTHER READING

Crossland S, Berkin L. Problem based review: the patient with 'palpitations'. Acute med. 2012;11(3):169–171. 2012; http://www.ncbi.nlm.nih.gov/pubmed/22993750
An interesting article tackling the diagnostic problem of palpitations

Thavendiranathan P, Bagai A, Khoo C, et al. Does this patient with palpitations have a cardiac arrhythmia? JAMA. 2009;302(19):2135–2143. http://www.ncbi.nlm.nih.gov/pubmed/19920238
A review helping the clinician identify those with palpitations who have underlying cardiac conditions

 For additional resources and to test your knowledge, visit the companion website at:

www.wiley.com/go/camm/cardiology

6 Cardiac Murmurs

Blair Merrick
Hammersmith Hospital, London, UK

6.1 DEFINITION

An additional noise produced by increased or turbulent blood flow.

6.2 CLASSIFICATION

Cardiac murmurs may be classified in numerous different ways; most commonly by their timing:

- **Systolic murmur:** occurs during ventricular contraction – between the 1st and 2nd heart sounds
- **Diastolic murmur:** occurs during ventricular relaxation – between the 2nd and 1st heart sounds
- **Continuous murmur:** can be heard in both systole and diastole

    For clinical practice their nature is highly important, i.e. benign or pathological:

- **Benign (innocent) murmur:** not related to underlying structural defect
- **Pathological murmur:** related to underlying structural defect

    Murmurs can also be categorized based on a number of additional features:

- Intensity (see Box 14.2, Chapter 14)
- Character
- Where they are heard loudest
- Accentuating and diminishing manoeuvres
- Radiation

Clinical Guide to Cardiology, First Edition. Edited by Christian F. Camm and A. John Camm.
© 2016 John Wiley & Sons, Ltd. Published 2016 by John Wiley & Sons, Ltd.
Companion website: www.wiley.com/go/camm/cardiology.

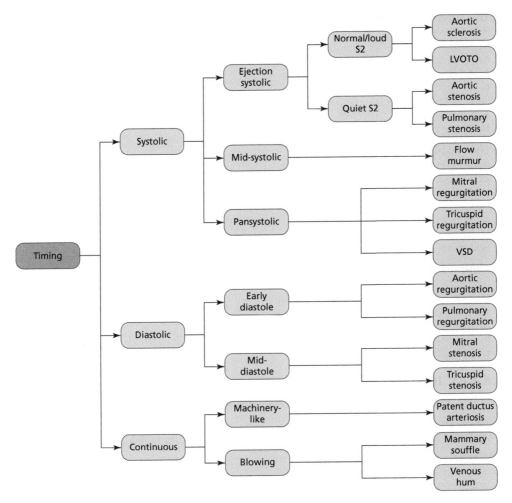

Figure 6.1 Flow-chart of potential underlying causes for murmurs based on timing.

Box 6.1   Murmur characteristics

- **Intensity:** systolic murmurs can be graded from 1–6 and diastolic murmurs from 1–4 based on volume and associated thrill (see Box 14.2 for more details)
- **Shape:** crescendo, decrescendo, crescendo–decrescendo, uniform
- **Loudest location:** four valve areas
- **Accentuating/diminishing manoeuvres:** inspiration, expiration, sitting the patient forward, moving the patient into the left lateral position, getting the patient to stand, squat, perform a valsalva manoeuvre
- **Radiation:** to the axilla, the carotid arteries, the apex or through to the back

6.3 DIFFERENTIALS LIST

'New' murmurs can either be truly novel, representing new or developing pathology in the patient, or previously recognized and representative of a more chronic process. Clinically, murmurs can either occur in patients who are stable or in those who are acutely ill.

In the unwell patient
1. Prosthetic valve dysfunction
2. Aortic dissection
3. Acute myocardial infarction:
   a. Acute ventricular septal rupture
   b. Acute mitral regurgitation
4. Infective endocarditis (IE):
   a. Native valve
   b. Prosthetic valve

In the stable patient
1. Aortic sclerosis
2. Aortic stenosis (AS)
3. Hypertrophic (obstructive) cardiomyopathy
4. Mitral regurgitation (MR)/mitral valve prolapse (MVP)
5. Aortic regurgitation
6. Mitral stenosis (MS)
7. Flow murmur

Diagnoses to consider
1. Tricuspid regurgitation
2. Murmur associated with prosthetic heart valve
3. Murmur associated with congenital heart disease:
   a. Septal defects
   b. Pulmonary regurgitation
   c. Coarctation of the aorta

6.4 KEY HISTORY FEATURES

(See Audio Podcast 6.1 at **www.wiley.com/go/camm/cardiology**)

General points
In any patient found to have a cardiac murmur, a thorough cardiovascular history is vital:

- **Potential cardiovascular symptoms:** chest pain, shortness of breath, palpitations, syncope, orthopnoea, peripheral oedema
- **Cardiovascular risk factors:** non-modifiable (age, sex, family history); modifiable (smoking history, BP, lipid disorders, diabetes)
- **Previous cardiovascular events:** myocardial infarction, stroke
- **Previous cardiac surgery:** coronary artery bypass grafting, valve replacement/repair etc.
- **Medications:** especially those taken for cardiovascular disease (e.g. antihypertensives, statins)

Unstable diagnosis 1
Diagnosis: Prosthetic valve dysfunction

Questions
a. Time of symptom onset

Patients with acute valvular insufficiency will have sudden onset of symptoms, e.g. dyspnoea, chest pain, syncope. In subacute insufficiency there will be a short history of worsening symptoms of heart failure.

b. Previous valve replacement?

Although uncommon, prosthetic valve dysfunction should be excluded. Patients may carry a card that gives details about their valve replacement, this is helpful as certain valves are normally associated with particular murmurs and thus may well be functioning normally.

Unstable diagnosis 2
Diagnosis: Aortic dissection

Questions
a. Pain history

Typically sudden-onset, severe pain, described as tearing or ripping, in the chest and/or the back (intrascapular). The location of the pain is related to the site of dissection, and can migrate as the dissection extends. However, pain is not severe in all cases and thus a high index of suspicion is needed.

b. History of hypertension?

Poorly controlled hypertension is the single biggest risk factor for dissection.

c. History of connective tissue disorder?

Patients with underlying connective tissue disorders are at higher risk of aortic dissection.

Unstable diagnosis 3
Diagnosis: Myocardial infarction

Questions
a. Are there any cardiac risk factors?

See Box 2.1.

b. Is there chest tightness or heaviness made worse with exertion?

This is a typical description of cardiac pain, however the character can be very variable. There may be radiation to either arm, the neck, the back or the jaw.

c. Are there associated autonomic symptoms?

Commonly nausea/vomiting and sweating.

Unstable diagnosis 4
Diagnosis: Infective endocarditis

Questions
a. Is there a history of symptoms of systemic infection?

Fevers, rigors or night sweats would be highly suspicious. Subacute IE can often present non-specifically, so ensure to also ask about unintentional weight loss, anorexia, lethargy and myalgia too.

b. Has the patient had any neurological symptoms?

IE is associated with neurological complications in 40% of cases, especially embolic strokes.

c. Does the patient have an underlying congenital heart defect, known valvular pathology or history of valve replacement?

Individuals with congenital heart disease, even if this has been surgically corrected, are at an increased risk of developing IE, as are those with a valvular abnormality. Prosthetic valve endocarditis can be differentiated into early (within 1 year) and late (after 1 year); this has implications for likely pathogens and patient outcomes.

d. Is there a history of intravenous drug use?

Typically results in right-sided valve endocarditis due to repeated injections with either dirty needles or through infected sites, e.g. groin abscesses or cellulitis.

Stable diagnosis 1
Diagnosis: Aortic sclerosis

Questions
a. What cardiovascular risk factors dose the patient have?

Aortic sclerosis is age-related degeneration of aortic valve function, and shares the same cardiac risk factors as atherosclerosis, e.g. age, hypertension etc.

b. Does the patient have any symptoms?

Aortic sclerosis is almost always detected incidentally in an asymptomatic patient, thus symptoms suggest alternative or co-existent pathology.

Stable diagnosis 2
Diagnosis: Aortic stenosis

Questions
a. Any angina-type pains, unexplained syncope or shortness of breath?

Associated symptoms in a patient with AS can help predict mortality (see Chapter 14), and thus the timeframe during which intervention may be needed.

b. Past history of rheumatic fever or abnormal aortic valve?

Both are risk factors for development of AS. Bicuspid (as opposed to the normal tri-leaflet) aortic valves are more likely to become stenotic, with this occurring at an earlier age (in the sixth decade rather than in their eighth decade).

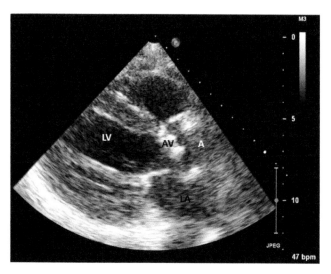

Figure 6.2 Heavily calcified aortic valve (AV) in a patient with severe aortic stenosis. There is concentric hypertrophy of the left ventricular (LV) wall and post-stenotic dilatation of the aorta (A). LA, left atrium.
Source: Harpreet Kaur Sahemey, Echocardiographer, Hammersmith Hospital.

Stable diagnosis 3
Diagnosis: Left ventricular outflow tract obstruction (LVOTO)

Questions
a. How old is the patient?

Younger patients are less likely to have degenerative changes to the aortic valve, and more likely to have congenital abnormalities such as H(O)CM (see Chapter 15) or coarctation of the aorta (see Chapter 18).

b. Any episodes of collapse on exertion?

This is a red flag for outflow obstruction, especially when there is little or no warning prior to the event. LVOTO prevents an increase in cardiac output to match an increased demand.

c. Episodes of chest pain (dull/pressure-like, central, worse on exertion)?

Outflow obstruction is frequently associated with angina due to poor coronary vessel perfusion.

d. Is there a family history of early cardiovascular disease (males <50 years old or females <55 years old) or sudden (cardiac) death?

Previous myocardial infarction or sudden death in first-degree male relative <50 years or female relatives <55 years suggests a strong family history for cardiovascular disease.

Stable diagnosis 4

Diagnosis: Mitral regurgitation/prolapse

Questions

a. Signs or symptoms of heart failure?

Ask about shortness of breath, lethargy, orthopnoea and paroxysmal nocturnal dyspnoea.

b. Past history of rheumatic fever or infective endocarditis?

Both can damage the mitral valve leading to regurgitation.

c. Is there a history of palpitations?

Atrial fibrillation commonly develops due to left atrial dilatation, it is important to identify this, as it is associated with a worse outcome.

d. Is there a history of connective tissue disease?

Individuals with such disorders are more likely to develop mitral valve prolapse.

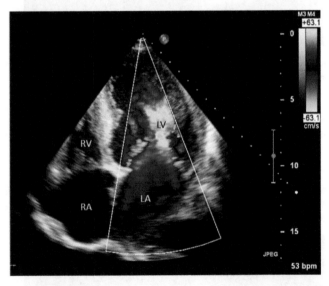

Figure 6.3 Mitral regurgitation. Doppler shows a jet of blood passing from the left ventricle (LV) into the left atrium (LA). RV, right ventricle; RA, right atrium.
Source: Harpreet Kaur Sahemey, Echocardiographer, Hammersmith Hospital.

Stable diagnosis 5

Diagnosis: Aortic regurgitation

Questions

a. Known aortic valve pathology?

Stenotic valves can become regurgitant when the calcification of the valve prevents the leaflets closing completely. Abnormal aortic valves, e.g. bicuspid, are also more likely to become regurgitant.

b. History of connective tissue disorder?

Patients with underlying connective tissue disorders such as Marfan's syndrome and Ehlers–Danlos (type IV) are more likely to get a regurgitant valve. Ankylosing spondylitis and tertiary syphilis can also result in aortic root dilatation leading to functional aortic regurgitation.

c. Past history of infective endocarditis?

Endocarditis can lead to the development of regurgitation which will remain after the infection is cleared.

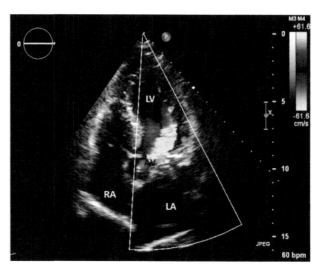

Figure 6.4 Aortic regurgitation, Doppler imaging shows a jet of blood directed back into the left ventricle (LV) from the aorta. AV, aortic valve; LA, left atrium; RA, right atrium.
Source: Harpreet Kaur Sahemey, Echocardiographer, Hammersmith Hospital.

Stable diagnosis 6
Diagnosis: Mitral stenosis

Questions:
a. Past history of rheumatic fever?

Risk factor for development of MS, and commonest cause of MS worldwide. The patient may not be aware they previously had rheumatic fever, so ensure to ask if they were born or lived in a country with a high incidence rate.

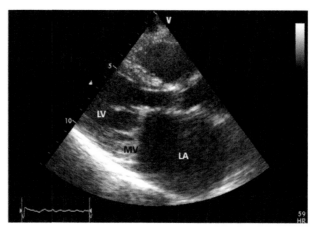

Figure 6.5 Mitral stenosis. The mitral valve (MV) is heavily calcified. The left atrium (LA) is dilated. LV, left ventricle.
Source: Harpreet Kaur Sahemey, Echocardiographer, Hammersmith Hospital.

Stable diagnosis 7
Diagnosis: Flow murmur

Questions:
a. Are there symptoms of precipitating conditions?

High-output states such as anaemia, hyperthyroidism or Paget's disease can lead to a flow murmur.

b. Could the patient be pregnant?

Pregnancy, in particular, is a high-output state often associated with a relative anaemia, and thus blood flow is more likely to be turbulent. Increased blood flow to the breasts during lactation can also produce a continuous murmur (mammary soufflé murmur).

c. Is the patient asymptomatic?

Young, fit individuals can have flow murmurs with normal anatomy.

Diagnosis to consider 1
Diagnosis: Tricuspid regurgitation

Questions
a. History of chronic lung disease?

Tricuspid regurgitation is most commonly secondary to right ventricular pressure overload, and this is most commonly secondary to chronic lung disease (pulmonary hypertension). It can also occur in primary pulmonary hypertension.

b. History of rheumatic heart disease or infective endocarditis?

Both can damage the tricuspid valve causing it to be regurgitant. Right-sided endocarditis is more common in intravenous drug users (IVDUs).

Diagnosis to consider 2
Diagnosis: Prosthetic heart valve

Questions
a. History of valve replacement?

Need to ask about position, e.g. aortic or mitral, type, e.g. tissue or metallic (and if metallic which subtype), and when it was inserted. Patient may carry a card that gives details about their valve replacement.

Diagnosis to consider 3
Diagnosis: Associated with congenital heart disease

Questions
a. Any paediatric history concerning their heart?

Patients may have been previously investigated for a murmur. If this was due to a small atrial septal defect (ASD) or ventricular septal defect (VSD) the decision may have been not to intervene, as the defect could potentially close naturally, or the risks of surgery outweighed the benefits.

b. Previous cardiac surgery to repair defect?

Surgical repair of a congenital heart defect may mean patient no longer has a murmur. However, certain procedures may leave the patient with a murmur, e.g. pulmonary regurgitation post repair of pulmonary stenosis; this is classically seen in patients who have had surgical repair of tetralogy of Fallot (for more detail see Chapter 18).

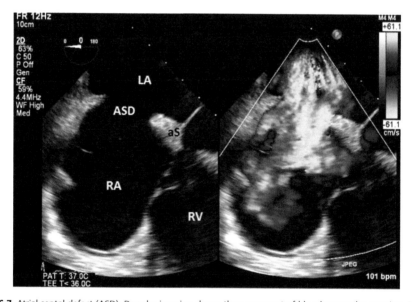

Figure 6.6 Ventricular septal defect (VSD), Doppler imaging shows the movement of blood across the opening. RV, right ventricle; RA, right atrium; vS, ventricular septum; LV, left ventricle; LA, left atrium.
Source: Harpreet Kaur Sahemey, Echocardiographer, Hammersmith Hospital.

Figure 6.7 Atrial septal defect (ASD), Doppler imaging shows the movement of blood across the opening. RA, right atrium; LA, left atrium; aS, atrial septum; RV, right ventricle.
Source: Harpreet Kaur Sahemey, Echocardiographer, Hammersmith Hospital.

6.5 KEY EXAMINATION FEATURES

This chapter covers a wide range of conditions in which a heart murmur may be present, many of which are rare. On finding a patient has a murmur; it is helpful to have in your mind what the underlying lesion (if indeed there is one) may be.

(See Audio Podcast 6.2 at **www.wiley.com/go/camm/cardiology**)

Unstable diagnosis 1
Diagnosis: Prosthetic valve dysfunction

Examination findings

a. General observation

Patient will be very unwell, may be unresponsive, have evidence of poor peripheral perfusion – look pale, feel cool.

b. Pulse

Tachycardic, weak or not palpable.

c. Blood pressure

Hypotensive, there may be a widened pulse pressure in aortic insufficiency.

d. Auscultation

Aortic insufficiency – early diastolic murmur in aortic area radiating down towards apex best heard in full expiration, loss of metallic A2 with prosthetic valve failure.

Mitral insufficiency – harsh pansystolic murmur loudest in mitral area, often radiates across praecordium and into axilla.

Unstable diagnosis 2
Diagnosis: Aortic dissection

Examination findings

a. General observation

Patient is likely to be very unwell and may be in extremis.

b. Pulse and blood pressure

The pulse may be tachycardic, weak or not palpable. Blood pressure will be low, classically there is a significant (>20 mmHg) difference in blood pressure between arms, however absence of this sign does not exclude dissection.

c. Auscultation of praecordium

Early diastolic murmur in aortic area if the aortic valve has been involved in the dissection (Stanford Type A). Rupture of the aorta in the pericardial sac leads to cardiac tamponade with associated muffled heart sounds.

d. Auscultation of lungs

Bilateral inspiratory crepitations as a result of pulmonary oedema.

e. Neurological examination

Focal neurological defects can arise due to involvement of the carotid arteries in the dissection.

f. Abdominal examination

May have abdominal pain due to involvement of gastrointestinal tract arteries or renal arteries, however, there will be little to find on clinical examination.

Unstable diagnosis 3
Diagnosis: Myocardial infarction (for full findings see Chapter 9)

Examination findings

a. General observation

Patient likely to be very unwell and in cardiogenic shock due to sudden haemodynamic changes – peripherally shut down, tachypnoeic, tachycardic and hypotensive.

b. JVP

Elevated due to back pressure on right side of the heart.

c. Auscultation of praecordium

Harsh pansystolic murmur loudest at the left sternal edge; may have loud P2 due to elevated pulmonary pressures.

d. Auscultation of lungs

Bilateral inspiratory crepitations as a result of pulmonary oedema.

Unstable diagnosis 4
Diagnosis: Infective endocarditis

Examination findings
a. General observation

In acute IE the patient is often very unwell; if subacute, there is often evidence of a long-standing illness, e.g. cachexia.

b. Hands (and feet)

Look for splinter haemorrhages (common, also seen in individuals with repeated nail trauma, e.g. gardeners), Janeway lesions (rare), Osler's nodes (rare), finger clubbing (rare). May feel warm peripherally due to vasodilatation.

c. Signs of sepsis

Likely to be tachycardic, may be bounding if profoundly septic, or weak if becoming peripherally shut down. Tachypnoea and hypotension may also occur.

d. Eyes

Roth spots may be visible on the retina using an ophthalmoscope. These are retinal haemorrhages that have a pale centre caused by embolic occlusion of retinal vessels.

e. Auscultation of praecordium

Murmur will be dependent on valve implicated and the nature of lesion. Most commonly the mitral valve is affected, leading to mitral regurgitation (pansystolic murmur), followed by the aortic valve, leading to aortic regurgitation (early diastolic murmur).

Box 6.2   Peripheral stigmata of infective endocarditis

- **Finger clubbing:** increase in soft tissue around the ends of the fingers (or toes) with loss of the nail bed angle (subacute endocarditis only)
- **Splinter haemorrhages:** linear haemorrhages in the finger or toenails
- **Janeway lesions:** non-tender erythematous macules on palms
- **Osler's nodes:** red, tender palpable nodules, often in finger pulps
- **Roth spots:** retinal haemorrhage with a pale centre, visible on fundoscopy

---

Stable diagnosis 1
Diagnosis: Aortic sclerosis

Examination findings
a. Auscultation of praecordium

Ejection systolic murmur loudest in the aortic area with no or minimal radiation to the carotids. It may radiate down towards apex of heart. A2 may be loud (or normal, but not soft) due to the calcified valve snapping shut.

Stable diagnosis 2
Diagnosis: Aortic stenosis

Examination findings

a. Pulse and blood pressure

In severe disease a central pulse (brachial or carotid) may be slow rising and/or flat and a narrow pulse pressure, i.e. small difference between the systolic and diastolic blood pressure.

b. Palpation of praecordium

A heave due to left ventricular hypertrophy may be felt, the apex beat is usually non-displaced, but can become more laterally displaced in advanced disease.

c. Auscultation of praecordium

Ejection systolic murmur loudest in the aortic area in full expiration, may radiate to the carotids. A2 may be normal or soft as stenotic valve fails to close fully.

d. Auscultation of lungs

Bilateral inspiratory crepitations may be heard as a result of pulmonary oedema if the aortic stenosis has culminated in left-sided heart failure.

Stable diagnosis 3

Diagnosis: Hypertrophic (obstructive) cardiomyopathy

Examination findings

a. Pulse

Causes rapid up and down pulsation.

b. Auscultation

Mid-systolic murmur at left sternal edge radiating up to aortic area and carotids and down to mitral area. Accentuated by valsalva manoeuvre (vs. reduced in AS).

Stable diagnosis 4

Diagnosis: Mitral regurgitation/prolapse

Examination findings

a. Pulse

May be irregularly irregular if atrial fibrillation is present – often occurs due to dilatation of the left atrium.

b. Palpation of praecordium

Apex beat may be laterally displaced due to left ventricular dilatation (most common cause of functional or secondary mitral regurgitation).

c. Auscultation of praecordium

MR – pansystolic murmur loudest in the mitral area +/- radiation into the axilla. The murmur is heard best in full expiration, and with the patient in the left lateral position.

MVP – midsystolic click followed by systolic murmur best heard in the mitral area. The click is caused by the prolapse of one of the valve leaflets.

d. Auscultation of lungs

Bilateral inspiratory crepitations may be heard as a result of pulmonary oedema.

e. Musculoskeletal examination

Evidence of connective tissue disorder (e.g. joint hypermobility, arachnodactyly, high-arched palate) may be apparent.

Stable diagnosis 5

Diagnosis: Aortic regurgitation

Examination findings

a. General observation

Long-standing severe AR can be associated with a number of eponymous signs (see Box 14.19). Many of these signs are due to the collapsing nature of the pulse and widened pulse pressure in AR.

b. Auscultation of praecordium

Early diastolic murmur, loudest in full expiration in the aortic area with radiation down towards the apex. Sitting the patient forward helps to accentuate the murmur. Often heard in conjunction with the ejection systolic murmur of aortic stenosis.

c. Musculoskeletal examination

Evidence of connective tissue disorder (e.g. joint hypermobility, arachnodactyly, high-arched palate) may be apparent.

Stable diagnosis 6

Diagnosis: Mitral stenosis

Examination findings

a. Pulse

Atrial fibrillation is more common in individuals with MS (50% of patients). AF also quickly leads to compromise in patients with MS, and thus it is important to identify and treat appropriately.

b. JVP

May be elevated if patient has developed right-sided heart failure.

c. Face

Can be associated with mitral facies – a rash across the cheeks that is pathognomic of mitral stenosis.

d. Auscultation of praecordium

Loud S1 with 'opening snap' and low, rumbling, mid to late diastolic murmur best heard in the mitral area with the patient in the left lateral position. As the valve becomes more calcified, S1 and the opening snap may disappear. If right-sided heart failure starts to develop may have a loud P2.

Stable diagnosis 7

Diagnosis: Flow murmur

Examination findings

a. General observation

Look for signs of thyrotoxicosis – weight loss, heat intolerance, tremor, lid retraction, or signs of thyroid eye disease. Does the patient look pale – may be anaemic?

b. Hands

Palmar erythema can occur in high-output states such as thyrotoxicosis and Paget's disease. Can have a fine tremor associated with thyrotoxicosis. Nails beds may be pale if patient is severely anaemic. In iron deficiency can see spooning of the nails (koilonychia).

c. Face

Conjunctival pallor may be seen if the patient is anaemic. Lid retraction and lid lag in hyperthyroidism, may also have proptosis due to thyroid eye disease. Angular cheilitis and glossitis can be seen in iron-deficiency states.

d. Auscultation of praecordium

Systolic murmur, loudest in either aortic or pulmonary area due to high flow rates across the valve.

Diagnosis to consider 1
Diagnosis: Tricuspid regurgitation

Examination findings
a. JVP

Elevated with a prominent 'v' wave.

b. Palpation of the praecordium

Right ventricular heave may be present.

c. Auscultation of the praecordium

High-pitched, pansystolic murmur loudest in the tricuspid area. The murmur is best heard in full inspiration. It is often associated with a loud P2 due to concurrent pulmonary hypertension.

d. Abdominal examination

Tender, pulsatile hepatomegaly can develop in right-sided heart failure due to back pressure of blood.

Diagnosis to consider 2
Diagnosis: Prosthetic heart valve

Examination findings
a. Inspection of the praecordium

Surgical scar as evidence for previous cardiac surgery. Aortic and mitral valves can be inserted via median sternotomy approach; mitral valves can also be inserted via lateral thoracotomy approach. Beware aortic valve replacement can now be accomplished by a catheter approach (i.e. no praecordial scars).

b. Auscultation of praecordium

Aortic valves – often result in a degree of outflow obstruction and soft systolic murmur which increases in intensity as cardiac output increases. Tissue valves produce closing sound similar to that of native valves, whereas metallic valves produce a loud metallic click (S2) on closure (absence of this is pathological). Some valves do not completely occlude the outflow tract and so may be associated with a quiet diastolic (regurgitant) murmur.

Mitral valves – often associated with short systolic murmur due to a degree of regurgitation, pansystolic murmurs are pathological. Tissue valves produce closing sound similar to that of native valves, whereas metallic valves produce a loud metallic click (S1) on closure.

Box 6.3   Types of metallic heart valve and associated murmur during normal function

1. **Bileaflet tilting disc:**
   - Commonest type of metallic prosthetic valve
   - Opening click should be quieter than closing click
   - Outflow obstruction causes mid-systolic (aortic position) or short diastolic (mitral position) murmur
2. **Single tilting disc:**
   - As with bileaflet valve, but a short diastolic murmur (aortic position) due to regurgitation
3. **Caged ball:**
   - No longer inserted, but a number of patients still have these valves
   - Loud opening click and followed by several clicks as ball bounces within cage
   - Quieter closing click
   - Ejection systolic murmur (aortic position)
   - Systolic murmur (mitral position) due to LVOT turbulence

---

Diagnosis to consider 3
Diagnosis: Murmur associated with congenital heart disease

Examination findings

a. Inspection of the praecordium

Surgical scar as evidence of previous cardiac surgery.

b. Auscultation of praecordium

ASD – may be associated with systolic flow murmur due to increased flow across the pulmonary valve and fixed splitting of S2.

VSD – may be associated with a harsh pansystolic murmur best heard at the left sternal edge. Smaller defects often produce louder murmurs.

Pulmonary regurgitation – post repair of tetralogy of Fallot, individuals commonly have pulmonary regurgitation, which is associated with a soft early diastolic murmur loudest in the pulmonary area.

Box 6.4 Scars seen after cardiac surgery

1. Median sternotomy: overlying sternum, evidence of open heart surgery (e.g. coronary artery bypass graft (CABG))

2. Lateral thoracotomy: in left axilla seen after minimally invasive replacement of mitral valve

3. Groin scars: overlying femoral arteries. Access site for transaortic valve implantation (TAVI), endovascular aneurysm repair (EVAR)

4. Vein harvest scars: leg vein harvested as a graft for CABG

6.6 KEY INVESTIGATIONS

Bedside tests

Table 6.1 Bedside tests of use in patients presenting with a murmur

Test	Justification	Potential result
Oxygen saturations	Simple, non-invasive test Helps guide need for oxygen therapy	Low if impaired oxygen diffusion, e.g. pulmonary oedema
ECG	May reveal evidence of previous infarction, hypertrophy or arrhythmias	Septal rupture: evidence of old cardiac events LVOTO: evidence of left ventricular hypertrophy MR/MS: evidence of atrial fibrillation

Blood tests

Table 6.2 Blood tests of use in patients presenting with a murmur

Test	Justification	Potential result
Full blood count	Investigate for inflammatory/infective diseases, anaemia	WCC may be raised in infective processes e.g. IE Hb low in anaemia
Renal function and electrolytes	Investigate for impaired kidney function	May have AKI if renal perfusion is reduced
Liver function tests	Investigate for liver injury	ALP elevated in Paget's disease (increased osteoblast activity) May be deranged in right heart failure due to backpressure on the liver
C-reactive protein	Investigate for inflammatory/infective diseases	Raised in infective processes, e.g. IE
Clotting profile	May be important if requiring urgent surgical management	Can be deranged in overwhelming sepsis
Group and save/ cross-match	May be important if requiring urgent surgical management	
Thyroid function tests	Assess thyroid status	High T4 + low TSH in primary hyperthyroidism
Blood cultures	Identify organism in infective diseases and provide antibiotic sensitivities	*Staphylococcus* or *Streptococcus* species most common causes of IE Any number of organisms may be identified in the septic patient
Cardiac enzymes (e.g. troponin I)	Look for evidence of cardiac infarction	Elevated if cardiac myocyte damage
Brain natriuretic peptide	Sensitive and specific marker of heart failure	Levels markedly elevated in heart failure, if low, very unlikely to be heart failure

Imaging

Table 6.3 Imaging modalities of use in patients presenting with a murmur

Test	Justification	Potential result
Chest X-ray	May show evidence of cardiac or respiratory pathology	Cardiomegaly, or enlargement of particular heart chambers, e.g. LA in MS Features of heart failure, e.g. pulmonary oedema Aortic root aneurysm which could be causing functional AR
Trans-thoracic echocardiogram	Formal assessment of ventricular and valvular function	Valvular stenosis or regurgitation – Doppler allows for assessment of severity based on flow across the valve (see Figures 6.3, 6.4, 6.5, 6.6, 6.7) Vegetations on the valves seen in IE (see Figure 6.8) Septal defect (see Figures 6.6, 6.7)

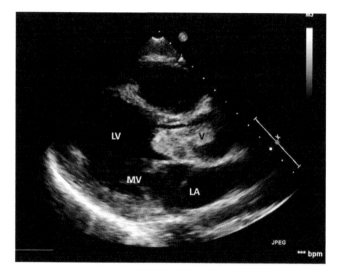

Figure 6.8   Vegetation (V) on aortic valve in a patient with infective endocarditis. LV, left ventricle; MV, mitral valve; LA, left atrium.
Source: Harpreet Kaur Sahemey, Echocardiographer, Hammersmith Hospital.

Special tests

Table 6.4   Specialist tests of use in patients presenting with a murmur

Test	Justification	Potential result
CT angiogram of aorta	Evaluate aorta for dissection	Intramural haematoma or intimal flap separating the two aortic channels (true and false lumens)
Transoesophageal echocardiogram	More sensitive in detecting valvular pathology especially if prosthetic valve Better visualization of posterior structures in heart – left atrium, left atrial appendage and descending aorta	Vegetations in IE Valvular stenosis or regurgitation
Coronary angiogram (PCI)	Assess for coronary artery disease which can be treated at the same time as valvular surgery	Narrowing of one or more of the coronary arteries
Cardiac MRI	Detailed assessment of heart muscle function and perfusion	Abnormal septal tissue in H(O)CM Areas of scar tissue post MI
Genetic testing	Identify genetic cause for disease	Defect in specific gene, e.g. fibrillin in Marfan's syndrome

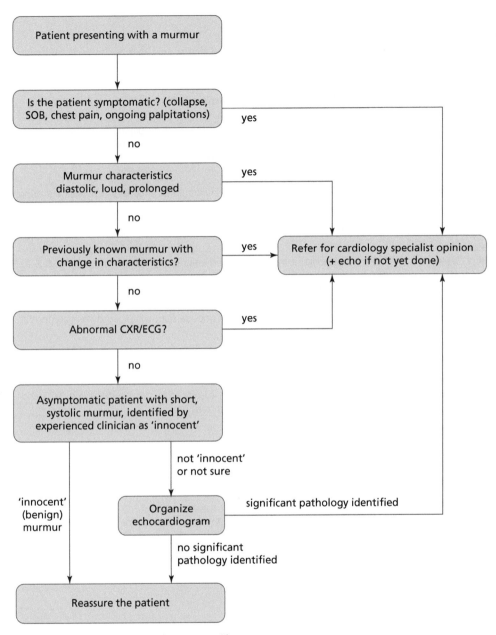

Figure 6.9 Work-up of a patient who presents with a murmur.

6.7 WHEN TO CALL A SENIOR

Situations
In the context of heart murmur, there are two key circumstances where a senior needs to be called:
A) In the acutely unwell patient
B) Where specialist follow-up is likely to be required

These two scenarios illustrate each situation:

1. Patient presenting with a fever and early diastolic murmur

2. Asymptomatic middle-aged gentleman found to have ejection systolic murmur, intensity 4/6 with radiation to the carotids, first identified when seen in pre-assessment clinic prior to elective laparoscopic cholecystectomy

What should be arranged by the time the senior arrives
Scenario 1

Infective endocarditis must be excluded in this patient, and is the working diagnosis until it has been excluded. In any unwell patient it is imperative to get help early, especially if the patient is deteriorating. Whilst waiting for their arrival the following should be arranged:

- Oxygen therapy titrated to keep saturations >94%
- Blood tests including FBC, U&Es, LFTs, CRP, blood cultures (minimum of three sets over one hour prior to commencing antibiotics), lactate and VBG
- IV access (ideally ×2)
- Empirical broad-spectrum antibiotics based on local hospital protocol after three sets of cultures have been taken
- Fluid challenge (e.g. 500 mL crystalloid) if hypotensive and volume replacement (e.g. 30 mL/kg) as required
- 12-lead ECG
- Portable chest X-ray
- Echocardiogram – cardiology SpR may be able to perform bedside scan whilst awaiting more formal assessment

Scenario 2

The patient is stable in this situation, and thus there is not the same urgency required as in scenario 1. However, the patient is scheduled on an operating list, this may need to be delayed to allow work-up of the murmur. As the patient was due to have an operation it is likely some investigations, e.g. ECG and bloods may have already been carried out. In addition, patient will need:

- Chest X-ray
- Echocardiogram
- Discussion with anaesthetist and cardiologist

What should be completed by the time the senior arrives
Scenario 1
- A full ABCDE assessment including results of a quick clinical examination
- The investigations and management as outlined, the length of time it takes for a senior to arrive will affect how far you will be able to progress

Scenario 2
- A full history and examination findings
- Results of previous investigations – there may be previous blood tests, ECGs or even echocardiograms available

KEY CLINICAL TRIALS

Key trial 6.1
Trial name: Mastering cardiac murmurs: the power of repetition.
Participants: 51 second year medical students in US medical school.
Intervention: A monitored group, who listened to 500 repetitions of four murmurs.
Control: No repetition of murmurs.
Outcome: Repetition significantly improved auscultatory proficiency in recognizing basic cardiac murmurs.
Reason for inclusion: Demonstrates murmur identification is improved through practice.
Reference: http://www.ncbi.nlm.nih.gov/pubmed/15302733.

Key Trial 6.2

Trial name: Intra-aortic balloon pump (IABP) support for ventricular septal rupture and acute mitral regurgitation.

Participants: 81 patients who developed either ventricular septal rupture (n = 55) or acute mitral regurgitation (n = 36) post MI.

Intervention: Bridging of patients to surgery with IABP.

Control: Best medical care prior to surgery.

Outcome: IABP reduced 30-day mortality (61% vs. 100%, p = <0.04).

Reason for inclusion: In shocked patients IABP bridging therapy to surgery offers survival benefit.

Reference: http://www.ncbi.nlm.nih.gov/pubmed/24035169.

GUIDELINES

ACC/AHA. Management of patients with valvular heart disease. 2006. http://content.onlinejacc.org/article.aspx?article id=1137806

ACC/AHA/ASE. Clinical application of echocardiography: summary article. 2003. https://circ.ahajournals.org/content/108/9/1146.full.pdf+html

FURTHER READING

Aboulhosn J, Child JS. Congenital heart disease for the adult cardiologist. Circulation. 2006;114:2412–2422. http://circ.ahajournals.org/content/114/22/2412.full.pdf+html

Comprehensive review on subtypes of left ventricular outflow tract obstruction.

Mokadam NA, Stout KK, Verrier ED. Management of acute regurgitation in left-sided cardiac valves. Tex Heart Inst J. 2011;38(1):9–19. http://www.ncbi.nlm.nih.gov/pubmed/21423463

Excellent summary on the diagnosis and management of left sided acute valvular insufficiency.

Garacholou SM, Karon BL, Shub C, et al. Aortic valve sclerosis and clinical outcomes: moving toward a definition. Am J Med. 2011;124(2):103–110. http://www.ncbi.nlm.nih.gov/pubmed/21295189

Good review article on aortic sclerosis.

 For additional resources and to test your knowledge, visit the companion website at:

www.wiley.com/go/camm/cardiology

7 Shock

Ji-Jian Chow

Imperial College Healthcare NHS Trust, London, UK

7.1 DEFINITION

Shock is the inability of the body to perfuse tissues with oxygen and nutrients causing end-organ dysfunction, and is usually characterized by alterations in basic observations of the patient.

7.2 DIAGNOSTIC ALGORITHM

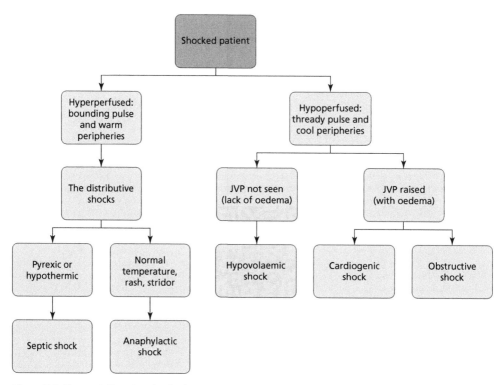

Figure 7.1 Diagnostic flow chart for shock.

Clinical Guide to Cardiology, First Edition. Edited by Christian F. Camm and A. John Camm.
© 2016 John Wiley & Sons, Ltd. Published 2016 by John Wiley & Sons, Ltd.
Companion website: www.wiley.com/go/camm/cardiology.

7.3 DIFFERENTIALS LIST

Dangerous diagnoses
All causes of shock are dangerous. However some are far more common, especially in the settings junior doctors encounter.

Common diagnoses
1. Hypovolaemic shock: circulating volume falls leading to poor tissue perfusion
2. Septic shock: infection leads to vasodilatation, a fall in blood pressure and poor tissue perfusion
3. Anaphylactic shock: a severe allergic reaction leads to vasodilatation, blood pressure falls and poor tissue perfusion
4. Cardiogenic shock: a pump failure leads to poor perfusion
5. Obstructive shock: a physical obstruction of the heart or great vessels, prevents blood flow and causes poor tissue perfusion

Diagnoses to consider
1. Neurogenic shock: loss of vasomotor tone below a neurological lesion causes pooling of blood and reduction in effective circulating volume
2. Endocrine shock: inadequate levels of the body's regulating steroids cause a distributive shock

(See Audio Podcast 7.1 at **www.wiley.com/go/camm/cardiology**)

7.4 KEY HISTORY FEATURES

History of a shocked patient is often difficult as the mental status is altered in many. Useful collateral histories may be taken from family members, bystanders and attending healthcare professionals.

Common diagnosis 1
Diagnosis: Hypovolaemic

Questions
a. Has there been significant bleeding?

History features could include abdominal pain or fractures of long bones after trauma. See Table 7.1 for further details.

b. Has the patient been dehydrated for a long period of time (poor intake)?

Particularly at risk are those who cannot eat and drink unassisted, or able people who are stranded in emergencies.

c. Have there been other increased outputs?

Examples include diarrhoea, vomiting, burns and perspiration.

Table 7.1 Sites in the adult body where significant haemorrhage can occur, with associated history and examination features

Site	Volume potential (mL)	History	Examination
Intracranial	1700, but brain usually tamponades. Shock usually does not occur	• Head injury • Loss of consciousness • Vomiting	• Surface injury to head • Boggy swellings of skull • Bilateral 'panda eyes' • Haemotympanum • Focal neurology
Chest	1500 (unilateral) 3000 (bilateral)	• Traumatic injury • Breathing difficulty • Chest pain (tearing to back)	• Deviated trachea • Engorged neck veins • Uneven expansion • Dullness to percussion • Reduced breath sounds • Reduced oximeter saturations
Abdomen	>5000	• Traumatic injury • Abdominal pain (tearing to back) • Distension above normal	• Flank/abdominal bruising • Distension • Tenderness • Pulsating masses
Pelvis	1500 5000 (if bleeding into retroperitoneal space)	• Traumatic injury • Pain in pelvis • Post-traumatic haematuria	• Bruising • Crepitus/tenderness over bony prominences • Reduction in anal tone • ALWAYS EXAMINE ABDOMEN
Long bones	Humerus – 750 Tibia – 750 Femur – 1500	• Traumatic injury • Pain	• Bruising • Tenderness • Deformity • Reduced range of motion
External	>5000	• High-velocity collisions • Gunshots • Stab wounds	• Evidence of wounds – puncture, laceration, crush and spinal transection

---

Box 7.1 Parkland formula for calculating fluid requirements (mL) in burns (first 24 hours)

4 x weight (kg) x % body surface area burned
50% of fluid over 8 hours
Remaining 50% of fluid over further 16 hours

Common diagnosis 2
Diagnosis: Septic

Questions
a. Has there been evidence of a fever or feeling febrile?

The observations taken at triage may not prove an objective temperature, but a good history of night sweats, rigors, or even feeling 'hot and cold' may suggest infective cause.

b. Are there any infective features?

These include productive cough, urinary symptoms, pustular wounds, signs of meningism.

c. Is there any risk of immune compromise?

Recent steroid use, chemotherapy or immune-compromising illness, such as AIDS, increase the risk of septic shock.

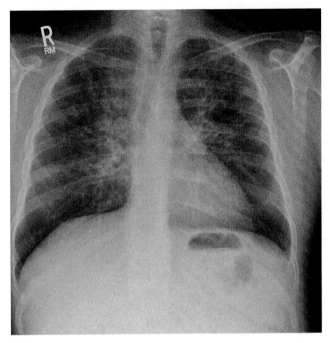

Figure 7.2 Pneumocystis pneumonia (PCP) – a potential cause of septic shock in immunocompromised patients. Source: Daniel Hughes, FY2 Doctor in Radiology, Queen Elizabeth Hospital, Woolwich.

Common diagnosis 3
Diagnosis: Anaphylactic

Questions
a. Are there known allergies?

An allergy bracelet or an autoinjector on their person may be a clue. Existing allergies may give clues as to new ones via recognized associations (see Table 7.2).

b. Has the patient noticed a new rash or itch?

Patients may have existing rashes; it is important to ask about this to determine whether the rash has had a recent onset.

c. Any difficulty breathing or the feeling of facial and oral swelling?

Patients may have baseline shortness of breath; it is important to ask about this before drawing conclusions from an examination.

d. Was there exposure to a new or known allergen?

Anaphylaxis can be a first presentation of a severe allergy. Some substances (e.g. penicillins) are known to be more allergenic than others, but in theory anything can be an allergen.

Table 7.2 A non-exhaustive sample of known allergic cross-reactions

Allergy	Associated allergens
Latex	Avocado, banana, chestnut, kiwi fruit, melon, tomato
Iodine contrast	Shellfish (relative risk 3.0)
	Eggs, milk, chocolate (relative risk 2.9)
	Strawberries and other fruit (relative risk 2.6)
	(Asthma – relative risk 2.2)
Penicillins	Cephalosporins (traditionally 10% cross-reactivity, however newer production methods and newer generations have figures as low as 1%)
	Carbapenems (45% cross-reactivity, but newer studies point to a figure closer to 10%)
Legumes	5% of legume-allergic persons are allergic to multiple legumes. Foods include:
	• Soya
	• Peas and chickpeas
	• Peanuts
	• Lentils
	• Beans

Common diagnosis 4
Diagnosis: Cardiogenic

Questions
a. Any cardiac history or risk factors?

The cardiac risk factors are covered in Chapter 10.

b. Chest pain/palpitations on presentation?

The commonest cause is acute MI. Other causes associated with chest pain/palpitations include myocarditis, aortic dissection, HOCM, tachyarrhythmia.

c. Any orthopnoea or leg swelling?

Previous poor ventricular function can contribute to acute cardiogenic shock and may indicate an undiagnosed cardiac history.

Common diagnosis 5
Diagnosis: Obstructive shock

Questions:
History features to suspect potential obstructive causes:
a. Tension pneumothorax – chest trauma
b. Pulmonary embolism – pain and swelling symptoms in leg, pro-coagulant states, pleuritic chest pain, history of venothrombotic disease
c. Constrictive pericarditis – recent myocardial infarction, connective tissue disease, history of renal failure
d. Pericardial tamponade – history as pericarditis, as well as: tearing back pain (aortic dissection), chest trauma, diagnostic procedures involving the heart (angiogram)

Box 7.2   Some causes of obstructive shock

1. Tension pneumothorax
2. Massive pulmonary embolism
3. Pericardial tamponade
4. Constrictive pericarditis

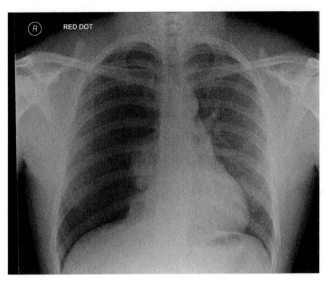

Figure 7.3 A large right-sided pneumothorax; if this begins to tension it could become a cause of obstructive shock.

Diagnosis to consider 1
Diagnosis: Neurogenic shock

Not to be confused with spinal shock, a term for the motor and sensory deficit following spinal cord transection with or without a circulatory component. Neurogenic shock is a type of distributive shock. In the early phase of a trauma scenario, neurogenic shock should be a diagnosis of exclusion.

Questions
a. Any significant trauma to the back or new-onset back pain?

Cervical and high thoracic lesions in particular risk neurogenic shock.

b. Any numbness or weakness below the traumatic lesion?

Pre-existing lesions should be accounted for before concluding anything from examination.

Diagnosis to consider 2
Diagnosis: Adrenal insufficiency

Insufficiency usually occurs after abrupt discontinuation of long-term or high-dose corticosteroid treatment, or when critically ill patients fail to meet their own steroid production demands.

Questions
a. Is there any history of corticosteroid use?

Patients with Addison's disease who have diarrhoea and vomiting may fail to absorb their corticosteroid medication.

b. Has the patient ever had tuberculosis or autoimmune disease?

Common causes of Addison's disease; patients may not realize they have the condition until their first crisis.

c. Are there signs of haemorrhage or sepsis?

Acute adrenal insufficiency can be caused by sudden haemorrhage, e.g. in pregnancy, or by sepsis (if meningococcal this is termed Waterhouse–Friderichsen syndrome).

Box 7.3   Addison's disease

Addison's disease results from destruction of the adrenal cortex leading to mineralo- and cortico-steroid deficiency. It has the following causes:

1. Autoimmune – 80% in the UK
2. Tuberculosis – the majority worldwide
3. Adrenal metastases – lung, breast and renal cancer
4. Lymphoma
5. Adrenal haemorrhage
6. Congenital late-onset adrenal hyperplasia

7.5 KEY EXAMINATION FEATURES

- **ABCDE:** shock is an emergency situation, this approach should be used to ensure thorough information gathering
- **Treatment:** problem-based initially, diagnosis-orientated as more information becomes available

Table 7.3 Generalized monitoring, examination and required actions that should be undertaken in patients with shock

	Monitor	Examine	Act
Airway		Look – physical obstructions	Airway adjuncts (as needed)
		Listen – snoring, stridor	
Breathing	Pulse oximetry	Look – chest expansion, trauma	Oxygen – use a bag if not
	Respiratory rate	Feel – tracheal deviation	making respiratory effort
		Percuss – assess resonance	
		Listen – air entry and added sounds	
Circulation	Blood pressure cuff	Look – fluid/blood loss, neck vein	IV access
	Cardiac monitor (if	distension, oedema	Take bloods (and ABG)
	unavailable, sats probe	Feel – pulses, peripheral warmth and	IV fluids (as needed)
	shows pulse rate)	capillary refill	
		Listen – heart sounds	
Disability	Thermometer	Look – pupils (reactivity/size)	Warm or cool patient as
	Blood glucose	Score – GCS or AVPU	needed
			Correct blood glucose if
			needed
Exposure	Urine output – catheter	Expose patient fully	Catheterize
	and urometer	Examine the abdomen	

Common diagnosis 1
Diagnosis: Hypovolaemic shock

Examination findings
a. Tachycardia and hypotension on the observation chart

If the patient can stand there are three criteria for postural hypotension: severe postural dizziness, pulse increment >30/min or systolic pressure drop >20 mmHg.

b. Signs of hypoperfusion

There may be cool peripheries, thready pulses and mottled skin.

c. Evidence of a low fluid status

Signs include non-visible JVP, dry mucous membranes, poor skin turgor, urine specific gravity >1.020.

d. Evidence of losses

Including burns, bleeding wounds, vomitus and diarrhoea. Do not miss internal losses – dull chests (haemothorax) and tender abdomens (internal bleeding).

Table 7.4 Classes of shock (haemorrhagic).

Parameter	Class			
	I	II	III	IV
Blood loss (mL)	<750	750–1500	1500–2000	>2000
Blood loss (%)	<15	15–30	30–40	>40
HR	<100	>100	>120	>140
BP	Normal	Normal	Low	Low
RR	14–20	20–30	30–40	>35
Urine output (mL/hr)	>30	20–30	5–15	Negligible
CNS symptoms	Normal	Anxious	Confused	Lethargic

Common diagnosis 2

Diagnosis: Septic shock

Examination findings

a. Initial hyperperfusion – when shock is more severe, peripheral shutdown will occur

The signs of hyperperfusion are warm, pink peripheries and a bounding pulse.

b. Systemic inflammatory response syndrome (SIRS) criteria with evidence of infection is sepsis

---

Box 7.4   Criteria for systemic inflammatory response (SIRS) – two or more required

1. Temperature: <36°C or >38°C
2. Heart Rate: >90 bpm
3. Respiration: >20 bpm or $PaCO_2$ <4.3 kPa
4. White Cells: <4 × 10^9/L or >12 × 10^9/L, or >10% bands

---

c. Sepsis with low blood pressure refractory to fluid resuscitation is septic shock

Generally the mean arterial pressure (MAP) is measured, and this should be above 65 mmHg.

Box 7.5   Estimating mean arterial pressure

$$\frac{1}{3}Systolic + \frac{2}{3}Diastolic$$

---

d. Evidence of infection – work from head to toe to find a source

See Box 7.6 for signs and symptoms that suggest an infective source.

Box 7.6   Finding an infective focus

- **Head:** headache, neck stiffness, rashes – possible meningitis
- **Respiratory:** poor air entry/expansion, dullness to percussion, crepitations – possible pneumonia
- **Cardiac:** new murmurs – possible endocarditis
- **Abdomen:** tenderness, guarding – commonly acute cholecystitis, appendicitis or diverticulitis
- **Pelvis and genitalia:** suprapubic tenderness, discolored and malodorous urine – possible UTI
- **Soft tissue and bone:** erythema, swelling, tenderness, hot to touch, evidence of pus – possible cellulitis, fasciitis or osteomyelitis

Common diagnosis 3
Diagnosis: Anaphylactic shock

Examination findings
a. Stridor and tissue swelling

Swelling mainly occurs in facial tissues, tongue (and larynx although this may not be easily seen). Stridor is probably the easiest to determine.

b. Rash, which the patient finds itchy

The allergic rash is red, hot or urticarial ('hives') – where the skin has palpable lumps.

c. Wheeze, high respiratory rate

The wheeze is generally polyphonic and widespread. The respiratory rate can be determined during your examination or from attached monitoring devices.

d. Initial hyperperfusion

Bounding pulses and warm peripheries, but, like the septic patient, in late stages there will be peripheral shutdown.

Common diagnosis 4
Diagnosis: Cardiogenic shock

Examination findings
a. Features of hypoperfusion

Cool peripheries and thready, tachycardic pulses

b. Signs of fluid overload

Patients may have a raised JVP, peripheral oedema or lung crepitations starting at the bases

c. S3/S4 gallop

*An S3 heart sound is associated with a '**Ken**tucky' rhythm and is caused by the rapid filling of a distended ventricle in acute heart failure. An S4 heart sound is associated with a 'Tenne**ssee**' rhythm and is caused by atrial contraction against a stiff ventricle. S4 is associated with hypertrophic ventricles.*

Common diagnosis 5
Diagnosis: Obstructive shock

Examination findings
a. Features of hypo-perfusion

Cool peripheries and thready, tachycardic pulses – similar to cardiogenic shock.

b. Features of an obstructive condition

- *Uneven chest expansion, hyper-resonant percussion unilaterally = tension pneumothorax*
- *Grossly raised JVP, muffled heart sounds = cardiac tamponade/constrictive pericarditis*
- *Signs and symptoms of DVT, right heart strain on ECG and respiratory alkalosis on ABG = massive pulmonary embolism*

Diagnosis to consider 1
Diagnosis: Neurogenic shock

Examination findings
a. Characteristic hypotension and bradycardia

However bradycardia can be seen in late stages of other types of shock and therefore neurogenic shock should be a diagnosis of exclusion.

b. Neurological deficits below the suspected lesion

Examine for the level where sensation and motor function are lost. This will approximate to the level of the spinal cord injury.

c. Warm, well perfused, dry skin below the suspected lesion

The hyper-perfusion of the skin below the lesion results from the loss of vascular tone – making it a distributive shock. The skin is dry due to the loss of innervation, reducing its ability to sweat.

Diagnosis to consider 2
Diagnosis: Adrenal insufficiency

Examination findings
a. Evidence of prior steroid use or adrenal insufficiency

- *Steroids in medication pack*
- *Medical information bracelet*
- *Hyper-pigmented skin creases*

7.6 KEY INVESTIGATIONS

Bedside

Table 7.5 Bedside tests of use in patients presenting with shock

Test	Justification	Potential results
Arterial blood gas	Allows early identification of several critical variables including: Respiratory function Acid–base balance Haemoglobin Lactate	pH – increasing derangement suggests increasingly severe pathology pO_2 – hypoxia seen in a range of respiratory pathologies pCO_2 – hypercapnia is especially seen in exacerbations of COPD, exhausted asthmatics Base excess (BE) – indicates the metabolic component of any alkalosis (high BE) or acidosis (low BE) Lactate – contributes to the BE and demonstrates anaerobic respiration (i.e. the undersupply of oxygen to tissues) Bicarbonate – contributes to the BE and the major buffer in the human body
Urine dip	Indicative of pregnancy, urine infection and hydration status	SG >1.020 – dehydrated hypovolaemia Positive beta-human chorionic gonadotrophin (hCG) – pregnancy (possibly ectopic in the shocked young woman) Leucocytes and nitrites – urine infection
Capillary glucose	May identify Addisonian or diabetic (high cardiovascular risk) patients	Addison's disease – low Diabetes – high
Electrocardiogram	The heart is involved in the pathophysiology of any shock subtype	Sinus tachycardia – common in most shock Atrial fibrillation – new respiratory pathology, new cardiac pathology or as a fast, non-perfusing rhythm ST segment changes – ischaemia, infarction or myocarditis Right ventricular strain – often indicative of massive PE

Blood tests

Table 7.6 Blood tests of use in patients presenting with shock.

Test	Justification	Potential results
Full blood count	Haemoglobin levels affect oxygen delivery and can indicate haemorrhage Low platelet levels are a risk factor for bleeding Raised WCC helps diagnose septic shock	WCC $<4 \times 10^9$/L or $>12 \times 10^9$/L – sepsis Normal Hb can be seen in early haemorrhage Low Hb can be seen in late haemorrhage and hampers survival in shock patients
Urea and electrolytes	Gives an indication regarding hydration status, renal function and electrolyte imbalance	High urea and creatinine – dehydration/renal failure Deranged potassium, magnesium, calcium – increases the risk of arrhythmia
Liver function tests	Existing liver disease can make upper GI bleed more likely Liver function becomes newly deranged in organ failure	High liver enzymes – liver disease The values may be low in established cirrhosis
CRP	A good indicator of inflammation	Sepsis – high
Clotting screen	A possible cause of haemorrhage and an indicator of organ failure if newly deranged	Haemorrhage – possibly high Multiple organ dysfunction – high
Group and save/ cross-match	Required in the haemorrhaging patient, or those with concurrent anaemia that compromises nutrient delivery further	

Imaging

Table 7.7 Blood tests of use in patients presenting with shock

Test	Justification	Potential results
Portable chest X-ray	A quick method to diagnose a wide range of pathologies	Cardiomegaly – in heart failure, pericardial effusion Consolidation – pneumonia Collapse – obstructing lesion in airway at any level Interstitial oedema – seen in heart failure Pleural effusion – may be associated with infection, malignancy or bilateral in heart failure Loss of lung markings, shifted mediastinum – a tension pneumothorax
Bedside ultrasound	Possible types include: **i.** FAST scan for haemorrhage **ii.** Echocardiography **iii.** Trauma chest ultrasound	Free fluid on the FAST scan – abdominal or pelvic bleeding, pericardial effusions Regional wall motion abnormalities on echocardiography – acute MI
Computed tomography	Progressing to CT requires full stabilization of the patient and will be a senior decision	CT head – intracranial bleeds CT chest – full trauma evaluation and identifying aortic dissections CT abdomen – intra-abdominal inflammation, abdominal aortic pathology and ischaemic bowel

Special

Table 7.8 Specialist tests of use in patients presenting with shock

Test	Justification	Potential results
Central venous line parameters	The central venous pressure and venous oxygen saturations provide two components of Early Goal-Directed Therapy, a strategy for septic shock	Target central venous pressure = 8–12 mmHg Target superior vena cava oxygen saturations = >70%
Invasive blood pressure	Via an arterial line, this is a must for patients needing inotropic support	High blood pressure – consider reducing inotropic support Low blood pressure – consider increasing inotropic support

(See Audio Podcast 7.2 at **www.wiley.com/go/camm/cardiology**)

7.7 WHEN TO CALL A SENIOR

Situations

All shocked patients should be seen by a senior at the earliest opportunity – they are, by definition, incredibly unwell. However making that phone call should NOT precede ABC assessment, leading to early life-saving interventions such as securing the airway, giving oxygen and fluids if appropriate.

In dire emergency, making contact can be a delegated task. One commonly used example is in the Cardiac Arrest or Medical Emergency Team call (2222 in UK hospitals). If the patient can be stabilized after examination enough for you to make a phone call, then extra information will allow your seniors to give advice and decide on the priority of the call.

In the following situations, you should not hesitate to make an emergency call:

- A patient making no respiratory effort or with no palpable pulse
- A patient with uncontrolled haemorrhage
- A patient with deteriorating vital signs despite maximal efforts to resuscitate with airway measures, oxygen and fluids

What should be completed by the time the senior arrives

You should have moved as far down the ABCDE pathway as possible. Priority one is completing the ABC cycle – problem finding is rapid and the consequences of inaction are severe.

> **Box 7.7** The sepsis six
>
> 1. High-flow oxygen
> 2. Fluid resuscitation
> 3. Blood cultures
> 4. Antibiotics
> 5. Measurement of serum lactate and haemoglobin
> 6. Measurement of urine output

(See Audio Podcast 7.3 at **www.wiley.com/go/camm/cardiology**)

KEY CLINICAL TRIALS

Key Trial 7.1

Trial Name: Early goal-directed therapy (EGDT) in the treatment of severe sepsis and septic shock.
Participants: 263 adult patients admitted with severe sepsis, septic shock or the sepsis syndrome.
Intervention: A protocol of goal driven interventions to be met in the first 6 hours.

Control: Standard practice – without protocol.

Outcome: EGDT reduced mortality at 28 days (49.2% vs. 33.3%) and 60 days (56.9% vs. 44.3%) post admission.

Reason for inclusion: A major trial that still influences practice in the management of shocked patients but has recently been called into question.

Reference: Rivers E, et al. Early goal-directed therapy in the treatment of severe sepsis and septic shock. N Engl J Med. 2001; 345:1368-1377. http://www.nejm.org/doi/full/10.1056/NEJMoa010307.

Key Trial 7.2

Trial Name: The ProCESS trial.

Participants: 1341 patients admitted with severe sepsis, septic shock or the sepsis syndrome.

Intervention: Protocol-driven early goal-directed therapy (either with or without a central venous catheter).

Control: Standard practice – without protocol.

Outcome: At 60 days, 90 days and 1 year there were no advantages to EGDT or protocoled care over usual care.

Reason for inclusion: It refutes the earlier trial on EGDT. Together the trials can be interpreted to demonstrate that protocols can be useful, but experienced clinical judgment should be exercised at all times.

Reference: The ProCESS investigators. A randomized trial of protocol-based care for early septic shock. N Engl J Med. 2014; 370:1683-1693. http://www.nejm.org/doi/full/10.1056/NEJMoa1401602.

Key Trial 7.3

Trial Name: SHOCK trial.

Participants: 302 patients with left ventricular failure and cardiogenic shock following acute MI.

Intervention: Early revascularization (within 6 hours of randomization).

Control: Medical therapy initially with revascularization as an option later in the clinical course.

Outcome: 30-day mortality was unchanged but significant survival benefits were seen at 6 months and 1 year with early revascularization.

Reason for inclusion: Demonstrates early therapy can greatly improve outcomes, which may only manifest in the long run, and influences current thought on early transport to cardiac catheterization laboratories.

Reference: Menon V, Fincke R. Cardiogenic shock: a summary of the randomized SHOCK trial. Congest Heart Fail. 2003;9(1):35-39. http://www.ncbi.nlm.nih.gov/pubmed/12556676.

GUIDELINES

The Surviving Sepsis Campaign. International guidelines for management of severe sepsis and septic shock. 2012. http://www.sccm.org/Documents/SSC-Guidelines.pdf

Resuscitation Council UK. Emergency treatment of anaphylactic reactions. 2008. http://www.resus.org.uk/pages/reaction.pdf

Resuscitation Council UK. Advanced Life Support. 2010. http://www.resus.org.uk/pages/als.pdf

FURTHER READING

Khalid L, Dhakam SH. A review of cardiogenic shock in acute myocardial infarction. Current Cardiology Review. 2008;4(1):34–40. http://www.ncbi.nlm.nih.gov/pubmed/19924275/
A review of cardiogenic shock – the majority of the treatments mentioned are higher level decisions but it is useful to have an awareness of them.

Myburgh JA, Mythen MG. Resuscitation fluids. N Engl J Med. 2013;369(13):1243–1251. http://www.ncbi.nlm.nih.gov/pubmed/24066745
A review of the omnipresent debate regarding fluid choice in resuscitation. Choosing the fluid used in resuscitation is a decision made by junior doctors frequently.

For additional resources and to test your knowledge, visit the companion website at:

www.wiley.com/go/camm/cardiology

8 Oedema

Sophie Maxwell
Walsall Manor Hospital, Walsall, UK

8.1 DEFINITION

Oedema is the abnormal increase in interstitial fluid which can develop in all bodily cavities, such as the lungs and abdomen. Oedema in the tissue peripheries presents as swelling.

8.2 DIAGNOSTIC ALGORITHM

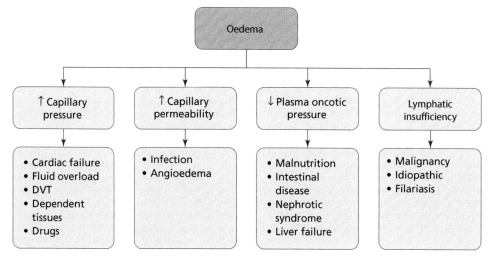

Figure 8.1 Flow chart detailing the pathophysiology of oedema.

8.3 DIFFERENTIALS LIST

Dangerous diagnoses
1. Deep vein thrombosis (DVT)
2. Angioedema
3. Nephrotic syndrome

Common diagnoses
1. Cardiac failure
2. Infection
3. Liver failure
4. Malnutrition/intestinal disease

Clinical Guide to Cardiology, First Edition. Edited by Christian F. Camm and A. John Camm.
© 2016 John Wiley & Sons, Ltd. Published 2016 by John Wiley & Sons, Ltd.
Companion website: www.wiley.com/go/camm/cardiology.

Diagnoses to consider
1. Drug related
2. Filariasis
3. Malignancy

8.4 KEY HISTORY FEATURES

(See Audio Podcast 8.1 at **www.wiley.com/go/camm/cardiology**)

Dangerous diagnosis 1
Diagnosis: DVT

Questions
a. Is the peripheral oedema unilateral?

Typically with DVT the swelling is unilateral; however, on rare occasions bilateral DVTs can be present.

b. Is there pain?

A DVT is usually very painful and the patient often presents with both pain and swelling.

c. Is there history of immobility/malignancy/pregnancy/family history of or previous DVT?

All of the above increase the risk of developing a DVT (some of these risks make up the Wells' score).

Dangerous diagnosis 2
Diagnosis: Angioedema

Questions
a. Is there a history of atopy?

In most cases there is a history of allergy, eczema, asthma or hayfever.

b. Is the patient on angiotensin-converting enzyme (ACE) inhibitors?

ACE inhibitors (in particular) can cause angioedema – even many years after being started.

c. Is the patient having difficulty breathing?

Angioedema of the larynx can be life threatening; in an attack patients experience difficulty swallowing and shortness of breath.

Dangerous diagnosis 3
Diagnosis: Nephrotic syndrome

Questions
a. Have there been changes to urine?

Excess protein in the urine can make it look frothy.

b. Any recent infections?

Glomerulonephritis, a leading cause of nephrotic syndrome can be post-streptococcal infection, such as a sore throat; a complication of nephrotic syndrome is also an increased susceptibility to infection.

c. Has the patient recently started any new medications?

Non-steroidal anti-inflammatory drugs (NSAIDs), gold, penicillamine and captopril have all been linked with causing nephrotic syndrome.

Box 8.1 Primary (idiopathic) causes of nephrotic syndrome

- Focal segmental glomerulosclerosis
- Minimal change glomerular disease
- Membranous glomerular disease
- Membranoproliferative glomerular disease (e.g. IgA nephropathy)

Box 8.2 Secondary causes of nephrotic syndrome

- Diabetes mellitus
- Systemic lupus erythematosus
- Amyloidosis
- Malignancy: lymphoma, myeloma
- Drugs
- Infections: hepatitis B, HIV, malaria, schistosomiasis
- Congenital: Alport's syndrome, nail patella syndrome

Common diagnosis 1
Diagnosis: Cardiac failure

Questions
a. Is the swelling bilateral?

Patients will complain of bilateral swelling in dependent areas, most commonly pedal (if long periods of time spent in bed, then sacral oedema will develop).

b. Is there a history of ischaemic heart disease?

The most common cause of cardiac failure is ischaemic heart disease; patients will often have a history of cardiac events and/or risk factors for ischaemic cardiac disease.

c. Has there been worsening exercise tolerance?

If the pedal oedema is part of congestive cardiac failure, the patient will often describe increased short-ness of breath on exertion.

Common diagnosis 2
Diagnosis: Infection

Questions
a. Is the swelling unilateral?

Soft tissue infection such as cellulitis is almost always unilateral.

b. Are there skin changes?

Patients will often present complaining of skin changes, such as increased redness, heat or tight, shiny skin.

c. Is there an obvious locus of infection?

Soft tissue oedema may stem from an obvious locus such as a wound, an ulcer or an insect bite, etc.

Common diagnosis 3
Diagnosis: Liver failure

Questions
a. How much alcohol does the patient drink in the average week?

Liver cirrhosis caused by alcohol abuse is a leading cause of liver-failure-based oedema.

b. Is there a history of foreign travel, intravenous drug use, unsafe sexual practice, recent tattoos?

Viral hepatitis is an important cause of liver failure.

Box 8.3   Causes of ascites

1. Liver cirrhosis
2. Heart failure
3. Hepatic vein occlusion (Budd–Chiari syndrome)
4. Constrictive pericarditis
5. Kwashiorkor (protein-energy malnutrition)
6. Nephrotic syndrome
7. Cancer
8. Infection (e.g. spontaneous bacterial peritonitis)

Common diagnosis 4
Diagnosis: Malnutrition/intestinal disease

Questions
a. Has there been a history of diarrhoea?

Chronic diarrhoea may suggest inflammatory bowel disease or coeliac disease, which may lead to the patient losing excess protein in their stool.

b. What does the patient eat?

Peripheral oedema due to low albumin is common in the elderly population who consume a diet low in protein due to ill health or anorexia.

Diagnosis to consider 1
Diagnosis: Drugs

Questions
a. Have any new medications been started?

Drugs such as calcium-channel blockers, NSAIDs and insulin can all cause peripheral oedema.

Diagnosis to consider 2
Diagnosis: Filariasis
   Lymphatic filariasis is a nematode (roundworm) infection caused mainly by *Wuchereria bancrofti* and *Brugia malayi*. More than 120 million people worldwide are affected by lymphatic filariasis.

Questions
a. Has the patient recently been abroad?

Filariasis is transmitted by mosquito bites, and occurs in Asia, Africa and South America.

Box 8.4   What is filariasis?

- Parasitic disease caused by roundworm species
- Can cause lymphatic oedema (*Wuchereria bancrofti*)
- Other species cause river blindness (*Onchocerca volvulus*)
- Diagnosis is dependent on species. *W. bancrofti* can be diagnosed on thick and thin films (blood must be drawn at night)

Diagnosis to consider 3
Diagnosis: Malignancy

Questions
a. Does the patient have a history suggestive of malignancy (e.g. fatigue, anorexia)?

Malignancy with lymph node involvement can cause lymphoedema in the peripheries, by obstructing the flow of lymph from the tissues; constitutional symptoms are common in malignancy.

b. Is there a history of surgery or radiotherapy for a previous malignancy?

Lymphoedema can be iatrogenic from lymph node removal or destruction from surgery or radiotherapy, respectively, to treat malignancy.

8.5 KEY EXAMINATION FEATURES

Dangerous diagnosis 1
Diagnosis: DVT

Examination findings
a. Warm, tender, swollen calf or thigh

Unilateral tenderness, particularly along the deep venous system when palpated.

b. Palpable mass in the abdomen/pelvis

An obstructing mass to the venous flow from the lower limbs can cause a DVT, malignancy also induces a hypercoagulable state.

c. Respiratory rate and oxygen saturation

A pulmonary embolus (PE) is the life-threatening complication of a DVT; it would usually present with increased respiratory rate and decreased oxygen saturations.

Dangerous diagnosis 2
Diagnosis: Angioedema

Examination findings
a. Stridor

The most important part of assessing a patient whom you suspect to have angioedema, is to ensure that their airway is not compromised by laryngeal oedema or spasm; if the upper airway is narrowed, an inspiratory stridor may occur.

b. Lip and tongue swelling

Facial swelling is classic in angioedema and particularly affects the mouth. If swelling is present lower down the airway, there may be respiratory compromise (it is important to carry out basic observations).

c. Rash

Patients with angioedema may develop a red urticarial rash.

Dangerous diagnosis 3
Diagnosis: Nephrotic syndrome

Examination findings
a. Periorbital oedema and swelling of the genitals

As well as oedema in the legs, the swelling is dependent with gravity and the genitals are often affected, typically pitting. Periorbital oedema develops as tissue resistance around the eyes is low.

b. Assess for DVT as described earlier

Nephrotic syndrome is a hypercoagulable state so DVT or PE could occur as a complication.

 (See Audio Podcast 8.2 at **www.wiley.com/go/camm/cardiology**)

Common diagnosis 1
Diagnosis: Cardiac failure

Examination findings
a. Bilateral pedal oedema, raised JVP and bi-basal crackles

Signs of fluid overload which are classic of cardiac failure. Peripheral oedema and an elevated JVP are more common in right-sided heart failure, and pulmonary oedema causing bi-basal crackles on auscultation is more common in left-sided failure.

b. Cool peripheries

This is an indicator that the heart is not pumping effectively enough. This sign may be elicited when examining the patient's hands or when you find you are unable to obtain an oxygen saturation recording.

c. Displaced apex, right ventricular heave, murmur on auscultation

A right ventricular heave can signify pulmonary hypertension, a murmur may highlight valvular disease, a displaced apex from left ventricular dilatation shows the outcome of cardiac failure.

Box 8.5   Framingham criteria for congestive cardiac failure

Diagnosis of CCF requires the presence of at least two major criteria, or one major criterion and two minor criteria.

Major criteria:
- Paroxysmal nocturnal dyspnoea
- Crepitations
- S3 gallop
- Cardiomegaly (cardiothoracic ratio >50% on CXR)
- Increased central venous pressure (>16 cmH_2O at right atrium)
- Weight loss >4.5 kg in 5 days in response to treatment
- Neck vein distension
- Acute pulmonary oedema
- Hepatojugular reflux

Minor criteria:
- Bilateral ankle oedema
- Dyspnoea on ordinary exertion
- Tachycardia (heart rate >120 bpm)
- Decrease in vital capacity by 1/3 from maximum for patient
- Nocturnal cough
- Hepatomegaly
- Pleural effusion

Common diagnosis 2
Diagnosis: Infection

Examination findings
a. Unilateral presentation of the four hallmarks of inflammation (calor, dolor, rubor, tumor)

Heat, pain, redness and swelling respectively; these features may surround an obvious locus of infection such as a wound, ulcer or insect bite.

b. Temperature

It is important to assess the temperature of the skin around any swelling, and also the patient's core body temperature.

Common diagnosis 3
Diagnosis: Liver failure

Examination findings
a. Peripheral signs of liver dysfunction

Jaundice, spider naevi and palmar erythema are signs of chronic liver failure which can be seen in severe disease or acute decompensation.

b. Ascites

Due to the low albumin content of the blood, fluid accumulates in the abdomen (ascites) as well as the peripheries.

c. Altered behaviour, confusion, reduced consciousness

In liver failure, cerebral oedema can develop causing varying degrees of hepatic encephalopathy.

Common diagnosis 4
Diagnosis: Malnutrition/intestinal disease

Examination findings
a. Low body mass index (BMI)

A nutritionally inadequate diet, or chronic diarrhoea from an underlying intestinal disease, will cause weight loss.

b. Abdominal tenderness on palpation

Particularly if there is underlying intestinal disease such as coeliac disease.

c. Signs of specific nutrient deficiencies

Malnourishment; an affected patient will also exhibit signs from other nutritional deficiencies such as a lack of iron or vitamin D (see Table 8.1).

Table 8.1 Signs related to deficiency of specific nutrients

Deficiency	Iron	B_{12}/folate	Vitamin D

Signs	Pale complexion
	Pale conjunctiva
	Koilonychia
	Leuconychia
	Angular stomatitis
		Glossitis
		Angular stomatitis
		Mood changes
		Peripheral neuropathy
		Subacute combined
		  degeneration of the
		  spinal cord
			Rickets (children)
			Osteomalacia (adults)
			Myalgia
			Proximal muscle weakness

Diagnosis to consider 1
Diagnosis: Drugs

Examination findings
There are often no specific examination findings if the cause of the patient's peripheral oedema is from a medication. The key in making this diagnosis is from the history. There may be outward signs of medication use, such as insulin injection marks, but it is often much easier to just ask the patient about new medications. Once the medication is withdrawn, the oedema should resolve.

Diagnosis to consider 2
Diagnosis: Filariasis

Examination findings
a. Elephantitis

This describes the gross swelling of the lower limbs as seen in chronic infection of lymphatic filarial disease.

b. Lymphadenopathy

During acute infection there may be fever accompanied by painful lymphadenopthy in the groin and axilla.

c. Hydrocoele

Gross hydrocoeles may be seen in male patients with chronic infection.

Diagnosis to consider 3
Diagnosis: Malignancy

Examination findings
a. Breast lump, abdominal/pelvic mass, etc.

If a patient develops lower limb oedema a thorough abdominal examination is crucial to exclude large intra-abdominal masses. If a female patient develops unilateral upper limb oedema, a breast examination should be conducted to exclude breast lumps.

b. Scarring

This may be from previous radiotherapy or surgery to treat malignancy. If the lymph nodes have been removed or damaged, there may be resulting oedema in that limb.

8.6 KEY INVESTIGATIONS

Bedside tests

Table 8.2 Bedside tests of use in patients presenting with oedema

Test	Justification	Potential result
ECG	Non-specific signs of cardiac and respiratory pathology	**Cardiac failure:** may highlight ischaemic heart disease **DVT/nephrotic syndrome:** right heart strain if complicated by PE
Oxygen saturations	Important in any acutely unwell patient	**Cardiac failure:** decreased in pulmonary oedema **Angioedema:** decreased in airway compromise **DVT/nephrotic syndrome:** decreased if complicated by PE
Temperature	Immediate result, painless	**Infection/filariasis:** may be raised
Blood pressure	Important in any acutely unwell patient	**Cardiac failure:** low with narrow pulse pressure

Blood tests

Table 8.3 Blood tests of use in patients presenting with oedema

Test	Justification	Potential result
Full blood count (FBC)	May show signs of infection or red cell changes suggestive of other causes	**Infection:** raised white cell count **Liver failure:** macrocytosis if alcohol induced **Nephrotic syndrome:** raised white cell count if superimposed infection **Iron deficiency:** microcytic anaemia
Urea and electrolytes (U+E)	Important to assess renal function to investigate nephrotic syndrome	**Nephrotic syndrome:** decreased renal function may occur
Liver function tests (LFTs)	Important to assess liver function to investigate liver failure	**Liver failure:** raised aspartate aminotransferase (AST) (although cirrhosis may have normal values) **Malnutrition:** low protein and albumin **Nephrotic syndrome:** albumin <25 g/L
Clotting	Measure of liver synthetic function	**Liver failure:** INR increased **Nephrotic syndrome:** clotting factors increased
B-type natriuretic peptide (BNP)	Suggestive of ventricular strain and dysfunction	**Cardiac failure:** increased
Hepatitis screen	If liver failure suspected, can indicate cause	**Hepatitis:** a positive viral screen
D-dimer	Sensitive marker of fibrin degradation (suggests clotting)	**DVT, infection, malignancy:** raised
Blood film	To diagnose filariasis	**Filariasis:** filariae can be seen on blood smear

Imaging

Table 8.4 Imaging modalities of use in patients presenting with oedema

Test	Justification	Potential result
Chest X-ray	May show signs of heart failure	**Cardiac failure:** May show cardiomegaly, pulmonary oedema
Echocardiography	To assess cardiac structure and function	**Cardiac failure:** right ventricular dysfunction (systemic oedema), left ventricular dysfunction (pulmonary oedema)
Venous Doppler ultrasound	Assessment of DVT	**DVT:** presence of clot in deep venous system
Liver ultrasound	To assess liver structure	**Cirrhosis:** small liver with heterogeneous texture and surface nodularity

Special tests

Table 8.5 Special investigations of use in patients presenting with oedema

Test	Justification	Result
Renal biopsy	To diagnose cause of nephrotic syndrome	**Nephrotic syndrome:** will show direct cause
Urinary protein and albumin:creatinine ratio (ACR)	Required for the diagnosis of nephrotic syndrome	**Nephrotic syndrome:** proteinuria >3 g/24hrs, ACR >300–350 mg/mmol

8.7 WHEN TO CALL A SENIOR

Situations
1. A patient with angioedema and airway compromise – this is a life-threatening situation and requires immediate attention
2. A patient with ongoing oedema that requires investigation

Flash pulmonary oedema can also be life threatening, but this is covered elsewhere in the book.

What should be arranged by the time the senior arrives
Situation 1
After your ABCD assessment and resuscitation following the ALS algorithm, the following should be arranged by the time your senior arrives on the scene:

• Basic blood tests
• Chest X-ray – ideally portable
• Urgent anaesthetic review if laryngeal compromise suspected

Situation 2
If the patient is stable, some ongoing investigations could take place as an outpatient. Before your senior arrives to review the patient, the following should be arranged:

• Basic blood test
• ECG
• Imaging, for example echocardiogram if suspected cardiac failure, venous Doppler if suspected DVT
• Urinalysis and ACR if nephrotic syndrome suspected

In the case of a DVT, if a clot is suspected, anticoagulation treatment should start without waiting for the result of a venous Doppler.

What should be completed by the time the senior arrives
Situation 1
As with any unwell patient, a thorough history should be taken, including a comprehensive past medical, drug and social history, if this is possible. If the patient is having difficulty breathing it may be more prudent to limit your history taking to the essentials. The patient should also be examined to assess the extent and location of the oedema. An ABCD assessment is paramount and directs immediate management. In angioedema it is important to monitor oxygen saturations as a reflection of airway compromise. In this instance it is important to contact your seniors early.

Situation 2
The junior doctor should be able to compile a list of differentials which can help direct choice of investigations based on history and examination findings. It would be pointless, for example, to organize an echocardiogram for a patient with unilateral, well defined ankle swelling surrounding an infected insect bite.

Simple investigations, such as the bedside tests outlined in Table 8.2 should be completed by the time a senior arrives, as these should be explained in your handover. Nursing staff will often be able to help with these tests whilst the history is being taken or the patient examined.

Blood can be taken before the senior arrives. Filling a variety of blood bottles such as haematology, biochemistry and clotting bottles can mean that extra blood tests can be added later without the need to take more blood. If the patient is acutely unwell, making sure they have venous access is important.

KEY CLINICAL TRIALS

Key trial 8.1
Trial name: RALES trial.
Participants: 1663 patients with severe heart failure and a left ventricular ejection fraction (LVEF) of <35%.
Intervention: 25 mg spironolactone daily.
Control: Placebo drug.
Outcome: Blockade of aldosterone receptors by spironolactone, in addition to standard therapy, substantially reduces the risk of both morbidity and death among patients with severe heart failure.
Reason for inclusion: Landmark trial in the treatment of cardiac failure.
Reference: Pitt B, Zannad F, Remme WJ, et. al. for the Randomized Aldactone Evaluation Study Investigators. The effect of spironolactone on morbidity and mortality in patients with severe heart failure. N Engl J Med. 1999; 341:709–717. http://www.nejm.org/doi/full/10.1056/NEJM199909023411001

GUIDELINES

NICE. Chronic heart failure: management of chronic heart failure in adults in primary and secondary care. 2010. http://www.nice.org.uk/guidance/CG108/chapter/introduction

NICE. Venous thromboembolism: reducing the risk: Reducing the risk of venous thromboembolism (deep vein thrombosis and pulmonary embolism) in patients admitted to hospital. 2010. http://www.nice.org.uk/guidance/CG092

FURTHER READING

Ely JW, et al. Approach to leg edema of unclear etiology. J Am Board Fam Med. 2006;19(2):148–160. http://www.jabfm.org/content/19/2/148.long.
An interesting review covering the diagnostic process for peripheral oedema of unknown cause.

 For additional resources and to test your knowledge, visit the companion website at:

www.wiley.com/go/camm/cardiology

PART 3
Conditions

9 Acute Coronary Syndrome

Nicholas Sunderland
King's College Hospital NHS Foundation Trust, London, UK

9.1 DEFINITION

Acute coronary syndrome (ACS) represents a collection of signs and symptoms that are characteristic of a single underlying pathology – myocardial ischaemia, with or without infarction.

> **Box 9.1**   Entities included in acute coronary syndrome (ACS)
>
> **1.** ST-segment-elevation myocardial infarction (STEMI)
> **2.** Non-ST-segment-elevation myocardial infarction (NSTEMI)
> **3.** Unstable angina (UA)

Acute myocardial infarction criteria
1. A rise and/or fall of cardiac biomarker (preferably cardiac troponin)
2. Plus, at least one of the following:
- **Symptoms:** cardiac ischaemia (e.g. chest pain)
- **New ECG changes:** ST segment, T-wave, left bundle branch block (LBBB), or development of pathological Q-waves
- **Imaging:** new loss of viable myocardium or regional wall motion abnormality
- **Thrombus:** identification of an intracoronary thrombus by angiography or autopsy

Prior myocardial infarction criteria:
- **ECG:** pathological Q-waves in the absence of non-ischaemic causes
- **Imaging:** region of loss of viable myocardium (thinned and fails to contract), in the absence of non-ischaemic causes
- **Pathology:** findings of a prior MI

(See Audio Podcast 9.1 at **www.wiley.com/go/camm/cardiology**)

9.2 UNDERLYING CONCEPTS

Hypoperfusion and myocardial ischaemia is the common end-point underlying the acute coronary syndrome. In the vast majority this is caused by atherosclerotic plaque rupture, however there are other causes (see Figure 9.1).

Clinical Guide to Cardiology, First Edition. Edited by Christian F. Camm and A. John Camm.
© 2016 John Wiley & Sons, Ltd. Published 2016 by John Wiley & Sons, Ltd.
Companion website: www.wiley.com/go/camm/cardiology.

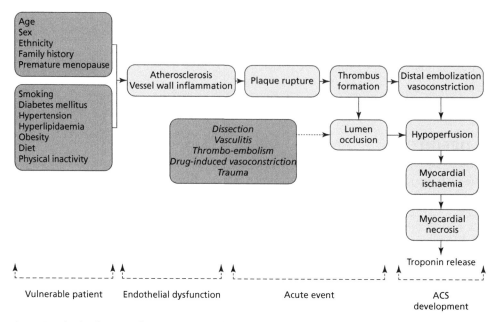

Figure 9.1 The development of acute coronary syndrome.

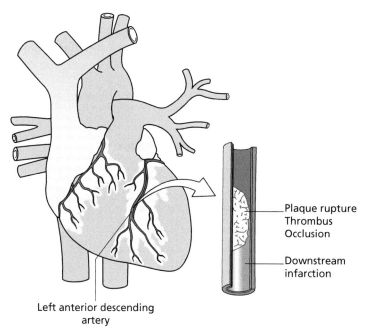

Figure 9.2 Diagram of coronary occlusion, due to an atherosclerotic plaque and associated thrombus, with downstream infarction.

Box 9.2   Definition of type 1 and type 2 myocardial infarctions

- **Type 1:** ischaemia due to a primary coronary event such as plaque erosion/rupture, fissuring or dissection
- **Type 2:** ischaemia due to either increased oxygen demand or decreased supply, e.g. coronary artery spasm, coronary microembolism, anaemia, arrhythmias, or hyper-/hypotension

Table 9.1 Pathophysiology vs. ACS presentation

Pathophysiology	Most likely outcome	MI type
Total occlusion of major coronary	STEMI	1
Partial occlusion of major coronary artery	NSTEMI	1
Total occlusion of minor coronary artery	NSTEMI	1
Increased oxygen demand or decreased supply (e.g. coronary artery spasm, anaemia, arrhythmias, hyper-/hypotension)	Unstable angina	2

Cardiac biomarkers
- **Necrosis:** results from ischaemia and leads to the release of cellular components into the bloodstream
- **Troponins:** cardiac troponins are regulatory proteins in the cardiac contractile apparatus and are the main biochemical marker used to measure the extent of myocardial damage
- **Other markers:** include creatine kinase and lactate dehydrogenase. Temporal profiles are shown in Figure 9.3

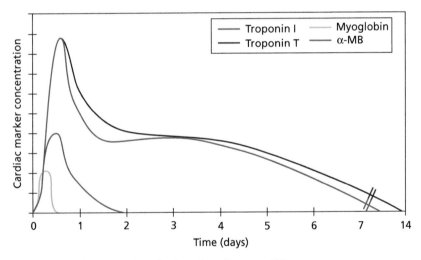

Figure 9.3 Cardiac markers: approximate levels vs. time of onset post MI.

- **Troponin timescale:** increase within 3–12 hours from the onset of chest pain, peak at 24–48 hours and return to baseline in 5–14 days
- **Diagnosis:** at least one value should be above the 99th percentile upper reference limit
- **Repetition:** including a second sample within 6 hours of presentation increases sensitivity to nearly 100%

Box 9.3 Factors that may exacerbate or precipitate ACS

1. Anaemia
2. Infection
3. Inflammation
4. Fever
5. Metabolic or endocrine (e.g. thyroid)

Cardiac anatomy

The main arteries supplying the heart:

1. Left anterior descending
2. Left circumflex
3. Right coronary

The regions supplied by each coronary artery are discussed in Chapter 28. The ECG leads representing each coronary artery are discussed in Chapter 19.

9.3 KEY DATA

Aetiology
1. Atherosclerosis and plaque rupture
2. Hypoperfusion
3. Coronary vasospasm
4. Coronary artery dissection

Risk factors
See Chapter 10.

Incidence
- **STEMI:** 7 per 10^4 per year
- **NSTEMI:** 13 per 10^4 per year

Mortality

Table 9.2 Mortality for acute coronary syndromes. Adapted from the ESC Guidelines for the management of acute coronary syndromes in patients presenting without persistent ST-segment elevation

ACS	Non ST-elevation	ST-elevation
In hospital	3–5%	7%
6-month mortality	12%	13%

9.4 CLINICAL TYPES

Pre-troponin
Initially, before a patient's troponin level is known, ACS should be classified, based on ECG findings, as:

- ACS with persistent (>15–20 minutes) ST elevation (STE-ACS)
- ACS without persistent ST elevation (NSTE-ACS)

Post-troponin
Three different ACS entities are commonly recognized:

1. Unstable angina (UA)
2. ST-elevation myocardial infarction
3. Non-ST-elevation myocardial infarction

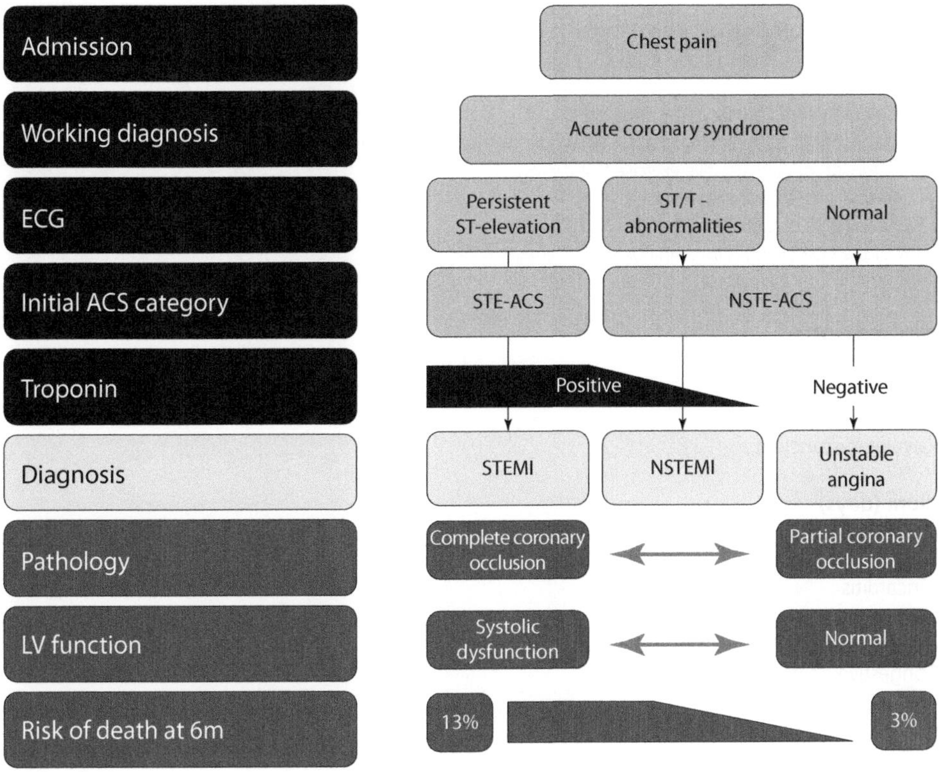

Figure 9.4 Diagnostic algorithm for differentiating different forms of ACS.

Box 9.4   Myocardial infarction vs. unstable angina

Definitions differ, but are defined by the serum concentration of cardiac markers:

- **ESC/ACC:** classify any troponin elevation as a myocardial infarction
- **BCS:** recognize a category 'ACS with myocyte necrosis' with mild troponin rises
- **WHO:** classify ACS with only mild troponin rises as 'unstable angina'

Use of troponin measurement to define myocardial damage has blurred distinctions. ACS can be thought of as a spectrum of myocyte damage.

Table 9.3 Features defining the clinical types of ACS

	Chest pain	Persistent ST elevation	Troponin rise
STEMI	✓	✓	✓
N-STEMI	✓	✗	✓
Unstable angina	✓	✗	✗

Box 9.5 Requirements in addition to chest pain needed to define unstable angina

Any one of:

1. Documentation of coronary artery disease:
   - History of MI, angina, ischaemic cardiomyopathy or resuscitated sudden cardiac death
   - History of, or new, positive exercise test
   - Known ≥50% coronary stenosis
   - Previous PCI or CABG
2. Any of the ECG changes listed in Box 9.8

Complications

Early (minutes–hours)
1. Arrhythmias
2. Cardiogenic shock
3. Valvular dysfunction

Medium (days)
1. Thrombus/emboli
2. Ventricular rupture
3. Pericarditis

Late (weeks–months)
1. Congestive heart failure
2. Dressler's syndrome
3. Ventricular aneurysm

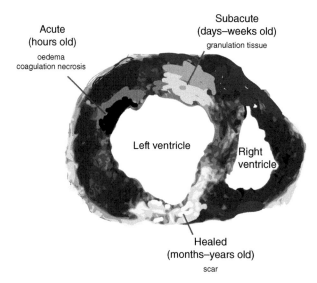

Figure 9.5 Cartoon representation of the pathological features following myocardial infarction.

(See Audio Podcast 9.2 at **www.wiley.com/go/camm/cardiology**)

9.5 PRESENTING FEATURES

Contrast the typical presenting features of angina (see Chapter 10) with those of an acute coronary syndrome.

Table 9.4 Typical features of cardiac chest pain

Site	Central, retrosternal, epigastric
Onset	Over seconds–minutes
Character	Dull, aching, heavy, pressure, crushing
Radiation	Left arm, neck, jaw, (right arm)
Associated symptoms	Autonomic symptoms: nausea, vomiting, sweating, SOB
	Heart failure symptoms: SOB, syncope, fatigue, altered mental state
	Other symptoms: palpitations
Timing	Constant, at rest, for >15–20 minutes
Exacerbating/ relieving factors	Does not respond to GTN*, does not resolve with rest
Severity	Usually severe, but can be variable

*N.B. Response to GTN should not be used to make a diagnosis.

Box 9.6 Atypical symptoms in ACS

Some patients present only with less typical symptoms:

- Nausea/vomiting
- Sweating
- Shortness of breath
- Fatigue
- Palpitations
- Syncope
- Altered mental state

Box 9.7 Patients more likely to present with atypical features of ACS

1. Diabetic
2. Chronic renal failure
3. Elderly
4. Dementia
5. Ethnic minority
6. Female

The physical examination is frequently normal; however, some features can be observed.

Features associated with ACS itself
- **Autonomic features:** pale, clammy skin
- **Dyskinetic cardiac impulse:** can be palpated occasionally in anterior wall MI

Signs suggesting exacerbating conditions
- **Anaemia:** pallor
- **Thyrotoxicosis:** sweating and tremor

Features associated with ACS complications
- **Arrhythmias:** tachycardia (VT) or bradycardia (heart block)
- **Congestive heart failure:** elevated JVP, low BP, breathlessness, fine inspiratory crackles, dull lung bases, peripheral oedema, ascites
- **Cardiogenic shock:** CCF findings, cool peripheries, low urine output, altered consciousness
- **Mitral regurgitation:** pansystolic murmur
- **Thrombus/emboli:** evidence of systemic emboli (e.g. stroke)

- **Ventricular rupture:** Beck's triad of low BP, raised JVP and quiet heart sounds indicating cardiac tamponade
- **Pericarditis:** pericardial friction rub, Beck's triad
- **Dressler's syndrome:** as for pericarditis
- **Ventricular aneurysm:** double apex beat, evidence of systemic embolism

9.6 DIFFERENTIALS

Non-atherosclerotic myocardial infarctions
1. Emboli
2. Vasculitis
3. Coronary artery spasm
4. Cocaine use
5. Congenital coronary anomalies
6. Coronary trauma

Conditions mimicking non-ST-elevation myocardial infarctions

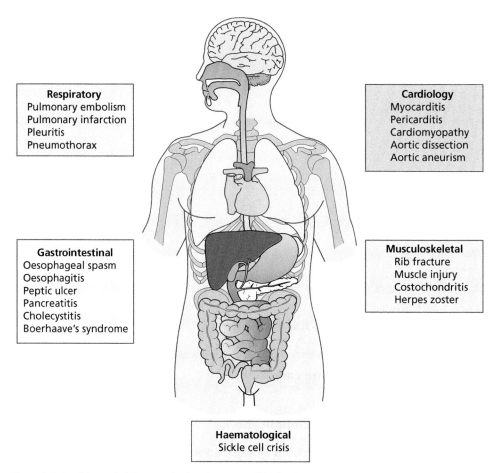

Respiratory
Pulmonary embolism
Pulmonary infarction
Pleuritis
Pneumothorax

Cardiology
Myocarditis
Pericarditis
Cardiomyopathy
Aortic dissection
Aortic aneurism

Gastrointestinal
Oesophageal spasm
Oesophagitis
Peptic ulcer
Pancreatitis
Cholecystitis
Boerhaave's syndrome

Musculoskeletal
Rib fracture
Muscle injury
Costochondritis
Herpes zoster

Haematological
Sickle cell crisis

Figure 9.6 Conditions mimicking non-ST-elevation myocardial infarctions.

9.7 KEY INVESTIGATIONS

Bedside tests

Table 9.5 Bedside tests of use in patients presenting with acute coronary syndrome

Test	Justification	Potential result
Oxygen saturations	Hypoxia will exacerbate cardiac ischaemia	Commonly normal Aim for 94–98% Low in PE
Blood glucose (capillary BM reading)	Should be checked in ALL patients presenting with reduced level of consciousness or syncope Hyperglycaemia is a poor prognostic indicator	Low – if cause of syncope or seizure High – hyperglycaemia >11 mmol/L should be treated
BP	BP reading in each arm	Normal Low if cardiogenic shock
ECG	Looking for changes characteristic of myocardial ischaemia Serial ECGs may demonstrate evolving events	**STEMI criteria:** >1 mm of ST elevation in contiguous limb leads or >2 mm in contiguous chest leads **NSTEMI/unstable angina:** see Box 9.8

Box 9.8 Potential ECG changes seen in NSTEMI

- Transient ST elevation/depression
- T-wave inversion
- Flat T-waves
- Pseudo-normalization of T-waves
- No ECG changes

Box 9.9 A normal ECG in ACS

1. A completely normal ECG does not exclude the possibility of NSTE ACS
2. Circumflex artery or right ventricular ischaemia may not have 12-lead ECG findings
   - These may be detected using leads V7–V9 and V3R/V4R, respectively

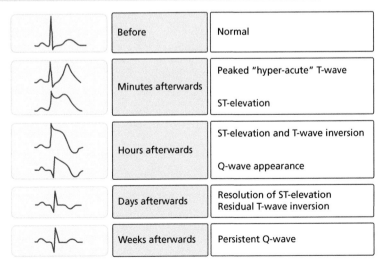

	Before	Normal
	Minutes afterwards	Peaked "hyper-acute" T-wave ST-elevation
	Hours afterwards	ST-elevation and T-wave inversion Q-wave appearance
	Days afterwards	Resolution of ST-elevation Residual T-wave inversion
	Weeks afterwards	Persistent Q-wave

Figure 9.7 ECG changes seen over time in ST-elevation myocardial infarction.

Blood tests

Table 9.6 Blood tests of use in patients presenting with acute coronary syndrome

Test	Justification	Potential result
Troponin	Cardiac troponins reflects myocardial cellular damage In the setting of myocardial ischaemia (chest pain, ECG changes, or new wall motion abnormalities) troponin elevation indicates MI	See Boxes 9.10 and 9.11 for non-ACS causes of an elevated troponin
FBC	Anaemia, sepsis and hyperthyroidism may precipitate an MI There may be a raised MCV with hyperthyroidism	WCC raised – potential sepsis Haemoglobin low – anaemia
U&E and LFTs	Coronary artery disease may be a marker for vascular disease in general Renovascular disease may result in renal impairment, important because: • May be starting an angiotensin-converting enzyme inhibitor (ACEi) • Contrast will be given during angiogram	Creatinine high – renal disease Hyperkalaemia – contraindication to starting an ACEi Electrolyte disturbances (especially K^+, Mg^{2+} and Ca^{2+}) may predispose to arrhythmias
Coagulation screen	The INR should be known before electively taking someone to the Cath Lab	High INR – potentially taking warfarin
Lipid profile	All ACS patients get high-dose statin therapy; this should be re-evaluated at 4–6 weeks	Low density lipoprotein (LDL)-cholesterol target: <1.8 mmol/L
Glycated haemoglobin (HbA1c)	Diabetes and poor glycaemic control is a risk factor for coronary artery disease	HbA1c >7.5% (59 mmol/mol) indicates poor glycaemic control

Box 9.10   Non-coronary cardiac causes of a raised troponin

1. Severe congestive cardiac failure
2. Hypertensive crisis
3. Arrhythmias (tachy- or brady-)
4. Myocarditis
5. Takotsubo cardiomyopathy
6. Cardiac contusion
7. Iatrogenic (e.g. ablation, pacing, cardioversion)
8. Aortic valve disease

Box 9.11 Non-cardiac causes of a raised troponin

1. Chronic or acute renal dysfunction
2. Pulmonary embolism
3. Severe pulmonary hypertension
4. Acute neurological disease, e.g. stroke or subarachnoid haemorrhage
5. Aortic dissection
6. Hypothyroidism
7. Infiltrative (e.g. amyloid, sarcoid, haemochromatosis, scleroderma)
8. Drug toxicity: adriamycin, 5-flurouracil, herceptin, snake venoms
9. Burns: especially if >30% total body surface area
10. Rhabdomyolysis
11. Sepsis

Imaging

Table 9.7 Imaging modalities of use in patients presenting with acute coronary syndrome

Test	Justification	Potential result
Chest X-ray	Heart failure Assessment for alternative diagnoses: pneumothorax, aortic dissection	Features of heart failure: A – alveolar shadowing B – Kerley B lines C – cardiomegaly D – upper lobe diversion E – effusions
Echocardiography	Functional assessment of the heart	Regional wall hypokinesis Reduced ejection fraction Valvular dysfunction Hypertrophy

Special tests

Table 9.8 Specialist tests of use in patients presenting with acute coronary syndrome

Test	Justification	Potential result
Myocardial perfusion scan – SPECT	Shows areas in the heart that have a decreased perfusion	Identifies areas amenable to revascularization
Angiography	Images the coronary arteries, looking at the luminal calibre Timing of angiography based on risk assessment (see Box 9.12)	Arterial occlusion and degree of stenosis
Cardiac MRI	Assessment of heart function using cine imaging Assessment of myocardial perfusion and viability in order to guide revascularization therapies	Infarcted regions will be shown by delayed uptake of gadolinium contrast
Coronary optical coherence tomography (OCT)	Uses near-infrared light to image the coronary artery walls. It is effectively 'optical ultrasound'	OCT can give very detailed pictures of atherosclerotic plaque/vessel wall morphology and stent positioning

Box 9.12   Timing of PCI in patients with ACS

- **Urgent (<2 hours):** if very high-risk patient, refractory pain or haemodynamic compromise
- **Early (<24 hours):** if GRACE score >140 and one high-risk criterion
- **Routine (<72 hours):** if one high-risk criterion, or recurrent symptoms

Risk scores

TIMI

The Thombolysis In Myocardial Infarction (TIMI) Study Group created the TIMI score to assess the risk of death and ischaemic events in patients with NSTEMI or unstable angina.

Table 9.9 TIMI Score following ACS event

Element	Points	Risk score	Risk of cardiac event by 14 days** (%)
Age ≥65 years	1	0/1	5
≥3 CAD risk factors*	1	2	8
Known CAD (stenosis ≥50%)	1	3	13
Aspirin use in the past 7 days	1	4	20
Recent severe angina (<24 hours)	1	5	26
Increased cardiac markers	1	6/7	41
ST-deviation ≥0.5 mm	1		
TOTAL (out of 7)			

*Coronary artery disease (CAD) risk factors = FH, hypertension, high cholesterol, DM, smoker)
**death, MI or urgent revascularization

GRACE

- The Global Registry of Acute Coronary Events (GRACE) is a database looking at ACS outcomes
- The GRACE risk score, derived from this database, predicts death and cardiovascular events, both in-hospital and at 6 months
- GRACE is not as simple as TIMI but can be calculated on-line:
  http://www.outcomes-umassmed.org/grace/acs_risk/acs_risk_content.html
- The components of the GRACE score are:
  a. Age
  b. Killip class
  c. Heart rate
  d. Systolic BP
  e. Serum creatinine
  f. ST-segment deviation
  g. Cardiac arrest at admission
  h. Elevated serum cardiac enzymes

Box 9.13   Killip classification

System to risk stratify post-acute MI patients based on heart failure symptoms

- **Class I:** no clinical signs of heart failure
- **Class II:** rales/crackles in the lungs, S3, elevated JVP
- **Class III:** frank acute pulmonary oedema
- **Class IV:** cardiogenic shock/hypotension (systolic BP <90 mmHg)

Table 9.10 GRACE risk score association with in-hospital and 6-month mortality. *Adapted from the ESC Guidelines for the management of acute coronary syndromes in patients presenting without persistent ST-segment elevation*

	In-hospital death	
Risk category	GRACE risk score	Death (%)
Low	≤108	<1
Intermediate	109–140	1–3
High	>140	>3
	6-month mortality	
Risk category	GRACE risk score	Death (%)
Low	≤88	<3
Intermediate	89–118	3–8
High	>118	>8

9.8 MANAGEMENT OPTIONS

(See Audio Podcast 9.3 at **www.wiley.com/go/camm/cardiology**)

Conservative

Conservative management focuses on improving modifiable risk factors and reducing disease progression:

- **Exercise:** organized programmes may increase tolerance
- **Smoking cessation:** nicotine replacement therapy improves success
- **Dietary:** Mediterranean diet has been shown to improve lipid profile

Medical

Table 9.11 Principles of medical management with acute coronary syndromes

Name	Management principles
STEMI	Rapid re-establishment of coronary perfusion with PCI or fibrolytic therapy Ongoing treatment with antiplatelets and anticoagulants
NSTEMI/unstable angina	Treatment with antipatelets and anticoagulants Coronary angiography based on risk stratification Follow-on PCI or referral for CABG based on angiographic findings

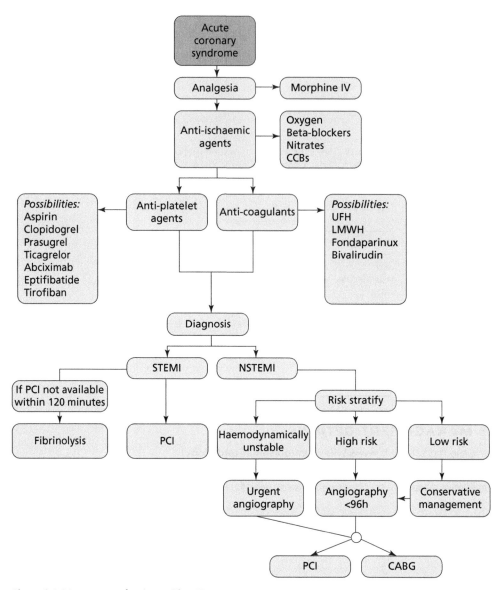

Figure 9.8 Management of patients with ACS.

Table 9.12 Common medications used in ACS management. N.B. Different combinations are used at different centres

	Management	Notes
Analgesia/ anti-ischaemic agents*	Morphine IV	Most effective analgesic Useful in the treatment of dyspnoea
	Nitrates PO/SL	GTN spray under the tongue – often most quickly available
	Oxygen	Do not routinely administer oxygen Aim for SpO$_2$ 94–98%, unless COPD in which case aim for SpO$_2$ 88–92%
	Beta-blocker	Routine beta-blockade in ACS patients improves mortality Contraindicated if in, or at high risk of, cardiogenic shock
	Nitrates IV	Good for relieving symptoms of angina and dyspnoea Contraindicated if BP <90 mmHg and if taking phosphodiesterase-5 (PDE-5) inhibitors
	Calcium-channel blocker	Useful if coronary artery spasm is suspected. Should only be used with caution with beta-blockers
Antiplatelet agents	Aspirin	Single loading dose of 300 mg; 75 mg maintenance dose Improves mortality
	Clopidogrel	Single loading dose of 600 mg; 75 mg maintenance dose if patients cannot be treated with ticagrelor or prasugrel Omeprazole decreases clopidogrel-induced platelet inhibition
	Prasugrel	Preferred over clopidogrel if the patient is diabetic. Indicated if there has been stent thrombosis on clopidogrel
	Ticagrelor	Recommended in patient at high risk of having had an ischaemic event. Clopidogrel should be stopped if this is used
	Abciximab Eptifibatide Tirofiban	GPIIb/IIIa inhibitors – recommended in combination with dual antiplatelet therapy during high-risk PCI if there is a low risk of bleeding and/or angiographic evidence of massive thrombus, slow re-flow or thrombotic complications
Anticoagulants	Unfractionated heparin (UFH)	A single bolus is commonly added to fondaparinux during PCI
	Low molecular weight heparin (LMWH)	Sometimes used instead of UFH
	Fondaparinux	The most favoured anticoagulant in terms of efficacy–safety profile
	Bivalirudin	Direct thrombin inhibitor sometimes used during PCI

*Anti-ischaemic drugs either decrease myocardial oxygen demand (by decreasing heart rate, lowering blood pressure, reducing preload, or reducing myocardial contractility) or increase myocardial oxygen supply (by inducing coronary vasodilatation).

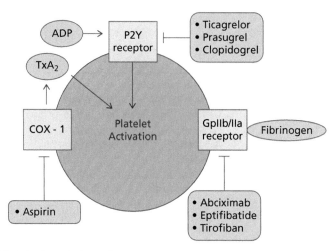

Figure 9.9 Simplified platelet activation pathway.

Invasive
- **PCI:** involves widening of coronary arteries from within using a balloon catheter +/− insertion of a stent to maintain patency (see Chapter 26)
- **CABG:** a surgical procedure in which vein grafts (legs) or arterial grafts (wrist or chest wall) are used to bypass coronary artery disease

STEMI
- **<12 hours post onset:** PCI reperfusion therapy is indicated in all patients with STEMI or new left bundle branch block (LBBB)
- **>12 hours post onset:** reperfusion therapy is indicated if there is evidence of ongoing ischaemia
- **120 minutes:** time frame from first medical contact for performing PCI for STEMI

Box 9.14   Multi-vessel disease in primary PCI

50% of STEMI patients have multi-vessel disease. Only the infarct-related artery should be treated unless:

1. There is cardiogenic shock and multiple critically stenosed arteries (>90%)
2. Highly unstable lesions are present
3. Persistent ischaemia after PCI to the affected artery

- **CABG:** not used routinely as the initial revascularization strategy; duration from symptom onset to final surgical result is too long

---

Box 9.15   When CABG is used as a primary revascularization strategy

When CABG is attempted in the primary setting:

1. Not possible to perform PCI
2. PCI has been attempted and failed

Surgical risks in this acute period are high; the patient will have received dual antiplatelet therapy increasing bleeding risks

NSTEMI/unstable angina
- **Revascularization:** dependent on clinical status, disease severity and lesion characteristics
- **<96 hours:** timeframe for revascularization in patients with high predicted mortality (e.g. GRACE score)
- **CABG/PCI:** the benefit from PCI is related to its early performance, whereas the benefit from CABG is greatest when performed after several days of medical stabilization
- **Multidisciplinary meeting (MDM):** centres should have regular MDMs (including cardiology and cardiothoracic surgery) to discuss the best strategy on a case-by-case basis

---

Box 9.16 Factors that would warrant an early invasive strategy (PCI within 24 hours) in patients with NSTE ACS

1. Increased cardiac biomarkers (troponin, CK-MB)
2. New ST segment depression
3. Signs or symptoms of congestive heart failure (rales on examination, hypoxia with pulmonary oedema on chest X-ray)
4. Haemodynamic instability
5. Sustained ventricular tachycardia or ventricular fibrillation
6. Recent coronary intervention within 6 months
7. Prior coronary artery bypass grafting
8. High TIMI risk score
9. Reduced left ventricular systolic function (EF <40%)
10. Recurrent angina at rest or with low-level activity
11. High-risk findings from non-invasive testing

Long-term treatment (the standard post-MI bundle)

Table 9.13 Long-term therapies used post-ACS

Therapy	Detail
Lifestyle education	Information regarding diet, smoking cessation and exercise from a specialist multidisciplinary team
Aspirin	Life-long
Clopidogrel (or prasugrel) (or ticagrelor)	Duration (1–12 months) depends on: • STEMI vs. NSTEMI vs. UA • Stent vs. no stent • Drug-eluting vs. bare-metal stent • Brand of stent
Proton-pump inhibitor (PPI)	Prophylaxis against drug-induced GI damage Do not give omeprazole with clopidogrel
Beta-blocker	Optimize dose to BP and HR Continue for at least 12 months
Statin	High-dose therapy initially Reduce dose in accordance with serum lipid levels
ACEi	Optimize dose to BP and renal function Continue life-long
Mineralocorticoid-receptor inhibitors	Consider post MI if severe LV systolic dysfunction is present Monitor renal function

(See Audio Podcast 9.4 at **www.wiley.com/go/camm/cardiology**)

KEY CLINICAL TRIALS

Key trial 9.1

Trial name: CURE.

Participants: Non-ST-elevation acute coronary syndrome.

Intervention: Combined aspirin (300 mg STAT and 75–150 mg daily) and clopidogrel (300 mg stat and 75 mg daily).

Control: Only aspirin (300 mg STAT and 75–150 mg daily).

Outcome: Combination therapy provided a further 2.1% absolute risk reduction (20% relative) in the combined end-point (cardiovascular death, stroke or myocardial infarction) in high-risk patients (electrocardiographic evidence of ischaemia or elevated cardiac markers) with non-ST-elevation acute coronary syndromes.

Reason for inclusion: Justification for dual antiplatelet therapy (DAPT) in NSTEMI.

Reference: Yusuf S, Zhao F, Mehta SR, et al. Effects of clopidogrel in addition to aspirin in patients with acute coronary syndromes without ST-segment elevation. N Engl J Med. 2001;345(7):494-502. http://www.ncbi.nlm.nih.gov/pubmed/11519503.

Key trial 9.2

Trial name: EPHESUS.

Participants: Patients 3–14 days post-myocardial infarction with LVEF $\leq$40% and features of heart failure.

Intervention: Eplerenone.

Control: Placebo.

Outcome: Eplerenone reduces all-cause mortality (RR 0.85) and mortality from cardiovascular causes and hospitalizations for cardiovascular issues (RR 0.87). Eplerenone increases risk of hyperkalaemia and gastrointestinal issues.

Reason for inclusion: Justification of long-term post-MI treatment.

Reference: Pitt B, Remme W, Zannad F, et al. Eplerenone, a selective aldosterone blocker, in patients with left ventricular dysfunction after myocardial infarction. N Engl J Med. 2003;348(14):1309-1321. http://www.ncbi.nlm.nih.gov/pubmed/12668699.

Key trial 9.3

Trial Name: COMMIT.

Participants: Patients presenting with ST elevation, ST depression or LBBB within 24 hours of a suspected MI.

Intervention: Used a 2×2 factorial design: (1) clopidogrel + aspirin; (2) metoprolol.

Control: (1) Aspirin alone; (2) placebo.

Outcome: Clopidogrel + aspirin: reduced death, reinfarction, or stroke (OR 0.91, 95%CI 0.86–0.97) with no increase in bleeding. Metoprolol: decreased risk of reinfarction (OR 0.82; 95%CI 0.72–0.92) and VF (OR 0.83; 95%CI 0.75–0.93), but increased risk of cardiogenic shock (OR 1.30; 95%CI 1.19–1.41). It had no effect on death from any cause (OR 0.99; 95%CI 0.92–1.05).

Reason for inclusion: Rationale for DAPT and beta-blockers post MI.

Reference: Chen ZM, Jiang LX, Chen YP, et al. Addition of clopidogrel to aspirin in 45,852 patients with acute myocardial infarction: randomised placebo-controlled trial. Lancet. 2005;366(9497):1607-1621. http://www.ncbi.nlm.nih.gov/pubmed/16271642.

GUIDELINES

European Society of Cardiology. ESC Guidelines for the management of acute myocardial infarction in patients presenting with ST-segment elevation. 2012. http://www.escardio.org/guidelines-surveys/esc-guidelines/GuidelinesDocuments/Guidelines_AMI_STEMI.pdf.

European Society of Cardiology. ESC Guidelines for the management of acute coronary syndromes in patients presenting without persistent ST-segment elevation. 2011. http://www.escardio.org/guidelines-surveys/esc-guidelines/guidelinesdocuments/guidelines-nste-acs-ft.pdf.

National Institute for Health and Clinical Excellence. Chest pain of recent onset (CG95). 2010. http://www.nice.org.uk/nicemedia/live/12947/47938/47938.pdf.

FURTHER READING

Bhatt DL, Hulot JS, Moliterno DJ, et al. Antiplatelet and anticoagulation therapy for acute coronary syndromes. Circ Res. 2014;114(12):1929–1943. http://www.ncbi.nlm.nih.gov/pubmed/24902976.
A recent review on the use of different anti-platelet therapies.

Barnett K, Feldman JA. Noninvasive imaging techniques to aid in the triage of patients with suspected acute coronary syndrome: a review. Emerg Med Clin North Am. 2005;23(4):977–998. http://www.ncbi.nlm.nih.gov/pubmed/16199334.
A review looking at imaging techniques of use when assessing patients with suspected ACS.

 For additional resources and to test your knowledge, visit the companion website at:

www.wiley.com/go/camm/cardiology

10 Stable Angina

Katie Glover

Guy's and St Thomas' NHS Foundation Trust, London, UK

10.1 DEFINITION

Symptom of chest discomfort or pain, due to myocardial ischaemia, which usually arises as a result of physical exertion or emotional stress.

10.2 UNDERLYING CONCEPTS

This chapter will focus on atherosclerotic angina in its stable form.

1. **Ischaemia:** results from reduced coronary flow that cannot meet myocardial oxygen demand
2. **Pain:** results from damage to the myocardium resulting from ischaemia
3. **Atherosclerotic plaques:** grow and progressively obstruct coronary arteries reducing coronary flow

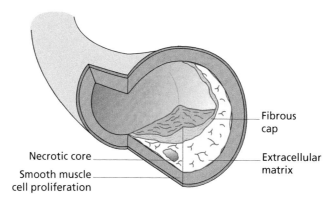

Figure 10.1 A partially occluded coronary artery.

(See Audio Podcast 10.1 and 10.2 at **www.wiley.com/go/camm/cardiology**)

10.3 KEY DATA

Diagnosis is primarily based on history and is therefore subjective. As such, prevalence and incidence are difficult to assess.

Aetiology/risk factors
Modifiable:

1. Smoking
2. Diabetes
3. Hypertension
4. Hypercholesterolaemia
5. Obesity
6. Low physical activity

Non-modifiable:

1. Increasing age
2. Male gender
3. Family history
4. Previous cardiovascular event

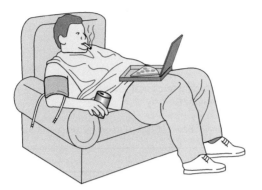

Figure 10.2   Modifiable and non-modifiable risk factors for coronary artery disease.

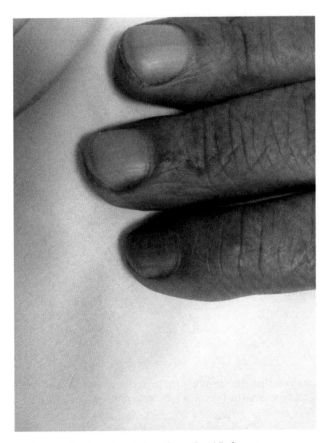

Figure 10.3 Right hand showing nicotine stains on the index and middle fingers.

Incidence
- 50 per 10^4 per year (in those over 40)

Prevalence
- Men >60 years: 2000 per 10^4
- Women >60 years: 1500 per 10^4

Mortality
- Annual mortality 2%
- Risk of mortality, MI or stroke 4.5%

10.4 CLINICAL TYPES

- Stable angina can be classified according to clinical severity
- Unstable angina is discussed in Chapter 9

Table 10.1 Classification of stable angina as based on clinical severity (Canadian Cardiovascular Society)

Grade	Definition
Class I	Angina results only from strenuous, rapid or prolonged exercise
Class II	Angina causing slight limitation provoked by ordinary (moderate) physical activity (e.g. walking or climbing stairs rapidly)
Class III	Angina causing marked limitation provoked by mild or ordinary physical activity (e.g. climbing one flight of stairs at normal pace)
Class IV	Inability to carry on any physical activity without angina symptoms and may be present at rest

---

Box 10.1 Types of angina

- Obstructive (atherosclerotic)
- Microvascular
- Prinzmetal
- Aortic stenosis
- Coronary artery bridging

(See Audio Podcast 10.3 at **www.wiley.com/go/camm/cardiology**)

10.5 PRESENTING FEATURES

On take (acute)
Primarily characterized by central chest pain (see Box 10.2).

Accompanying symptoms
- Shortness of breath
- Fatigue
- Nausea
- Sweating
- Restlessness

Commonly presents during exertional or stressful situations, after heavy meals, in cold temperatures and early in the morning. Rapidly relieved by buccal or sublingual nitrates.

Signs
Often physical examination is normal. Potential findings include:

- Tachycardia
- Tachypnoea
- Autonomic features: cold, pale and sweaty

Box 10.2 Pain

- **Site:** usually retrosternal or in the anterior chest
- **Character:** pressure, tightness, heaviness or aching sensation
- **Radiation:** epigastrium, neck, jaw, shoulder blades or arms
- **Timing:** commonly lasts less than 10 minutes
- **Severity:** variable; no relation to disease process

In clinic (chronic)
Patients will present with similar features as in the acute setting. In addition, the following questions should be asked to all patients with angina:

1. What brings on the pain (triggers)?
2. How far can you walk before the pain comes on (threshold)?
3. How often do you use your GTN spray (symptom density)?
4. Can you walk as far as you could 2 months ago (stability)?

Physical examination is often normal, however associated signs include:

1. **Lipid disorder:** cutaneous xanthomata, xanthelesma and corneal arcus (signs of peripheral lipid deposition)
2. **Arterial stenosis:** plaque formation in other arteries can result in bruits (e.g. carotid/renal)
3. **Murmurs:** may be heard if there is underlying valvular disease
4. **Hypertension:** predisposing factor in the development of cardiovascular disease
5. **Smoking related:** nicotine staining around finger tips (Figure 10.3)

10.6 DIFFERENTIALS

Most common
1. Musculoskeletal (e.g. intercostal muscle spasm, costochondritis)
2. Gastro-oesophageal reflux disorder (GORD)
3. Oesophageal spasm
4. Psychogenic – anxiety and depression

Less common but dangerous
1. Pulmonary embolus
2. Aortic dissection
3. Acute coronary syndrome

Not to miss
1. Herpes Zoster – shingles
2. Pericarditis
3. Pneumothorax

10.7 KEY INVESTIGATIONS

Bedside

Table 10.2 Bedside tests in patients with suspected stable angina

Investigation	Justification	Potential result
Blood pressure	Risk factor for left ventricular hypertrophy and coronary artery disease	Normal or raised
ECG	To look for ischaemic changes	See Box 10.3

Box 10.3   ECG findings in stable angina

1. Often normal
2. Current changes:
   - ST-segment depression
   - T-wave flattening and/or inversion
3. Pre-existing cardiovascular disease:
   - Q-waves due to old infarction
   - Large QRS-complex amplitude due to LV hypertrophy

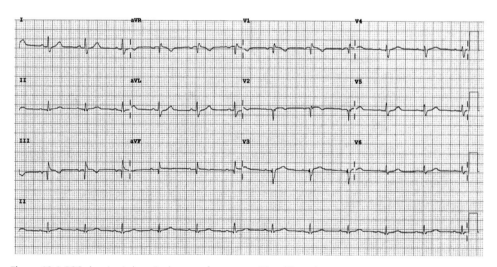

Figure 10.4 ECG showing ischaemic changes of someone with stable angina.

Blood tests

Table 10.3 Blood tests in patients with suspected stable angina

Investigation	Justification	Potential Result
Full blood count	Anaemia can result in myocardial ischaemia	Low Hb level
Thyroid function (if clinically indicated)	Hyperthyroidism can result in myocardial ischaemia	High T3/T4, low thyroid-stimulating hormone (TSH)
Troponin (if uncertain of diagnosis)	Rule out myocardial infarction Should be taken 8–12 hours post chest pain	Angina (stable/unstable): normal Myocardial infarction: raised
Lipid profile	Assess for lipid risk factors	High LDL/cholesterol Low HDL
Glucose	Assess for diabetes (risk factor)	Diabetes: high glucose

Imaging

Table 10.4 Imaging modalities of use in patients with suspected stable angina

Investigation	Justification	Expected result
Chest X-ray	Often routinely performed but of little diagnostic value	Normal

Special tests

Table 10.5 Special tests to be considered in patients with suspected stable angina

Investigation	Justification	Potential results
Stress echocardiography	Low cost, safe, widely available	Previous MI: regional wall motion abnormalities
Exercise ECG	Should not be used to diagnose or exclude stable angina	Provocation of chest pain with associated ST-segment/T-wave changes
Calcium scoring (cardiac CT)	High score associated with higher cardiovascular (CV) event rate	Calcium in coronary arteries – correlates with atherosclerosis
Technetium scan – myocardial perfusion imaging	Can show reversible ischaemia	Ischaemic myocardium
CT coronary angiogram	High sensitivity and specificity for CAD. Can be used to exclude PE and dissection	Coronary artery stenosis
Coronary angiography	Useful if diagnosis is unclear especially if revascularization is being considered	Used to delineate anatomy and stenosis
Cardiac MRI	Can assess function, perfusion and viability, excellent detail	Coronary artery disease: artery stenosis Ischaemia: reduced tissue perfusion

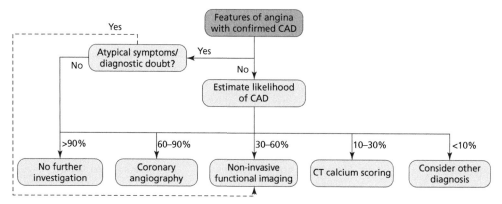

Figure 10.5 Investigations for stable angina.
Source: NICE 2010. Reproduced with permission of NICE.

10.8 MANAGEMENT OPTIONS

Conservative

Conservative management is focused on improving modifiable risk factors and reducing the progression of angina symptoms:

- **Smoking cessation:** nicotine replacement therapy
- **Dietary:** Mediterranean diet has been shown to improve lipid profile
- **Exercise**: organized programmes may increase exercise tolerance

(See Audio Podcast 10.4 at **www.wiley.com/go/camm/cardiology**)

Box 10.4 Recommendations on daily diet in stable angina

- <5 g of salt
- 30–45 g of fibre
- 200 g of fruit (2–3 servings)
- 200 g of vegetables (2–3 servings)
- Alcohol limited to 20 g (men) or 10 g (women)

Medical

1. **Symptom relief:** short-acting nitrates (e.g. GTN spray)
2. **Symptom control (attempt in order):**
   a. Beta-blocker **or** calcium-channel blocker (CCB)
   b. Beta-blocker **and** CCB
   c. Alternative medication
   d. Beta-blocker or CCB + alternative medications

N.B. Only add a third medication when symptoms not controlled and patient is waiting for revascularization or it is not appropriate

3. **Co-morbidity treatment:**
   a. Hypertension (see Chapter 16)
   b. Diabetes
   c. Hyperlipidaemia (e.g. statins)

Box 10.5   Alternative medications of use in stable angina

1. **Long-acting nitrates:** especially if good symptom relief with GTN
2. **Nicorandil:** can be used if contraindications to other drugs
3. **Ranolazine:** can reduce frequency of symptoms
4. **Ivabradine:** used if contraindication to beta-blockers

Invasive
Revascularization therapy (see Chapter 26):

1. Coronary artery bypass graft (CABG)
2. Primary coronary intervention (PCI)

KEY CLINICAL TRIALS

Key trial 10.1
Trial name: COURAGE.
Participants: 2200 patients with stable coronary artery disease.
Intervention: Percutaneous coronary intervention.
Control: Optimal medical therapy alone.
Outcome: Treatment with PCI was not associated with a difference in death or MI compared with medical therapy alone.
Reason for inclusion: To highlight the preference for medical therapy over surgical intervention in the treatment of stable angina.
Reference: Shaw LJ, Berman DS, Maron DJ, et al. Optimal medical therapy with or without percutaneous coronary intervention to reduce ischemic burden: results from the Clinical Outcomes Utilizing Revascularization and Aggressive Drug Evaluation (COURAGE) trial nuclear substudy. Circulation. 2008;117(10):1283–1291. http://www.ncbi.nlm.nih.gov/pubmed/18268144.

Key trial 10.2
Trial name: ACTION trial.
Participants: 7600 patients with stable symptomatic angina.
Intervention: Addition of nifedipine to the basic angina treatment regime (beta-blockers, nitrates).
Control: Placebo.
Outcome: Addition of nifedipine has no effect on major cardiovascular event free survival but is safe and reduces the need for coronary angiography and other interventions.
Reason for inclusion: To highlight controversy and debate around medications in chronic stable angina.
Reference: Poole-Wilson PA, Lubsen J, Kirwan B, et al. Effect of long-acting nifedipine on mortality and cardiovascular morbidity in patients with stable angina requiring treatment (ACTION trial): randomised controlled trial. http://www.ncbi.nlm.nih.gov/pubmed/?term=15351192.

GUIDELINES

European Society of Cardiology. Guidelines on CVD prevention in clinical practice. 2012. http://www.escardio.org/guidelines-surveys/esc-guidelines/GuidelinesDocuments/guidelines-CVD-prevention.pdf

European Society of Cardiology. Guidelines on the management of stable coronary artery disease. 2013. http://eurheartj.oxfordjournals.org/content/34/38/2949.full.pdf

NICE. Chest pain of recent onset: Assessment and diagnosis of recent onset chest pain or discomfort of suspected cardiac origin. 2010. http://guidance.nice.org.uk/cg95

NICE. Management of stable angina. 2011. http://guidance.nice.org.uk/CG126

FURTHER READING

Campeau, L. Letter: Grading of angina pectoris. Circulation. 1976;54(3):522–523. http://www.ncbi.nlm.nih.gov/pubmed/947585
Widely used, well known classification of stable angina
Pellicori P, Costanzo P, Joseph AC, et al. Medical management of stable coronary atherosclerosis. Curr Atheroscler Rep. 2013;15(4):313.
A modern review discussing the management of stable angina

 For additional resources and to test your knowledge, visit the companion website at:

www.wiley.com/go/camm/cardiology

11 Heart Failure

Arvind Singhal
Chelsea and Westminster Hospital NHS Foundation Trust, London, UK

11.1 DEFINITION

An abnormality of cardiac structure or function preventing delivery of sufficient oxygen to meet tissue demands.

11.2 UNDERLYING CONCEPTS

- **Reduced cardiac output:** prevents sufficient oxygenated blood reaching tissues
- **Frank–Starling mechanism:** ventricular contraction increases as the ventricle is stretched, up to a critical point. Beyond this, contraction is less efficient

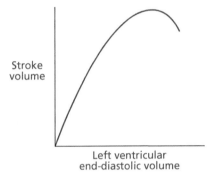

Stroke volume

Left ventricular end-diastolic volume

Figure 11.1 The Frank–Starling curve.

- **Compensatory mechanisms:** these mechanisms include:
  - a. **Sympathetic activation:** causes tachycardia and vasoconstriction to maintain perfusion, but causes strain and increased myocardial metabolic demand in the long term
  - b. **Renin–angiotensin–aldosterone (RAA) system:** activation results in increase in blood pressure through vasoconstriction and fluid retention

---

Box 11.1 Common terms describing ventricular size/function

- **End-diastolic volume (EDV):** the volume of blood in the ventricle at the end of relaxation
- **End-systolic volume (ESV):** the volume of blood in the ventricle at the end of contraction
- **Stroke volume (SV):** the volume of blood ejected from the ventricle during systole. SV = EDV − ESV
- **Ejection fraction (EF):** the fraction of volume removed from the ventricle during systole. EF = SV/EDV

Clinical Guide to Cardiology, First Edition. Edited by Christian F. Camm and A. John Camm.
© 2016 John Wiley & Sons, Ltd. Published 2016 by John Wiley & Sons, Ltd.
Companion website: www.wiley.com/go/camm/cardiology.

- **Preload:** fluid retention through the RAA system increases left ventricular end-diastolic volume
- **Afterload:** increased systemic vasoconstriction improves systemic blood pressure but forces the heart to pump against a greater pressure
- **Decompensation:** without treatment, heart failure results in a downwards spiral of fluid retention and reduced cardiac function

(See Audio Podcast 11.1 at **www.wiley.com/go/camm/cardiology**)

11.3 CLINICAL TYPES

Heart failure may be divided along two separate axes.

Systolic vs. diastolic failure
Systolic dysfunction
- Failure of the pump action of the heart
- During systole, the heart is unable to eject sufficient blood
- Defined by the ejection fraction
- Also called heart failure with reduced ejection fraction (HF-REF)

Diastolic dysfunction
- Heart failure symptoms when the ejection fraction is normal
- Cardiac output is insufficient due to inadequate ventricular filling during diastole
- Also called heart failure with preserved ejection fraction (HF-PEF)

Left-sided vs. right-sided failure
- Heart failure can be divided by which ventricle is primarily affected
- Usually heart failure is 'biventricular', since left-ventricular failure is more common and leads to right-ventricular failure

11.4 HEART FAILURE WITH REDUCED EJECTION FRACTION

Key data
Aetiology – left ventricular
1. Ischaemic heart disease/previous MI (see Chapter 9)
2. Cardiomyopathy (see Chapter 15)
3. Hypertension (see Chapter 16)
4. Valvular heart disease (see Chapter 14)
5. Arrhythmia (see Chapter 13)

Box 11.2   Causes of high-output heart failure

1. Anaemia
2. Hyperthyroidism
3. Paget's disease of the bone
4. Pregnancy
5. Arteriovenous fistula
6. Web beriberi (vitamin B1 deficiency)

Aetiology – right ventricular
Most commonly secondary to left-sided heart failure. Causes of selective right-sided failure include:

1. Pulmonary hypertension
2. Right ventricular ischaemia/infarction
3. Tricuspid or pulmonary valve disease

Box 11.3   Causes of pulmonary hypertension

1. Chronic lung disease
2. Pulmonary embolism
3. Connective tissue disease
4. Primary dysfunction of the pulmonary vessels

Incidence
- Male: 3.6 per 10^4 per year
- Female: 2.2 per 10^4 per year

Prevalence
- Male: 90 per 10^4
- Female: 70 per 10^4

Mortality
- 30–40% mortality within first year
- 10% mortality per year thereafter

Presenting features

Table 11.1   Presenting features of heart failure

	Features of left-sided heart failure	Features of right-sided heart failure
History	Shortness of breath (cardinal feature, see Table 11.2) Orthopnoea (shortness of breath lying flat) Paroxysmal nocturnal dyspnoea (PND) – waking up at night severely short of breath Palpitations – LV dilatation is arrhythmogenic Non-specific symptoms: fatigue, loss of appetite, cough	Swollen ankles Weight gain Abdominal distension Bloated feeling
Examination	Tachycardia Tachypnoea Bi-basal crepitations Laterally displaced apex beat Dullness to percussion and reduced breath sounds in bases (pleural effusion) 3rd and/or 4th heart sound (gallop rhythm) Murmur (heart failure may be secondary to valvular disease, or mitral regurgitation may be secondary to a dilated LV)	Raised JVP Dependent oedema Ascites Hepatomegaly Right-sided murmur (e.g. tricuspid regurgitation)

Table 11.2   New York Heart Association classification of heart failure. Adapted from ESC Heart Failure Guidelines 2012

Class I	Ordinary physical activity does not cause undue breathlessness or fatigue
Class II	Comfortable at rest, but ordinary physical activity results in undue breathlessness or fatigue
Class III	Comfortable at rest, but less than ordinary physical activity results in undue breathlessness or fatigue
Class IV	Symptoms at rest may be present. Any physical activity results in increased breathlessness

Differentials
Most common
1. COPD
2. Anaemia
3. Chronic renal failure
4. Asthma
5. Pulmonary embolism

Uncommon, but dangerous
1. Acute respiratory distress syndrome (ARDS)
2. Pericardial tamponade/constrictive pericarditis

Not to miss
1. Pulmonary fibrosis
2. Nephrotic syndrome

Key investigations
Bedside

Table 11.3 Bedside tests in patients with suspected heart failure

Test	Justification	Expected result
ABG	Important in patients with acute SOB. Gauge severity using PaO_2, and important for differentials, e.g. COPD	Low PaO_2 in severe pulmonary oedema
Blood pressure	Hypertension is a potential cause and exacerbating factor of heart failure. Hypotension may indicate severe heart failure or overtreatment	Hypertension or hypotension
ECG	ECG may reveal cause of heart failure. Normal ECG makes heart failure less likely	See Table 11.4

Table 11.4 Potential ECG findings in heart failure

ECG feature	What it may suggest	Why it is important
Q-waves, T-wave inversion	Previous MI, ischaemic heart disease	Secondary prevention, suggests ischaemic aetiology
High voltage in praecordial QRS	LVH	May suggest long-standing hypertension
Irregular rhythm, tachycardia	Arrhythmias, e.g. AF, VT	Consider anticoagulation +/- cardioversion/ICD if appropriate
Bradycardia	SA/AV node disease, over beta-blockade	May be an indication for pacing/limit use of beta-blocker
Broad QRS preceded by p-waves	Bundle branch block	Suggests cardiac dysynchrony, may be indication for CRT

Blood tests

Table 11.5 Blood tests of use in patients with suspected heart failure

Blood test	Justification	Potential result
FBC	Anaemia can mimic and exacerbate heart failure	Low haemoglobin
Renal function tests	Establish baseline renal function Renal impairment may limit use of ACEIs/ARBs and MRAs/diuretics may be less effective and require higher doses	Renal failure: raised urea and creatinine
Electrolytes	Electrolyte imbalance can cause arrhythmia Hyperkalaemia may limit use of ACEIs/ARBs and MRAs Hypokalaemia may limit use of diuretics	Hyperkalaemia, hypokalaemia, hyponatraemia
Brain natriuretic peptide (BNP)	Sensitive marker for heart failure	<100 pg/mL in untreated patients makes heart failure unlikely, higher levels may suggest a degree of heart failure
LFTs	RVF can result in congestive liver disease. Fluid retention may be caused by liver disease. Oedema may be caused by hypoalbuminaemia	Low albumin and raised transaminase enzymes, bilirubin and alkaline phosphatase (ALP) possible in both RVF and primary liver disease
TFTs	Thyroid disease can mimic and exacerbate heart failure	Hyperthyroidism: low TSH and high T3 and T4 Hypothyroidism: high TSH and low T3 and T4
HbA1c	May indicate poor glycaemic control	Poor control: HbA1c >48 mmol/mol

---

Box 11.4   Other causes of a raised BNP

- Left heart strain:

  a. Left ventricular hypertrophy
  b. Tachycardia/tachyarrhythmia
  c. Myocardial ischaemia

- Right heart strain:

  a. Pulmonary embolism
  b. COPD
  c. Restrictive lung disease

- Other:

  a. Sepsis
  b. Liver cirrhosis
  c. Diabetes
  d. Renal failure

(See Audio Podcast 11.2 at **www.wiley.com/go/camm/cardiology**)

Imaging

Table 11.6 Imaging modalities of use in patients with suspected heart failure

Test	Justification	Potential result
Chest X-ray	Heart failure can develop a series of findings on CXR May reveal alternative pulmonary pathology	Features of left-heart failure (see Box 11.5)
Echocardiography	Definitive imaging modality required when investigating heart failure	Systolic dysfunction: defined by LVEF Diastolic dysfunction: impaired relaxation of the ventricle

Box 11.5   Chest X-ray features of heart failure (ABCDE)

- **A**lveolar oedema (bat's wings appearance)
- Kerley **B** lines (short horizontal lines near peripheries representing interlobular septa)
- **C**ardiomegaly (cardiac shadow is >50% of chest diameter in PA film)
- **D**iversion of the upper lobes
- Pleural **E**ffusions

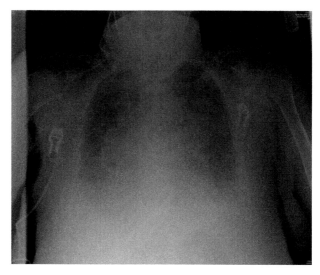

Figure 11.2 Chest radiograph showing pulmonary oedema. Note the presence of cardiomegaly, bilateral pleural effusions and 'bat's wing' appearance of the hili.

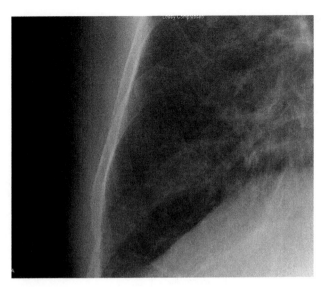

Figure 11.3 Enlarged chest radiograph showing Kerley B lines. These are short horizontal lines seen at the periphery of the radiograph and are a feature of pulmonary oedema.

Special investigations

Table 11.7 Special investigations of potential use in patients with suspected heart failure

Test	Justification	Potential result
Ambulatory ECG monitoring	Heart failure can increase risk of arrhythmias. Should consider if patient considered high risk	Ectopics, atrial fibrillation
Cardiac MRI	If suspicion of inflammatory/infiltrative disease or cardiomyopathy Scar tissue may be seen as delayed gadolinium enhancement	Specific findings on MRI (see Chapter 22)
Coronary angiography	If suspicion of ischaemic heart disease aetiology	Coronary artery stenosis
Endomyocardial biopsy	For histological diagnosis of inflammatory/infiltrative disease or cardiomyopathy (see Chapter 15)	Diagnostic appearance on microscopy (see Chapter 15)

Diagnostic algorithm

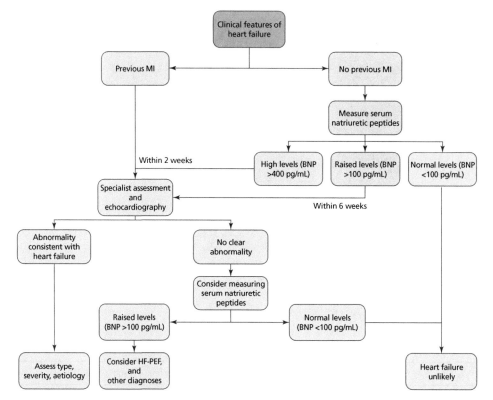

Figure 11.4 Diagnostic algorithm for heart failure.
Source: NICE 2010. Reproduced with permission of NICE.

Management options
Conservative
Conservative measures aim to reduce the risk of further disease progression or complications.

1. Patient education
2. Smoking cessation
3. Abstention from alcohol if alcohol is likely cause (e.g. alcohol-related cardiomyopathy, AF)
4. Vaccination:
   - Annual influenza vaccination
   - Pneumococcal (only one required)
5. Salt and fluid restriction – the evidence for this is unclear

Medical

Medical management aims to improve symptoms and decrease mortality in patients with heart failure

Angiotensin-converting enzyme inhibitors (ACE inhibitors):
1. Effective in reducing mortality and hospitalization for heart failure
2. Should be given to all patients with systolic heart failure (LVEF <40%)
3. Practical points:
   - Start with a low dose, slowly up-titrate (e.g. double dose every 2 weeks)
   - Monitor K^+ and creatinine
4. If not tolerated (e.g. due to cough) then an angiotensin II receptor blocker (ARB) can be used instead

Beta-blockers:
1. Reduce the risk of sudden cardiac death and overall mortality in heart failure
2. Should be attempted in all patients with systolic heart failure (LVEF <40%)
3. Practical points:
   - Start with a low dose and slowly up-titrate
   - Monitor heart rate and blood pressure
   - Review use of other heart-rate slowing drugs, e.g. non-DHP calcium-channel blockers

Loop diuretics:
1. Mainstay of symptomatic management of fluid overload
2. Recommended to relieve dyspnoea and oedema regardless of LVEF
3. No mortality benefit
4. Aim for lowest dose that achieves euvolaemia (patient's 'dry weight')

Second-line drugs – should be started by a specialist:
1. Mineralocorticoid-receptor antagonists (MRAs)
2. Ivabradine
3. Hydralazine with nitrates
4. Digoxin

Invasive
Implantable cardioverter-defibrillators (ICDs):
- Heart failure increases risk of sudden cardiac death, potentially due to ventricular arrhythmias
- Indications – see Box 11.6

Box 11.6   Indications for ICD insertion in heart failure patients

- **Primary prevention:** symptomatic heart failure with LVEF <35% despite optimal medical therapy
- **Secondary prevention:** ventricular tachycardia/fibrillation regardless of LVEF

Cardiac resynchronization therapy (CRT):
- Bundle branch block can result in asynchronous, less efficient, ventricular contraction

Box 11.7   Indications for CRT in heart failure patients

Both:

- Symptomatic heart failure
- LVEF <30% despite optimal therapy

And either of:

- LBBB morphology and QRS >130 ms
- RBBB morphology and QRS >150 ms

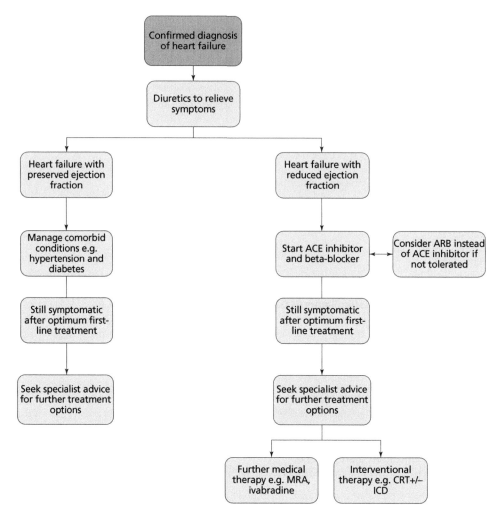

Figure 11.5 Flow chart for the management of heart failure.
Source: NICE 2010. Reproduced with permission of NICE.

Acute pulmonary oedema

Table 11.8 Emergency management in a patient presenting with acute pulmonary oedema

Category	Management
Airways	Ensure airway is patent
Breathing	Sit patient upright
	Measure oxygen saturation
	Deliver oxygen *if hypoxaemic* (S_aO_2 <90%)
	Check for tension pneumothorax
Circulation	Measure heart rate and blood pressure
	Gain IV access
	Look for signs of cardiac tamponade
Investigations	12-lead ECG – acute MI or arrhythmia precipitant?
	Keep on ECG monitor
	ABG if hypoxaemic
	CXR if stable
Early management	IV diuretics such as furosemide:
	• Acutely venodilate as well as cause diuresis
	• e.g. 40–80 mg furosemide IV bolus or 2.5 times usual oral dose
	IV nitrate infusion (e.g. GTN):
	• Titrated to systolic blood pressure – maintain >100 mmHg
	• Vasodilators reduce preload and afterload
	IV opiate (e.g. morphine):
	• May relieve anxiety and dyspnoea, reduce sympathetic drive and venodilate
	• Administer with anti-emetic (e.g. metoclopramide)

(See Audio Podcast 11.3, 11.4 and 11.5 at **www.wiley.com/go/camm/cardiology**)

11.5 HEART FAILURE WITH PRESERVED EJECTION FRACTION (HF-PEF)

Key data
Aetiology
Thought to be a result of left-ventricular stiffening and impaired relaxation in diastole.

> **Box 11.8**   Risk factors for the development of heart failure with a preserved ejection fraction
>
> **1.** Long-standing hypertension
> **2.** Female sex
> **3.** Left ventricular outflow tract obstruction (e.g. aortic stenosis)
> **4.** Diabetes mellitus
> **5.** Old age

Incidence
- Approximately one third of new cases of heart failure
- Predominant form in patients developing heart failure at >70 years

Diagnosis
- ESC guidelines require:
  - **a.** Signs and symptoms typical of heart failure
  - **b.** Normal or only mildly reduced LVEF with LV not dilated
  - **c.** Evidence of structural heart disease (e.g. LV hypertrophy) and/or diastolic dysfunction
- Potential non-cardiac causes of symptoms, such as anaemia or COPD, should be excluded first

Management

- No treatment reduces morbidity or mortality
- Diuretics may improve dyspnoea and oedema
- Treat risk factors and co-morbidities, e.g. hypertension, diabetes and ischaemic heart disease

KEY CLINICAL TRIALS

Key trial 11.1

Trial name: The SOLVD-treatment trial.

Participants: 2569 patients with symptomatic heart failure and LVEF ≤35%.

Intervention: Treatment with the ACE inhibitor in addition to conventional treatment.

Control: Placebo in addition to conventional treatment.

Outcome: 16% relative risk reduction (RRR) in all-cause mortality, 22% RRR in death from heart failure in treatment group compared with placebo.

Reason for inclusion: One of the key early trials proving the prognostic benefit of ACE inhibitors in all symptomatic patients with HF-REF.

Reference: The SOLVD Investigators. Effect of enalapril on survival in patients with reduced left ventricular ejection fractions and congestive heart failure. N Engl J Med. 1991;325:293–302. http://www.nejm.org/doi/full/10.1056/NEJM199108013250501.

Key trial 11.2

Trial name: The CIBIS II trial.

Participants: 2647 patients with NYHA class III–IV heart failure with LVEF ≤35%.

Intervention: Treatment with a beta-blocker (bisopropol) in addition to conventional treatment.

Control: Placebo in addition to conventional treatment.

Outcome: 34% relative risk reduction (RRR) in all-cause mortality and 44% RRR in sudden death in treatment group compared with placebo.

Reason for inclusion: One of the key early trials demonstrating a significant mortality benefit from beta-blockade in patients with symptomatic heart failure with reduced ejection fraction.

Reference: CIBIS-II Investigators and Committees. The Cardiac Insufficiency Bisoprolol Study II (CIBIS-II): a randomised trial. Lancet. 1999;353(9146):9–13. http://www.thelancet.com/journals/lancet/article/PIIS0140-6736(98)11181-9/abstract.

Key trial 11.3

Trial name: The EMPHASIS-HF trial.

Participants: 2737 patients with NYHA class II heart failure and LVEF ≤35%.

Intervention: Treatment with the mineralocorticoid receptor antagonist in addition to conventional treatment.

Control: Placebo in addition to conventional treatment.

Outcome: 24% relative risk reduction (RRR) in all-cause mortality, 37% RRR in cardiovascular death or heart failure hospitalization in treatment group.

Reason for inclusion: A key recent trial that demonstrates the prognostic benefit of MRAs when added to patients already taking ACE inhibitors and beta-blockers.

Reference: Annad F, McMurray JJ, Krum H, et al. Eplerenone in patients with systolic heart failure and mild symptoms. N Engl J Med. 2011; 364:11–21. http://www.nejm.org/doi/full/10.1056/NEJMoa1009492.

GUIDELINES

European Society of Cardiology (ESC). Guidelines for the diagnosis and treatment of acute and chronic heart failure. 2012. http://eurheartj.oxfordjournals.org/content/33/14/1787

National Institute of Health and Clinical Excellence (NICE). Management of chronic heart failure in adults in primary and secondary care. 2010. http://www.nice.org.uk/cg108

FURTHER READING

Gheorghiade M, Pang PS. Acute heart failure syndromes. J Am Coll Cardiol. 2009;53(7):557–573. http://www.sciencedirect.com/science/article/pii/S0735109708037960

A review of the pathophysiology, diagnosis and management of acute heart failure.

Shchekochikhin D, Schrier RW, Lindenfeld J. Cardiorenal syndrome: pathophysiology and treatment. Curr Cardiol Rep. 2013;15(7):380. http://www.ncbi.nlm.nih.gov/pubmed/23700289

A review of the pathophysiology and approach to management of cardiorenal syndrome

Mant J, et al. Systematic review and individual patient data meta-analysis of diagnosis of heart failure, with modelling of implications of different diagnostic strategies in primary care. Health Technology Assessment 2009;13(32).

A review of the evidence of clinical examination and investigation of heart failure. This provides rationale for the NICE diagnostic algorithm of heart failure.

 For additional resources and to test your knowledge, visit the companion website at:

www.wiley.com/go/camm/cardiology

12 Infective Endocarditis

Nicholas Sunderland

Kings College Hospital NHS Foundation Trust, London, UK

12.1 DEFINITION

Infection of the endocardium, predominantly heart valves or other intracardiac devices/material.

12.2 UNDERLYING CONCEPTS

1. **Heart valves:** fibrous structures covered by valvular endothelium
2. **Endothelium:** intact endothelium is resistant to bacterial colonization
3. **Damage:** valvular endothelium may become damaged, promoting microorganism attachment
4. **Transient bacteraemia:** the source for the infecting microorganism
5. **Pathogen characteristics:** those that decrease immune system effectiveness (e.g. formation of a biofilm) are most pathogenic
6. **Biofilm:** a matrix of extracellular polymeric substance (mainly polysaccharide and protein) produced by certain microorganisms

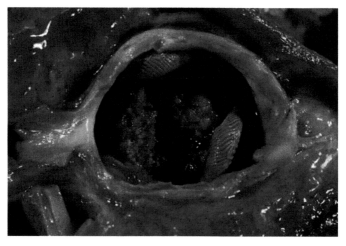

Figure 12.1 Aortic valve vegetation from infective endocarditis.
Source: Mr Gopal Soppa, Academic Clinical Lecturer in Cardiothoracic Surgery, St. George's University of London.

> **Box 12.1**   Causes of valvular endothelial damage
>
> 1. Iatrogenic – from instrumentation by electrodes or catheters
> 2. Repeated injection of solid material in intravenous drug users
> 3. 'Jet lesions' created by turbulent blood flow
> 4. Chronic inflammation, e.g. in rheumatic heart disease
> 5. Age-related degeneration

Clinical Guide to Cardiology, First Edition. Edited by Christian F. Camm and A. John Camm.
© 2016 John Wiley & Sons, Ltd. Published 2016 by John Wiley & Sons, Ltd.
Companion website: www.wiley.com/go/camm/cardiology.

Box 12.2   Causes of transient bacteraemia

1. Dental procedures
2. Invasive surgery (e.g. gastrointestinal)
3. Systemic infection
4. IV drug abuse
5. Colon cancer (associated with *Streptococcus bovis*)

12.3 KEY DATA

Aetiology
- Native valves (80%)
- Prosthetic valves (20%)

Microbiology:

1. *Staphylococcus aureus* (26%)
2. Oral (Viridans group) streptococci (18%)
3. *Streptococcus bovis/Streptococcus equinus* complex (13%)
4. Coagulase-negative staphylococci (10%)
5. *Enterococcus* spp. (10%)
6. Culture-negative endocarditis (9%)

Box 12.3   Causes of culture-negative endocarditis

1. HACEK organisms:
   a. *Haemophilus* species
   b. *Aggregatibacter* (formerly *Actinobacillus*)
   c. *Cardiobacterium hominis*
   d. *Eikenella corrodens*
   e. *Kingella kingae*
2. Other bacteria:
   a. *Coxiella burnetii*
   b. *Bartonella* species
   c. *Brucella* species
3. Fungi:
   a. *Candida* species
   b. *Aspergillus* species
4. Non-infective:
   a. Libman–Sacks (SLE)
   b. Carcinoid

Incidence
- 1 per 10^4 per year

Mortality
- In-hospital mortality rate: 10–50% (dependent on organism)
- 5-year mortality 40%

Table 12.1 Predictors of poor outcome in patients with IE (adapted from ESC Guidelines on infective endocarditis)

Category	Detail
Patient characteristics	Older age
	Prosthetic valve IE
	Diabetes mellitus
Presence of IE complications	Heart failure
	Renal failure
	Stroke
	Septic shock
Microorganism	*Staphylococcus aureus*
	Fungi
	Gram-negative bacilli
Echocardiographic findings	Periannular complications
	Severe left-sided valve regurgitation
	Low left ventricular ejection fraction
	Large vegetations
	Severe prosthetic dysfunction

12.4 CLINICAL TYPES

According to mode of acquisition

1. Healthcare-associated:
   a. Nosocomial (hospitalized >48 hours prior to onset)
   b. Non-nosocomial (hospitalized <48 hours prior to onset in someone from a healthcare facility)
2. Community-acquired (hospitalized <48 hours prior to signs and symptoms)
3. Intravenous drugs abuse-associated

Table 12.2 Causes of IE broken down by microorganism and mode of acquisition (adapted from http://www.nejm.org/doi/full/10.1056/NEJMcp1206782)

Pathogen	Overall	Native valve (80%)				Prosthetic valve (20%)	
		Community acquired (55%)	Healthcare associated (20%)		Drug abusers (5%)	Mid-term infection (2–12 months post) (5%)	Late infection (>12 months post) (15%)
			Nosocomial (15%)	Non-nosocomial (5%)			
Staphylococcus aureus	26%	20–22%	44–47%	25–42%	68–81%	7%	25%
Coagulase-negative staphylococci	10%	4–6%	12–15%	15–25%	0–3%	27%	9%
Enterococcus	10%	9%	6–14%	17–42%	4–5%	7%	20%
Oral streptococci	18%	26–28%	7–11%	0–6%	4–10%	7%	11%
Streptococcus bovis	13%	10–18%	3%	3–8%	0–1%	7%	9%

According to presentation

1. Acute (days)
2. Subacute (weeks)
3. Chronic (months)

 (See Audio Podcast 12.1 at **www.wiley.com/go/camm/cardiology)**

12.5 PRESENTING FEATURES

Table 12.3   Common presenting features of IE (adapted from Richet *et al.* J Antimicrob Chemother. 2008;62(6):1434–1440)

Symptoms/signs	Acute	Chronic presentation
Fever* (80%)	✓	✓
New murmur (48%)	✓	✓
Embolic phenomenon (30%)	✓	✓
Haematuria (25%)	✓	✓
Worsening of an existing murmur (20%)	✓	✓
Splenomegaly (11%)	✗	✓
Clubbing (10%)	✓	✓
Splinter haemorrhages (8%)	✓	✓
Janeway's lesions (5%)	✓	✓
Roth's spots (5%)	✓	✓
Conjunctival haemorrhages (5%)	✓	✓
Osler's nodes (<5%)	✗	✓

*Elderly patients may not mount a febrile response to infection.

Box 12.4   Less common features of IE

- Abscesses: cerebral, renal, splenic and vertebral
- Arthritides (migrating)
- Discitis
- Heart failure (unexplained)
- Meningitis
- Peripheral arterial occlusion (acute)
- Pulmonary emboli (septic)
- Renal failure
- Stroke
- Weight loss

Box 12.5   Bottom line on IE

Suspect IE in anyone with fever plus either:

- Risk factors for IE
- No obvious infective source

Picture	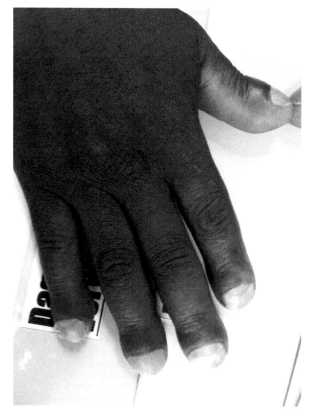 Janeway (palms)	Osler's nodes (finger pads)	Splinter haemorrhages (nail bed)
Sign	Janeway lesions	Osler's nodes	Splinter haemorrhages
Location	Palms	Finger pulps	Nail beds
Comments	Microabscesses due to septic emboli Non tender	Immune complex deposition leading to an inflammatory response Tender	Non specific

Figure 12.2 Hand signs of infective endocarditis.

Figure 12.3 Clubbing.
Source: Patrick Jahns, King's College Hospital NHS Foundation Trust.

Complications

Table 12.4 Complications of IE (adapted from ESC IE Guidelines, 2009)

Category	Details
Heart failure (60%)	Pulmonary oedema
	Cardiogenic shock
Uncontrolled infection	Persistent infection (>7–10 days)
	Septic shock
Neurological complications (20–40%)	Transient ischaemic attack
	Silent cerebral embolism
	Brain abscess
	Mycotic aneurysm
	Meningitis
Renal failure (30%)	Immune complex glomerulonephritis
	Renal infarction
	Hypoperfusion (heart failure, septic shock)
	Antibiotic toxicity
Periannular complications (10–40%)	Perivalvular abscesses
	Pseudoaneurysms
	Fistulae
Rheumatic complications (15%)	Arthralgia and arthritis
	Spondylodiscitis

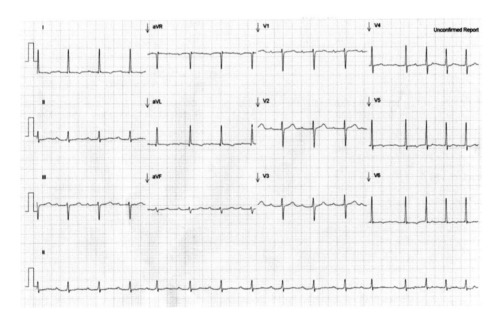

Figure 12.4 First-degree heart block.

12.6 DIFFERENTIALS

Most common
1. Common infective diseases + unrelated murmur/flow murmur
2. Causes of a pyrexia of unknown origin (PUO)
3. Systemic neoplasms (especially adenocarcinomas, sarcomas)

Box 12.6   Rarer organisms to consider as causes of pyrexia of unknown origin (PUO)

- *Brucella*
- Lyme disease
- TB
- Malaria
- Hepatitis
- Fungi

Less common but dangerous
- Lymphoma + benign murmur

Not to miss
1. Rarer organisms (culture negatives) in the immunocompromised
2. Atrial myxoma

12.7 KEY INVESTIGATIONS

Bedside tests

Table 12.5   Bedside tests for IE

Test	Justification	Potential result
Oxygen saturation	Useful in any patient with breathlessness	May be low due to pulmonary oedema (valvular incompetence)
ECG (daily)	Paravalvular abscess extension can affect the AV node	Paravavlular abscess – prolonged PR interval Coronary emboli – ischaemic changes (Chapter 9) Heart failure – widened QRS duration
Blood pressure	Incompetent valves/heart failure can affect blood pressure	Wide pulse pressure – aortic regurgitation Hypotension – heart failure
Urine dip	Renal embolic phenomenon	Haematuria

Blood tests

Table 12.6   Blood tests for IE

Test	Justification/comments	Potential result
FBC	Useful in any infection (WCC) Useful in any chronic disease (Hb)	Leucocytosis and anaemia in 50% of cases
Urea and electrolytes	IE can affect renal function Baseline – nephrotoxic antibiotic use	Elevated creatinine and urea (renal failure – uncommon)
Blood cultures	Useful in any infection, take **before** antibiotics Three samples from different peripheral sites	If positive, provides evidence for IE and refines treatment options If negative, should repeat blood cultures, and consider culture-negative causes
CRP/ESR	Useful in any infection	Elevated in 60% of cases

Repeat FBC, CRP/ESR and U&E regularly to assess the response to treatment and monitor for complications.

Imaging

Table 12.7 Imaging modalities of use in IE

Test	Justification/comments	Potential result
Trans-thoracic echocardiogram (TTE)*	Structural and functional cardiac assessment Should be performed first, but cannot rule out IE	Vegetations, valvular regurgitation, paravalvular abscess, dehiscence of the prosthesis, pseudoaneurysms, fistulas
Transoesophageal echocardiogram (TOE)*	Higher sensitivity and specificity than TTE Best practice to undertake this test in all patients suspected of IE	As above
CT cardiac/head	To examine for IE complications. Should be undertaken if cerebral infarction or infectious complications suspected	Stroke, mycotic aneurysms, intracardiac abscesses

*Repeat TTE/TOE within 7–10 days if initially negative but IE is still clinically suspected.

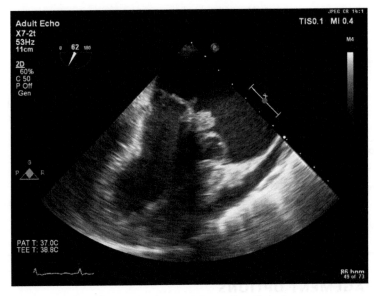

Figure 12.5 Trans-thoracic echocardiogram showing vegetation on the mitral valve.

Special tests

Table 12.8 Special tests for IE

Test	Justification/comments	Potential result
Serological tests	Unusual/culture-negative cause of IE can be diagnosed by this method	May be positive for *Bartonella* sp., *Coxiella burnetii* or *Brucella* sp.
Anti-nuclear antibodies	Rheumatological conditions can cause febrile episodes which may mimic IE	Positive in many rheumatological conditions

Table 12.9 Modified Duke's criteria for the diagnosis of IE (adapted from Li *et al.* Clin Infect Dis. 2000;30(4):633–638)

Major criteria	Microorganisms: • Typical microorganisms from two blood culture sets • Persistently positive blood cultures • One set of blood cultures/IgG serology positive for *C. burnetii* Endocardial involvement: • Vegetation, abscess, new dehiscence of prosthetic valve • New valvular regurgitation
Minor criteria	Predisposition: • Underlying heart condition/valve replacement • Intravenous drug use Immunological phenomenon: • Glomerulonephritis • Osler's nodes • Roth's spots • Rheumatic fever Fever >38°C Vascular phenomenon: • Major arterial emboli • Septic pulmonary infarcts • Mycotic aneurysm • Intracranial haemorrhage • Conjunctival haemorrhage • Janeway's lesions Microbiological evidence: • Positive blood culture but with no major clinical criterion met • Serological evidence of active infection with an organism consistent with IE
Definite diagnosis	Two major, one major and three minor, or five minor criteria
Possible diagnosis	One major criterion and one minor criterion or three minor criteria
Rejected diagnosis	• Firmly established alternative diagnosis • Resolution of IE-like syndrome with antibiotic therapy for ≤4 days • No pathological evidence of IE at surgery/autopsy, with antibiotic therapy for ≤4 days • Criteria for possible infective endocarditis not met

12.8 MANAGEMENT OPTIONS

Treatment should involve a multidisciplinary team with expertise in cardiology, cardiac surgery and infectious diseases.

Conservative

Supportive management, fluids and nutrition are key elements.

Medical
Empirical antibiotic treatment

Table 12.10 Empirical antibiotic treatment of IE (adapted from ESC IE Guidelines, 2009) – always take note of local guidelines

Antibiotic	Route	Duration (weeks)
Native valves or prosthetic valves (≥12 months post-surgery)		
Ampicillin-sulbactam	IV	4–6
OR		
Co-amoxiclav + gentamicin	IV	4–6
OR		
Vancomycin	IV	4–6
+ gentamicin	IV or PO	4–6
+ ciprofloxacin		
Prosthetic valves (early, <12 months post-surgery)		
Vancomycin	IV	6
+ gentamicin	IV	2
+ rifampin	PO	6

Specific antibiotic treatment
- Antibiotic sensitivity analysis will determine long-term treatment
- Always discuss long-term treatment with microbiology/infectious diseases
- Involve other relevant specialities based on complications

Anticoagulation
Patients already taking antithrombotics can generally continue these whilst being treated for infective endocarditis providing there are no haemorrhagic complications. IE in itself is not an indication for anti-coagulation.

Table 12.11 Use of antiplatelets/anticoagulants in IE (adapted from the ESC IE Guidelines, 2009)

Patient/situation	Action
Not currently taking aspirin	No antiplatelet agents
Currently taking aspirin for other indications	If no bleeding, aspirin can continue
Ischemic and non-haemorrhagic stroke complication, and already taking oral anticoagulants	Replace anticoagulant with heparin for 2 weeks

Prophylaxis
Antibiotic prophylaxis is no longer routinely recommended in patients with previous IE or risk factors for IE.

 (See Audio Podcast 12.2 at **www.wiley.com/go/camm/cardiology**)

Invasive

Table 12.12 Timing of surgery in patients with left-sided, native-valve infective endocarditis. Emergency = within 24 hours, urgent = within days, elective = after 1–2 weeks of antibiotic therapy (adapted from ESC IE Guidelines, 2009)

Indication		Timing of surgery
Heart failure	Refractory pulmonary oedema/cardiogenic shock	Emergency
	Severe acute regurgitation/obstruction and persistent heart failure/haemodynamic instability	Urgent
	Severe regurgitation and heart failure easily controlled with medical treatment	Elective
Uncontrolled infection	Locally uncontrolled infection (abscess, valve dehiscence, aneurysm)	Urgent
	Persistent fever and positive blood cultures for >5–7 days	Urgent
	Fungi or multidrug-resistant organism	Elective
Prevention of embolism	Large vegetations (>10 mm in length) after one or more embolic episodes	Urgent
	Large vegetations (>10 mm in length) and other poor predictors (heart failure, persistent infection or abscess)	Urgent
	Very large vegetations (>15 mm): surgery preferred if native valve preservation is feasible	Urgent

(See Audio Podcast 12.3 at **www.wiley.com/go/camm/cardiology**)

KEY CLINICAL TRIALS

Key trial 12.1
Trial name: Early surgery versus conventional treatment for infective endocarditis.
Participants: 76 patients with left-sided infective endocarditis, severe valve disease and large vegetations, but no indications for emergency surgery.
Intervention: Early surgery (within 48 hours).
Control: Conventional treatment.
Outcome: Surgery reduced embolic events (3% vs. 23%).
Reason for inclusion: Embolic events can be devastating, especially stroke. Recognition of people who are most at risk of embolization is important as surgery may be of benefit.
Reference: Kang D-H, Kim Y-J, Kim S-H, et al. Early surgery versus conventional treatment for infective endocarditis. N Engl J Med. 2012;366:2466–2473. http://www.ncbi.nlm.nih.gov/pubmed/22738096.

Key trial 12.2
Trial name: Effect of aspirin on the risk of embolic events in infective endocarditis.
Participants: 115 patients with native valve or prosthetic valve endocarditis without contraindication to aspirin.
Intervention: Aspirin (325 mg/day) for 4 weeks.
Control: Placebo.
Outcome: There was no significant difference in the embolic events between aspirin and placebo (28% vs. 20%).
Reason for inclusion: Aspirin is not specifically indicated in infective endocarditis.
Reference (Including URL): Chan KL, Dumesnil JG, Cujec B, et al. A randomized trial of aspirin on the risk of embolic events in patients with infective endocarditis. J Am Coll Cardiol 2003;42:775–780. http://www.ncbi.nlm.nih.gov/pubmed/12957419.

GUIDELINES

European Society of Cardiology. Guidelines on the prevention, diagnosis, and treatment of infective endocarditis (new version 2009). 2009. http://www.ncbi.nlm.nih.gov/pubmed/19713420

National Institute for Health and Clinical Excellence. Prophylaxis against infective endocarditis: antimicrobial prophylaxis against infective endocarditis in adults and children undergoing interventional procedures. 2008. http://www.nice.org.uk/nicemedia/pdf/CG64NICEguidance.pdf

FURTHER READING

Hoen B, Duval X. Clinical practice. Infective endocarditis. N Engl J Med. 2013;368(15):1425–1433. http://www.nejm.org/doi/full/10.1056/NEJMcp1206782.
   A comprehensive review of infective endocarditis published in the New England Journal of Medicine.
Li JS, Sexton DJ, Mick N, et al. Proposed modifications to the Duke criteria for the diagnosis of infective endocarditis. Clin Infect Dis 2000;30:633–8. http://www.ncbi.nlm.nih.gov/pubmed/10770721.
   Modifications to the Duke criteria.

 For additional resources and to test your knowledge, visit the companion website at:

www.wiley.com/go/camm/cardiology

13 Arrhythmias

Christian F. Camm

John Radcliffe Hospital, Oxford, UK

13.1 DEFINITION

A group of conditions characterized by abnormal electrical activity in the heart.

13.2 UNDERLYING CONCEPTS

- **Bradycardia:** slow heart rate (<60 bpm)
- **Tachycardia:** fast heart rate (>100 bpm)
- **Re-entrant circuit:** where a depolarization utilizes an abnormal conduction pathway (e.g. an accessory pathway) to allow for the depolarization to repeatedly re-enter areas of the heart
- **Automaticity:** the property of cardiac myocytes to spontaneously initiate an impulse. Unusual automaticity causes escape rhythms (ectopic beats) and can arise from anywhere in the heart

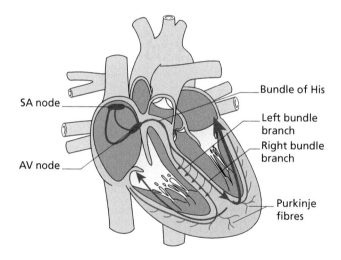

Figure 13.1 Normal conduction within the heart.

13.3 CLINICAL TYPES

Atrial

- Atrial fibrillation
- Atrial flutter
- Atrial tachycardia

Clinical Guide to Cardiology, First Edition. Edited by Christian F. Camm and A. John Camm.
© 2016 John Wiley & Sons, Ltd. Published 2016 by John Wiley & Sons, Ltd.
Companion website: www.wiley.com/go/camm/cardiology.

Nodal
- Atrioventricular re-entrant tachycardia (AVRT)
- Atrioventricular nodal re-entrant tachycardia (AVNRT)

Ventricular
- Ventricular tachycardia
- Ventricular fibrillation

13.4 ATRIAL FIBRILLATION

Key data

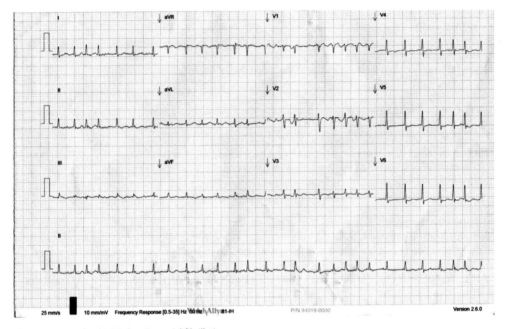

Figure 13.2 12-lead ECG showing atrial fibrillation.

Definition
A cardiac arrhythmia in which there is uncoordinated atrial activation resulting in decreased atrial mechanical function.

Aetiology
Most common:

1. Hypertension
2. Ischaemic heart disease
3. Heart failure
4. Valvular heart disease (e.g. rheumatic)
5. Idiopathic/lone AF

Not to forget:

1. Thyroid disease
2. Pneumonia/infection
3. Alcohol
4. Sepsis

Incidence
- Increases with age
- **<50 years old:** 5 per 10^4 per year
- **>80 years old:** 200 per 10^4 per year

Prevalence
- **Total:** 200 per 10^4 total prevalence
- **<60 years old:** 70 per 10^4 of patients
- **>85 years old:** 1000 per 10^4 of patients

Mortality
- Limited direct mortality resulting from AF
- **Overall:** two-fold increase in rate of mortality against age-matched controls
- **Stroke:** major concern with AF is the formation of thrombi in the atria leading to systemic thromboembolism
- **Heart failure:** two-fold increase in rate of development of heart failure

---

Box 13.1   Formation of thromboemboli in atrial fibrillation

The formation of thrombus relates to Virchow's triad, all of which are affected in AF:

1. **Haemodynamic:** static blood in the left atrium and the left atrial appendage
2. **Endothelium:** atrial endothelium is damaged leading to collagen exposure, triggering coagulation cascade
3. **Hypercoagulability:** increased platelet activation and abnormalities in factors IX and X

Pathophysiology
1. Increased atrial pressure: atrial pressure increases in line with any rise in intracardiac pressure or outflow obstruction (e.g. mitral stenosis). Intracardiac pressure is most commonly increased by systemic hypertension
2. Atrial dilatation: occurs as a result of raised intra-atrial pressure and increases the area for ectopic circuits to form
3. Trigger: ectopic atrial tissue within the pulmonary veins triggers repetitive atrial depolarization
4. Atrial fibrosis: occurs as a result of ischaemia, aging or persistent dilatation. Variable fibrosis provides non-homogeneity to refractory periods within the atria

Clinical types
AF is primarily divided based on duration of the arrhythmia and ability to return to sinus rhythm:

1. **Paroxysmal:** spontaneous return to sinus rhythm without need for intervention
2. **Persistent:** return to sinus rhythm possible following intervention
3. **Long-standing persistent:** arrhythmia lasting longer than 1 year without return to sinus rhythm
4. **Permanent:** sinus rhythm is not achievable even with intervention, or intervention is no longer considered

Presenting features
Atrial fibrillation is often asymptomatic. An irregularly irregular tachycardia may be the only indication.

Table 13.1 Presenting features of atrial fibrillation

Group	Symptoms	Signs	Acute presentation	Chronic presentation
Arrhythmia	Palpitations	Irregular pulse Tachycardia	Yes	Yes
Heart failure	Dyspnoea Orthopnoea Fatigue	Peripheral oedema	Yes	Yes
Ischaemia	Chest pain	Clammy, sweaty appearance	Yes	Yes
Thrombosis	Neurological changes Limb pain Abdominal pain	Focal neurology Cold, pale limbs	Yes	No

Differentials
Atrial fibrillation is by far the most common cause of an irregularly irregular rhythm. Differentials are not common.

Most common
1. Ectopic beats (atrial or ventricular origin)
2. Atrial flutter with variable block
3. Multifocal atrial tachycardia

Dangerous
Wolff–Parkinson–White syndrome (WPW): if occurring with AF can cause 'pre-exited AF'; an irregular wide-complex rapid tachycardia which is very dangerous.

Key investigations
Bedside

Table 13.2 Bedside tests of use in patients with AF

Test	Justification	Potential result
Oxygen saturations	Useful in any patient with breathlessness	May be low if atrial fibrillation has caused pulmonary oedema due to heart failure
ECG	Vital in any arrhythmia	Any irregularly irregular rhythm of ventricular depolarization is the key feature. No P-waves are present (see Figure 13.2)
Blood pressure	Hypertension is a cause for atrial fibrillation	May be high, however hypertension is common in many patients and this does not rule out other causes

Blood tests

Table 13.3 Blood tests of use in patients with AF

Test	Justification	Potential result
Full blood count	Anaemia increases cardiac output required to perfuse tissues, thus increasing heart failure symptoms	Low haemoglobin
Clotting	Many patients with atrial fibrillation are anticoagulated	Warfarin should provide an INR of 2–3 in atrial fibrillation INR is not a reliable marker of clotting when patient is on novel oral anticoagulants
Thyroid function	Hyperthyroidism is an uncommon but important cause of atrial fibrillation	Hyperthyroid: T_3/T_4 raised, TSH may be lowered
Troponin	Marker of cardiac damage Infarction is an important cause of new-onset AF AF with a fast ventricular rate may cause infarction	May be raised

Imaging

Table 13.4 Imaging modalities of use in patients with AF

Test	Justification	Potential result
Chest X-ray	May see evidence of cardiac disease	Signs of heart failure (see Chapter 11) Calcified valves
Trans-thoracic echocardiography	May demonstrate structural pathology as a cause for AF	Structural defects such as hypertrophic obstructive cardiomyopathy or valve disease May indicate poor LV function
Transoesophageal echocardiography	Required if AF duration is >48 hours to exclude an atrial thrombus prior to cardioversion	Thrombus within the left atrium/appendage

Special tests

Table 13.5 Special tests of use in patients with AF

Test	Justification	Potential result
24-hour Holter monitor	Provides an estimate of AF burden/duration and more definitive diagnosis	As with 12-lead ECG

Management options
Conservative
Conservative measures including avoidance of known trigger factors should be considered in all patients.

Box 13.2   Atrial fibrillation trigger factors

1. Obesity
2. Alcohol
3. Caffeine
4. Emotional stress
5. Sleep apnoea
6. Exercise

Medical
Treatment of causative factors:

1. Hypertension
2. Thyroid dysfunction
3. Weight gain

Medical cardioversion: conversion to sinus rhythm is ideal treatment and should be attempted in all patients with recent onset AF. Medical cardioversion can be attempted with:

1. Flecainide/profafenone – not to be used in patients with structural heart disease
2. Amiodarone

Rate control: this should be considered in older patients or in those with long-standing AF that have little chance of reverting to sinus rhythm. Agents of choice include:

1. Beta-blockers
2. Rate-limiting CCBs
3. Amiodarone
4. Digoxin – as monotherapy only for relatively sedentary patients

Rhythm control: maintenance of sinus rhythm following cardioversion (rhythm control) should be considered in young patients and those with paroxysmal AF. This should be the first-line treatment option:

1. Flecainide: initial dose of 50 mg BD
2. Sotalol: initial dose of 40 mg BD
3. Amiodarone: see Box 13.3
4. Dronedarone: initial dose 400 mg BD

Box 13.3   Dosing amiodarone

- First week: 200 mg TDS
- Second week: 200 mg BD
- Maintenance: 200 mg OD

Selection of any particular agent is dependent on level of heart disease and other factors.

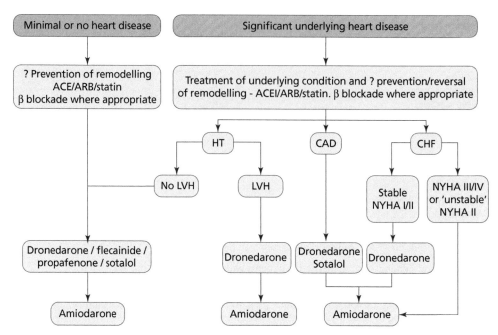

Figure 13.3 ESC rhythm control flow chart.
Source: Camm 2012. reproduced with permission of Oxford University Press. CAD, coronary artery disease; CHF, congestive heart failure; HT, hypertension; LVH, left ventricular hypertrophy.

Invasive
Invasive therapy includes the use of electricity to cardiovert the patient back to sinus rhythm (DC cardioversion), and procedures to prevent recurrence of AF in the future.

Reversion to sinus rhythm – DC cardioversion:
1. Performed under general anaesthetic (requires anaesthetist) or sedation
2. Either transoesophageal echocardiogram or anticoagulation for 3 weeks are required to rule out atrial thrombus
3. Energy levels:
    a. Monophasic – 200 J first shock, 360 J for subsequent shocks
    b. Biphasic – 150 J first shock, 200 J for subsequent shocks

Prevention of further events – pulmonary vein isolation (PVI) ablation:
• Elective procedure (see Chapter 29 for details)

Adjunct therapy
Anticoagulation therapy is required in many patients with AF. However, due to the increased risk of bleeding, therapy is based on risk stratification for thromboembolism.

Table 13.6 CHA_2DS_2VASc score, used to assess thrombotic risk in patients with AF

Letter	Detail	Points
C	Congestive heart failure	1
H	Hypertension (>140 mmHg systolic)	1
A	Age ≥75 years	2
D	Diabetes mellitus	1
S	Stroke/TIA	2
V	Vascular disease	1
A	Age 65–74 years	1
Sc	Sex category = female	1

Table 13.7 HAS-BLED score, used to assess bleeding risk in patients with AF

Letter	Detail	Points
H	Hypertension	1
A	Abnormal liver/renal function (1 point each)	1
S	Stroke	1
B	Bleeding history	1
L	Labile INRs	1
E	Elderly (>65 years)	1
D	Drugs/alcohol (1 point each)	1

Treatment options include:

- **Low risk of thrombosis (CHA_2DS_2VASc = 0):** no anticoagulation therapy
- **Moderate risk (CHA_2DS_2VASc = 1):** should consider anticoagulation
- **High risk of thrombosis (CHA_2DS_2VASc ≥2):** warfarin (target INR 2–3) or novel oral anticoagulants (e.g. dabigitran). See Chapter 36

For thromboprophylaxis in AF, antiplatelet agents such as aspirin are not appropriate or effective.

(See Audio Podcast 13.1 at **www.wiley.com/go/camm/cardiology**)

Table 13.8 Novel oral anticoagulants

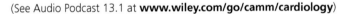

NOAC	Target	Standard Dose	Half-life	Metabolism/excretion
Dabigatran	Factor IIa	150 mg BD	12–17 hours	80% urine
Rivaroxaban	Factor Xa	20 mg OD	7–11 hours	66% hepatic
Apixaban	Factor Xa	5 mg BD	12 hours	75% biliary

13.5 ATRIAL FLUTTER

Atrial flutter and AF have significant overlap are often seen in the same patient groups. As a result there is significant overlap in their presentation, investigation and management. Only areas that differ between AF and atrial flutter are described in this section; for other aspects, please refer to the AF section (13.4).

Key data

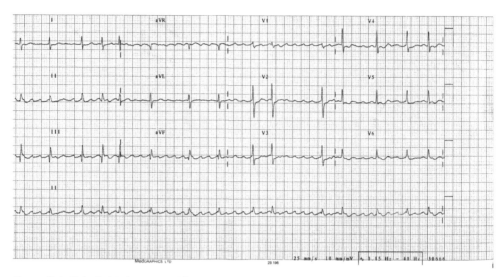

Figure 13.4 12-lead ECG showing atrial flutter.

Definition
Atrial flutter is an arrhythmia where there is regular atrial activation at approximately 300 bpm. There is variable conduction to the ventricles through the AV node.

Aetiology
Aetiological factors are the same as for AF.

Incidence
- **<60 years old:** 1 per 10^4 per year
- **>60 years old:** 50 per 10^4 per year

Prevalence
Acute, paroxysmal condition with a prevalence that is difficult to calculate.

Mortality
As with AF.

Pathophysiology
1. Re-entrant circuit: development of a circuit within the atria allows for rapid and stereotyped atrial depolarization. The rate of atrial depolarization in atrial flutter is normally 300 beats per minute
2. Location dependent: the re-entrant circuit is typically located in the right atrium and moves anti-clockwise always involving a strip of atrial tissue between the inferior vena cava and tricuspid valve
3. AV block: the atrioventricular node (AVN) blocks a variable proportion of atrial depolarization leading to a slower rate of ventricular depolarization

Clinical types
Common flutter:

- Anticlockwise macro re-entrant (90%)
- Negative flutter waves in II, III and aVF, positive in V1

Uncommon flutter:

- Clockwise macro re-entrant (10%)
- Positive flutter waves in II, III and aVF, negative in V1

Presenting features
As with AF, although normally presents with a regular pulse.

Differentials
1. Focal atrial tachycardias
2. AVNRT
3. AVRT

Key investigations
Investigations as for AF. Specific ECG findings include:

- 'Saw-tooth' F-wave demonstrating atrial depolarization
- Ventricular depolarization may occur at 1:1 with each atrial depolarization. However, more commonly, two to four atrial depolarizations occur for every ventricular beat
- Occasionally variable AV block leads to an irregular ventricular depolarization rate

Management options
- Management is as with AF
- However, PVI ablation is not used to treat atrial flutter. Instead ablation of the cavo-tricuspid isthmus is attempted to prevent further flutter episodes

13.6 SUPRAVENTRICULAR TACHYCARDIAS

Key data

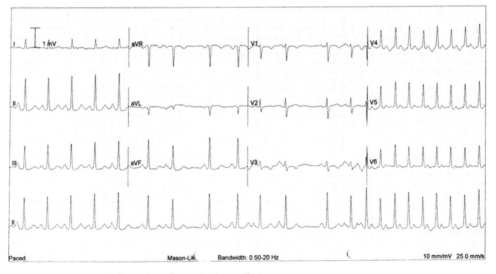

Figure 13.5 Supraventricular tachycardia starting in a patient.

Definition
An arrhythmia consisting of a rapid heart rate other than atrial fibrillation or flutter originating at or above the AV node.

Aetiology
Usually occurs in young healthy adults. Re-entrant circuit is normally present from birth but may not become apparent until adult life.

Incidence
- 5 per 10^4 per year

Prevalence
- 22 per 10^4

Mortality
Low cause of mortality if treated promptly.

Clinical types
Atrioventricular nodal re-entrant tachycardia (AVNRT)
Re-entrant circuit is located within the AVN which has two pathways with different conduction properties:

1. **Fast pathway:** fast conduction velocity, long refractory period
2. **Slow pathway:** slow conduction velocity, fast refractory period

Atrioventricular re-entrant tachycardia
Re-entrant circuit utilizes accessory connections between the atria and ventricles. Conduction still relies on the AVN to complete the circuit.

Box 13.4   Other types of supraventricular arrhythmia

- Sinus tachycardia
- Focal atrial tachycardia
- Multifocal atrial tachycardia

Presenting features

Table 13.9 Presenting features of supraventricular arrhythmias

Group	Symptoms	Examination	Acute	Chronic
Arrhythmia	Palpitations	Regular, tachycardic pulse	Yes	No
Heart failure	Dyspnoea Orthopnoea Fatigue	Peripheral oedema	Yes	No
Ischaemia	Chest pain	Sweating Nausea	Yes	No
Decreased cardiac output	Syncope Pre-syncope	Low blood pressure	Yes	No

Differentials
Most common
1. Atrial flutter
2. Atrial tachycardia

Dangerous
1. Ventricular tachycardia

Key investigations
Bedside

Table 13.10 Bedside investigations of use in patients with supraventricular tachycardia

Test	Justification	Potential result
Oxygen saturations	Useful in any breathless patient	May be low if tachycardia has caused pulmonary oedema due to low cardiac output
ECG (see Figure 13.5)	Vital in any arrhythmia	Regular narrow QRS complex during symptoms

Blood tests

Table 13.11 Blood tests of use in patients with supraventricular tachycardia

Test	Justification	Potential result
Full blood count	Anaemia increases cardiac output required to perfuse tissues, thus increasing heart failure symptoms	Low haemoglobin
Troponin	Marker of cardiac damage. Should be considered if patient complains of chest pain; infarction can occur due to high heart rate	May be high
Thyroid function	Hyperthyroidism is an uncommon but important trigger of supraventricular tachycardias	Hyperthyroid: T_3/T_4 raised, TSH may be lowered

Imaging

Table 13.12 Imaging modalities of use in patients with supraventricular tachycardia

Test	Justification	Potential result
Chest X-ray	May see evidence of cardiac disease	Signs of heart failure (see Chapter 11) Calcified valves
Trans-thoracic echocardiography	May demonstrate structural pathology as a cause for accessory pathways	Ebstein's anomaly Hypertrophic cardiomyopathy

Box 13.5 Box 13.5 Ebstein's anomaly

- Congenital heart defect
- Septal leaflet of the tricuspid valve is displaced towards apex of the right ventricle
- Causes enlargement of the aorta
- Is associated with Wolff–Parkinson–White syndrome

Special tests

Table 13.13 Special tests of use in patients with supraventricular tachycardia

Test	Justification	Potential result
24-hour Holter monitor	Provides an estimate of SVT burden/duration and more definitive diagnosis	As with 12-lead ECG

Management options

Conservative

Conservative measures should be attempted prior to further interventions. Options include:

1. Do nothing: if arrhythmic episodes are infrequent and well tolerated. This is not applicable if ventricular pre-excitation occurs

2. Vagal manoeuvres: stimulation of the vagus nerve causes slowing of conduction through the AV-node. Manoeuvres include:

  a. Valsalva manoeuvre
  b. Carotid sinus massage
  c. Head immersion in cold water

(See Audio Podcast 13.2 at **www.wiley.com/go/camm/cardiology**)

Medical

Medical therapy can be considered for termination of the tachycardia. The aim is to stop conduction through the AV node and interrupt re-entry.

Adenosine: IV administration of a rapid bolus. Requires a large vein and good access. Patients should be warned of temporary flushing and chest pain associated with the injection

For longterm treatment, oral medication can be used:

1. Beta-blocker: initial dose of 50 mg BD, more useful in preventing recurrence than stopping the SVT itself

2. Flecainide: initial dose of 50 mg BD

Invasive

1. DC cardioversion: this is uncommon as most are treated successfully with medical therapy. Should primarily be considered when a fast tachycardia is present that is compromising blood pressure. Normally performed under general anaesthetic

2. Radiofrequency ablation: this is successful in preventing further episodes in 95% of cases

13.7 VENTRICULAR TACHYCARDIA

Key data

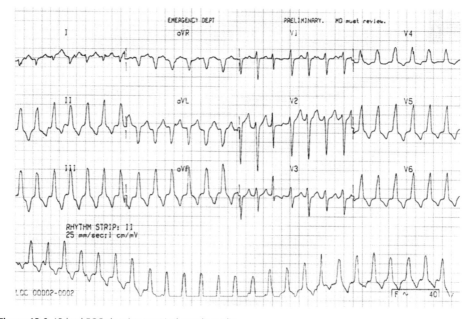

Figure 13.6 12-lead ECG showing ventricular tachycardia.

Definition
- **Ventricular tachycardia:** a tachycardia with three or more consecutive beats that originate from the ventricles, independent of atrial or AV nodal conduction
- **Torsades de pointes:** a form of polymorphic ventricular tachycardia with characteristic beat-to-beat changes in the QRS complex
- **Ventricular flutter:** monomorphic, regular arrhythmia of ventricular origin with no isoelectric interval between QRS complexes

---

Box 13.6   Terms in ventricular tachycardia

- **Accelerated idioventricular rhythm**: ventricular rhythm <100 bpm
- **Sustained VT**: VT lasting longer than 30 seconds
- **Monomorphic**: QRS complexes have a single morphology
- **Multiple monomorphic**: QRS complexes have more than one morphology in different episodes
- **Pleomorphic**: QRS complexes have more than one morphology during the same episode but are not continuously changing
- **Polymorphic**: constantly changing QRS complexes during the episode

---

Aetiology
1. Previous myocardial infarction
2. Structural:
   a. Non-ischaemic cardiomyopathy
   b. Infiltrative disease (e.g. sarcoid, amyloid)
   c. Arrhythmogenic right ventricular cardiomyopathy
3. Inherited ion-channel abnormalities:
   a. Long QT syndrome
   b. Brugada syndrome
4. Drugs (see Table 13.14)
5. Electrolyte disturbances
6. Infection:
   a. Viral myocarditis
   b. Chagas disease
   c. Lyme disease
7. Others:
   a. Tension pneumothorax
   b. Cardiac tamponade
   c. Pulmonary embolus

Box 13.7   Electrolyte disturbances predisposing to VT

- Hyperkalaemia
- Hypokalaemia
- Hypomagnesaemia
- Hypocalcaemia

Table 13.14 Drugs recognized to cause prolongation of the QT (see: www.crediblemeds.org)

Drug class	Specific drugs
Antiarrhythmics	Amiodarone
	Disopyramide
	Dofetilide
	Ibutilid
	Procainamide
	Quinidine
	Sotalol
Antibiotics	Chloroquine
	Clarithromycin
	Erythromycin
	Halofantrine
	Pentamidine
	Sparfloxacin
Antipsychotics	Chlorpromazine
	Haloperidol
	Mesoridazine
	Pimozide
	Thioridazine
Antiemetics	Domperidone
	Droperidol
Antihistamines	Terfenadine
	Astemizole
	Diphenhydramine
Calcium-channel blockers	Bepridil
	Lidoflazine
Opiates	Methadone
	Levomethadyl

Incidence

Epidemiology of ventricular tachycardia is not well categorized due to overlap with VF and the high prevalence of sudden death following development of the arrhythmia. This provides a rough estimate of incidence.

- **Sudden death incidence**: 5.3 per 10^4 per year

Prevalence

Sustained VT is an acute and paroxysmal condition and thus prevalence is not accurately recorded.

- **Non-sustained VT:** 200 per 10^4

Mortality

Mortality from VT is high and (along with VF) accounts for the majority of sudden cardiac death.

Pathophysiology

Ventricular tachycardia may result from one of several possible mechanisms:

1. A re-entry circuit: an area of scar tissue allows for a re-entrant circuit to develop and a tachycardia to initiate

2. Focus: an area of the ventricle acts as a focus of depolarization

3. Electrical abnormalities: ion channel or electrolyte abnormality causes electrophysiological changes within the ventricle (e.g. Brugada or long QT syndromes) making depolarization easier

Clinical types
Ventricular tachycardia can be classified according to the morphology of QRS complex amplitude:

- **Monomorphic:** all QRS complexes are the same amplitude and morphology; this suggests a stable pattern of inappropriate depolarization
- **Polymorphic:** QRS complexes vary in amplitude and morphology suggesting a shifting focus and changing pattern of inappropriate depolarization

VT can also be classified based on the clinical state of the patient.

Haemodynamic compromise:
- Ventricular tachycardia causes rapid and ineffective contraction of the ventricles
- In many patients this prevents appropriate cardiac output
- A pulse may be absent and/or the patient may be hypotensive

No haemodynamic compromise:
- Occasionally ventricular tachycardia maintains a sufficient cardiac output to be tolerated by the patient without becoming significantly hypotensive

Presenting features

Table 13.15 Presenting features of ventricular tachycardia

Group	Symptoms	Examination	Acute	Chronic
Haemodynamic compromise	Decreased consciousness	Lack of pulse Hypotension	Yes	No
Arrhythmia	Palpitations	Rapid pulse	Yes	Yes
Ischaemia	Chest pain	Sweating Nausea	Yes	No

Differentials
1. Supraventricular tachycardia with bundle branch block
2. Pre-excited atrial tachycardia or fibrillation
3. Hyperkalaemia

These are the other cause of a wide QRS-complex tachycardia. However, a wide QRS-complex tachycardia should be treated in the first instance as VT.

Key investigations
Investigations may be important in VT, but should not delay the initiation of treatment. If haemodynamic compromise is present, follow hospital protocol for dealing with peri-arrest scenarios.

Bedside

Table 13.16 Bedside tests of use in patients with ventricular tachycardia

Test	Justification	Potential result
Oxygen saturations	Should be performed in all peri-arrest patients	May be low
ECG	Vital in any arrhythmia. A repeat ECG should be taken after resolution of the arrhythmia to assess for underlying cause	A wide QRS-complex tachycardia Post arrhythmia ECG may show Q-waves suggesting previous infarction, or QT prolongation
Blood pressure	Assessment of haemodynamic compromise	Hypotensive if haemodynamic compromise

Blood tests

Table 13.17 Blood tests of use in patients with ventricular tachycardia

Test	Justification	Potential result
Electrolytes	Electrolyte disturbances are a reversible cause for VT	Hyper-/hypokalaemia Hypomagnesaemia Hypocalcaemia
Troponin	Marker of cardiac damage. Infarction is an important cause of new-onset VT Rapid VT may cause infarction	Infarction: raised

Imaging

Table 13.18 Imaging modalities of use in patients with ventricular tachycardia

Test	Justification	Potential result
Chest X-ray	May show tension pneumothorax	Area without lung markings at the periphery. However, CXR should not be needed to identify this
Trans-thoracic echocardiogram	May show cardiac tamponade	Infarction: regional wall motion abnormalities Tamponade: pericardial effusion compressing the heart

Special tests
Additional tests are likely to be useful in the setting of patients having chronic runs of VT.

Table 13.19 Special investigations of use in patients with ventricular tachycardia

Test	Justification	Potential result
24-hour Holter monitor	Provides an estimate of VT burden/duration and more definitive diagnosis	As with 12-lead ECG
Ventricular mapping	May locate specific area(s) of the ventricle(s) which are triggering the VT	May locate source of VT, likely to either be a specific ectopic focus or an area of ventricular scarring
Coronary angiogram	To assess for underlying coronary artery disease	Coronary artery stenosis

Management options
If patient is haemodynamically compromised or does not have a pulse, follow hospital protocol for peri-arrest and arrest scenarios respectively. DC cardioversion is likely to be needed.

Conservative
Conservative therapy is rarely appropriate due to potential for sudden cardiac death or emergent haemo-dynamic compromise during VT episodes.

Medical
Medical treatment may be appropriate for stable patients. Cardioverting agents of choice include:

1. **Lidocaine:** 1.5 mg/kg given over 10 minutes is modestly successful and has few side effects
2. **Amiodarone:** 300 mg over 30 minutes through a central vein followed by 900 mg over 24 hours

Longer-term medical treatment may be considered if the VT develops in a heart without structural abnormalities. Beta-blockers are the agent of choice.

Invasive
- **DC cardioversion:** this is the method of choice for returning the patient to sinus rhythm if unstable, or if medical therapy has failed
- **Mapping and ablation:** the focus for development of VT can be established using electrophysiolog-ical mapping (Table 13.19). If a focus if found, ablation can be attempted

13.8 OTHER ARRHYTHMIAS TO BE AWARE OF

Multifocal atrial tachycardia
- An irregular tachycardia characterized by three or more different P-wave morphologies
- Most common cause is underlying pulmonary disease, however, electrolyte abnormalities and digoxin toxicity are also recognized aetiologies
- Treatment involves targeting the underlying condition and calcium-channel blockers
- There is no role for cardioversion or ablation

Ventricular fibrillation
- Uncoordinated electrical activity within the ventricles preventing organized contraction
- Mechanism is unclear but may involve either re-entrant circuits or focal mechanisms
- Treatment is a medical emergency and should prompt a cardiac arrest call
- Treatment should be according to Resuscitation Council (UK) guidelines

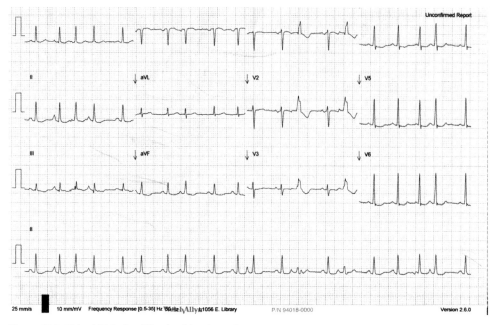

Figure 13.7 12-lead ECG of multifocal atrial tachycardia.

 (See Audio Podcast 13.3 at **www.wiley.com/go/camm/cardiology**)

KEY CLINICAL TRIALS

Key trial 13.1

Trial name: Acute treatment of recent-onset atrial fibrillation and flutter with a tailored dosing regimen of intravenous amiodarone.

Participants: 50 patients with recent onset AF or atrial flutter.

Intervention: Amiodarone.

Control: Digoxin.

Outcome: Increase cardioversion to sinus rhythm in amiodarone group (92% vs. 71%, p = 0.005). Heart rate was decreased faster and to a greater extent in amiodarone group at 1 and 8 hours (p < 0.05).

Reason for inclusion: Evidence for the use of amiodarone over digoxin when attempting to cardiovert patients with atrial fibrillation.

Reference: Hou ZY, Chang MS, Chen CY, et al. Acute treatment of recent-onset atrial fibrillation and flutter with a tailored dosing regimen of intravenous amiodarone: a randomized, digoxin controlled study. Eur Heart J. 1995;16:521–528.

Key trial 13.2

Trial name: AFFIRM.

Participants: 4000 patients with atrial fibrillation with a high risk of stroke or death.

Intervention: Rhythm-control strategies.

Control: Rate-control strategies.

Outcome: There was no difference in mortality between the two groups at 5 years (23.8% vs. 21.3%, p = 0.08). Increased hospitalization and adverse events in the rhythm-control group.

Reason for inclusion: Evidence to suggest that both rate- and rhythm-control strategies provide a similar benefit to the patient.

Reference: Wyse DG, Waldo AL, DiMarco JP, et al., for The Atrial Fibrillation Follow-up Investigation of Rhythm Management (AFFIRM) Investigators. A comparison of rate control and rhythm control in patients with atrial fibrillation. N Engl J Med. 2002;347:1825–1833.

Key trial 13.3

Trial name: AFASAK.

Participants: 1007 patients with chronic non-rheumatic atrial fibrillation.

Intervention: Warfarin (n = 335).

Control: Aspirin (n = 336) or placebo (n = 336).

Outcome: Decreased thromboembolic complications in warfarin group (warfarin = 5, aspirin = 20, placebo = 21).

Reason for inclusion: Treatment with warfarin decreases thromboembolic risk.

Reference: Petersen P, Boysen G, Godtfredsen J, et al. Placebo-controlled, randomized trial of warfarin and aspirin for prevention of thromboembolic complications in chronic atrial fibrillation: the Copenhagen AFASAK study. Lancet. 1989;1:175–179.

Key trial 13.4

Trial name: Amiodarone as compared with lidocaine for shock-resistant ventricular fibrillation.

Participants: 347 patients with out-of-hospital ventricular fibrillation resistant to three shocks.

Intervention: Amiodarone.

Control: Lidocaine.

Outcome: Increased survival to hospital in amiodarone group (22.8% vs. 12.0%, p = 0.009).

Reason for inclusion: Evidence for the use of amiodarone over other antiarrhythmic agents in VF arrests.

Reference: Dorian P, Cass D, Schwartz B, et al. Amiodarone as compared with lidocaine for shock-resistant ventricular fibrillation. N Engl J Med. 2002;346:884–890.

Key trial 13.5

Trial name: MADIT II.

Participants: 1200 patients with previous MI and LVEF ≤30%.

Intervention: Implantable cardioverting defibrillator (n = 742).

Control: Conventional medical therapy (n = 490).

Outcome: Decreased mortality in those in the ICD group at 20 months (14.2% vs. 19.8%, p = 0.016). The survival benefit from ICD implantation was similar in subgroup analyses for age, sex, ejection fraction and NYHA class.

Reason for inclusion: Evidence for the use of ICDs in those with reduced LVEF following myocardial infarction. Also confirms the role of VF in the mortality of such patients.

Reference: Moss AJ, Zareba W, Hall WJ, et al., for the Multicenter Automatic Defibrillator Implantation Trial II (MADIT II) Investigators. Prophylactic implantation of a defibrillator in patients with myocardial infarction and reduced ejection fraction. N Engl J Med. 2002;346:877–883.

GUIDELINES

European Society of Cardiology. Guidelines for the management of atrial fibrillation. 2010. http://www.escardio.org/guidelines-surveys/esc-guidelines/Pages/atrial-fibrillation.aspx.

European Society of Cardiology. 2012 focused update of the ESC guidelines for the management of atrial fibrillation. 2012. http://www.escardio.org/guidelines-surveys/esc-guidelines/Pages/atrial-fibrillation.aspx.

European Society of Cardiology/American College of Cardiology/American Heart Association. ACC/AHA/ESC guidelines for the management of patients with supraventricular arrhythmias. 2003. http://www.escardio.org/guidelines-surveys/esc-guidelines/Pages/supraventricular-arrhythmias.aspx.

European Society of Cardiology/American College of Cardiology/American Heart Association. ACC/AHA/ESC 2006 guidelines for management of patients with ventricular arrhythmias and the prevention of sudden cardiac death. 2006. http://www.escardio.org/guidelines-surveys/esc-guidelines/Pages/ventricular-arrhythmias-and-prevention-sudden-cardiac-death.aspx.

FURTHER READING

Heeringa J, van der Kuip DAM, Hofman A, et al. Prevalence, incidence and lifetime risk of atrial fibrillation: the Rotterdam study. http://eurheartj.oxfordjournals.org/content/27/8/949.full.

A key study establishing the epidemiology of atrial fibrillation.

Lip GYH, et al. ABC of atrial fibrillation: aetiology, pathology, and clinical features. BMJ. 1995;311:1425.
  An important, although slightly dated, review on atrial fibrillation.
Kannankeril P, Roden DM, Dabar D. Drug-induced long QT syndrome. Pharmacol Rev. 2010;62(4):760–781.
  http://www.ncbi.nlm.nih.gov/pmc/articles/PMC2993258/.
  A detailed but simple review on long-QT syndrome.

 For additional resources and to test your knowledge, visit the companion website at:

www.wiley.com/go/camm/cardiology

14 Valvular Heart Disease

Yang Chen
Imperial College Healthcare NHS Trust, London, UK

14.1 DEFINITION

Pathology related to abnormalities of the cardiac valves.

14.2 UNDERLYING CONCEPTS

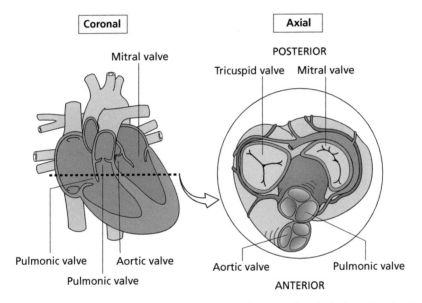

Figure 14.1 Diagrammatic representation of heart chamber and valves. Note the mitral valve is the only valve with two leaflets.

1. **Stenosis:** failure of a valve to open completely, impeding forward flow
2. **Regurgitation:** failure of a valve to close completely, allowing reversed flow
3. **Mixed valve disease:** both stenosis and regurgitation are present; overall effect depends on the severity of each lesion
4. **Prolapse:** a specific cause of regurgitation, usually mitral

---

Box 14.1   Factors determining the clinical consequences of valve dysfunction

1. The valve involved
2. The degree of impairment
3. The speed at which it develops
4. The effectiveness of compensatory mechanisms

Clinical Guide to Cardiology, First Edition. Edited by Christian F. Camm and A. John Camm.
© 2016 John Wiley & Sons, Ltd. Published 2016 by John Wiley & Sons, Ltd.
Companion website: www.wiley.com/go/camm/cardiology.

5. Two complications of valve dysfunction:
  • **Decompensation:** the development of heart failure leading to congestion of the pulmonary and/or systemic venous system (see Chapter 11)
  • **Infective endocarditis** (see Chapter 12)
6. **Cause of murmurs:** arise because of one of three different reasons:
  • Blood flow across an abnormal structure (valvular heart disease)
  • Increased flow across a normal structure (flow murmur)
  • Flow through a shunt with sufficient pressure gradient (VSD)

Box 14.2   Levine Scale of Murmur Intensity

1. Lowest intensity – difficult to hear even by experts
2. Low intensity – difficult, but usually audible to all listeners
3. Medium intensity, no thrill – easy to hear even by inexperienced listeners
4. Medium intensity, with thrill
5. Loud intensity, with thrill – audible even with the stethoscope placed partially on the chest
6. Loudest intensity with thrill – audible even with the stethoscope raised above the chest

N.B. Ease of detecting a murmur clinically does not correlate to severity in many cases.

 (See Audio Podcast 14.1 at **www.wiley.com/go/camm/cardiology**)

14.3 CLINICAL TYPES

The bulk of the clinical burden of valvular lesions relate to the left-sided (mitral and aortic) valves.

Mitral valve:
• Mitral regurgitation
• Mitral stenosis

Aortic valve:
• Aortic regurgitation
• Aortic stenosis

Others:
• Outflow tract obstruction (e.g. H(O)CM)
• Pulmonary stenosis
• Tricuspid regurgitation/valve disease
• Prosthetic heart valves
• Innocent murmur

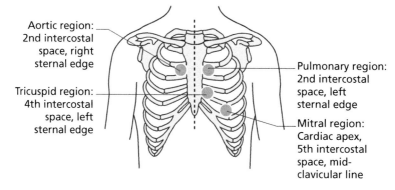

Figure 14.2 Auscultation locations for cardiac valves.

14.4 MITRAL REGURGITATION (MR)

Pathophysiology
1. **Mitral valve:** positioned between the left atrium and the left ventricle
2. **Mitral regurgitation:** retrograde flow of blood from the left ventricle to the left atrium
3. **Mitral prolapse:** involves thickening of leaflets via proteoglycan deposition; when ventricles contract, abnormal bulging of one or both leaflets of the mitral valve occurs, allowing backflow of blood into atrium

Acute MR
- **Rapid onset:** little enlargement of the left atrium (LA), ventricles are unable to expel sudden increase in volume
- **Volume overload:** causes increased LA and pulmonary venous pressures
- **Pulmonary oedema (acute):** results from increased pulmonary venous pressure

Chronic MR
- **Slow onset:** causes gradual enlargement of the LA
- **Accommodation:** volume overload occurs with little rise in LA pressure
- **Dilatation:** LV and LA dilated due to chronic volume overload
- **Heart failure (HF):** eventual result of ventricular dilatation
- **Atrial fibrillation (AF):** increased risk with dilated LA
- **Asymptomatic:** symptoms are absent or slowly progressive over years

Key data
Aetiology
Acute:
1. **Infective endocarditis:** leaflet disruption
2. **Myocardial infarction:** papillary muscle dysfunction can occur following infarction
3. **Trauma:** typically blunt trauma from a steering wheel in road traffic collisions

Chronic:
1. **Functional:** dilatation of annulus due to enlargement of LV
2. **Calcification:** particularly if diabetic
3. **Prolapse:** usually asymptomatic unless severe. Multifactorial aetiology with genetic predisposition
4. **Cusp degeneration:** age-related degeneration
5. **Rheumatic heart disease:** chronic occurrence after acute rheumatic fever

---

Box 14.3   Causes of functional mitral regurgitation

1. Ischaemic heart disease
2. Dilated cardiomyopathy
3. Aortic insufficiency

(See Audio Podcast 14.2 at **www.wiley.com/go/camm/cardiology**)

Prevalence
- 17 per 10^4
- 50 per 10^4 when >65 years

Mortality (5-year)
- 14–33%

Box 14.4   Predictors of poor outcome in mitral regurgitation

1. Increasing age
2. Accompanying AF
3. Severity of MR
4. Pulmonary hypertension
5. LV end-systolic dilatation >40 mm
6. Increased LV end-systolic diameter
7. LVEF <50%

Presenting features

Table 14.1 Potential presenting features of mitral regurgitation

	Signs	Symptoms
Acute	Bi-basal crepitations: may extend apically Irregularly irregular pulse	SOB Sense of impending doom Palpitations
Chronic	Bi-basal crepitations: extending apically Pleural effusion Irregularly irregular pulse Thrusting, displaced apex beat Murmur (see Table 14.2)	Fatigue SOB Orthopnoea

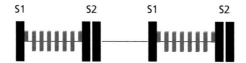

Figure 14.3 Auscultatory findings in mitral regurgitation.

Table 14.2 Murmur characteristics of mitral regurgitation

Location	Apex
Radiation	Axilla
Timing	Pansystolic
Pitch	Constant
Manoeuvres	Rolled to left Breath held in end-expiration
Additional sounds	Soft S1 and loud S2: due to pulmonary hypertension S3: sign of fluid overload Mid-systolic click: occurs in mitral prolapse
Additional markers of severity	AF Loud S2 RV heave Signs of decompensation (see Chapter 11)

Differentials

There are very limited differentials for a pansystolic murmur:

1. Ventricular septal defect (VSD)
2. Tricuspid regurgitation (TR)

See Chapter 6.

(See Audio Podcast 14.3 at **www.wiley.com/go/camm/cardiology**)

Key investigations

Bedside

Table 14.3 Bedside tests in patients with suspected MR

Test	Justification	Potential result
ABG	Important in acutely SOB patients Outline severity using PaO_2, pH etc.	Low PaO_2 if MR becomes decompensated Exhaustion can cause hypercapnia and acidosis
Blood pressure	Hypertension is a potential cause and exacerbating factor of MR	Elevated BP is common; its presence does not exclude other causes
ECG	MR can induce non-specific ECG changes	See Box 14.5

Box 14.5   ECG features suggestive of MR

1. Prolonged P-wave (P-mitrale): LA enlargement
2. Large QRS complexes (V1 and V6): LV hypertrophy
3. Peaked P-wave (P-pulmonale): RA enlargement
4. Irregular rhythm: atrial fibrillation
5. Q-waves: previous infarction

Blood tests

Table 14.4 Blood tests in patients with suspected MR

Test	Justification	Potential result
Full blood count	Anaemia can precipitate a flow murmur/exacerbate existing murmurs	Low Hb defines anaemia Common in older patients
Thyroid function tests	Hyperthyroidism can precipitate a flow murmur/exacerbate existing murmurs	Hyperthyroid: TSH low
Urea and electrolytes	Renal function may dictate suitability of treatments	Renal disease: creatinine elevated
Glucose and cholesterol	Screen for underlying CVD risk factors	Elevated if patient has undiagnosed diabetes or hypercholesterolaemia

Imaging

Table 14.5 Imaging modalities of use in patients with suspected MR

Test	Justification	Potential result
Chest X-ray	Look for evidence of end-organ damage Look for evidence of decompensation	Increased cardiothoracic ratio Signs of pulmonary oedema (see Box 11.5)
Trans-thoracic echocardiogram	Assessment of severity of regurgitation and presence of concomitant stenosis Can be done at bedside if patient acutely breathless	Regurgitant flow visualized through the mitral valve
Transoesophageal echocardiogram	Accurate assessment of feasibility of repair	Valve leaflet and surrounding structures visualized

Box 14.6   Grades of mitral regurgitation

- **Grade 1:** mild regurgitation
- **Grade 2:** moderate regurgitation
- **Grade 3:** moderate to severe regurgitation
- **Grade 4:** severe

Special tests

Table 14.6 Special tests used to investigate MR

Test	Justification/comments	Potential result
Cardiac catheterization	Coronary artery disease may be managed surgically at time of valvular repair/replacement	Complete or partial occlusion of a major coronary artery

Management options
Conservative
1. Patient education regarding oral hygiene
2. Salt restriction if mild symptoms of pulmonary oedema develop
3. Surveillance with echocardiography in asymptomatic patients

Medical
Medical therapies aim to manage complications arising from mitral regurgitation:

1. If pulmonary oedema is present then consider acute HF therapy (Chapter 11)
2. Once stable, consider long-term HF therapy as appropriate (Chapter11)
3. If AF present, treat as appropriate (Chapter 13)

Invasive
Invasive therapy aims to repair or replace the affected valve.

Box 14.7 Indications for invasive treatment in mitral regurgitation

1. Acute severe MR
2. High likelihood of durable repair
3. Asymptomatic + 1 of:
   - LVEF<60%, LV end-systolic diameter (LVESD) ≥45 mm, new-onset AF, systolic pulmonary pressure >50 mmHg, flail leaflet
4. Symptoms of heart failure + 1 of:
   - LVEF>30% + LVESD <55 mm, LVEF <30% refractory to medical therapy

Table 14.7 Invasive options for the management of mitral regurgitation

	Mitral valve repair	Mitral valve replacement
Surgical approach	Median sternotomy	Median sternotomy
Technique	Repair of a ruptured chorda or repair of a leaflet	Either tissue or mechanical valve
Advantages	Lower operative mortality	Tissue – no warfarin Mechanical – long lasting
Disadvantages	Restricted to certain patients	Tissue – lasts 5–10 years Mechanical – need for anticoagulation

14.5 MITRAL STENOSIS (MS)

Pathophysiology
1. **Pressure:** increased LA pressure is required to force blood across narrowed opening
2. **LA dilatation:** occurs as a result of increased pressure
3. **Atrial contraction:** important in maintaining flow across stenotic valve
4. **AF:** dilated LA increases risk of AF, onset of which may precipitate acute symptoms
5. **Pulmonary pressure:** hypertension develops secondary to increased LA pressure
6. **Cor pulmonale:** RV hypertrophy and RV failure eventually develops

Box 14.8 Potential (but rare) mass effects of an enlarged LA

1. **Ortner's syndrome:** compression of the recurrent laryngeal nerve causing a hoarse voice
2. **Dysphagia:** due to compression of the oesophagus
3. **Left lung collapse:** compression of left main bronchus

Key data
Aetiology
1. **Rheumatic heart disease:** chronic occurrence after acute rheumatic fever
2. **Degenerative:** severe mitral annulus calcification

Other causes are rare:

- **Congenital:** isolated or with atrial septal defect (Lutembacher's syndrome)
- **Rheumatic:** rheumatoid arthritis, systemic lupus erythematosus
- **Malignant carcinoid tumour:** carcinoids within the lungs cause left-sided valve lesions
- **Endocardial fibroelastosis**
- **Mucopolysaccharidoses:** Hurler's syndrome
- **Liposomal storage disorders:** Fabry's disease

- **Whipple's disease:** infection with *T. whipplei*
- **Iatrogenic:** rare (early artificial valve designs, e.g. Starr–Edwards)

Prevalence
- 1 per 10^4 (1:2 male:female ratio)

Mortality
- Survival in asymptomatic patients usually at least 10 years
- Progression is highly variable

Box 14.9   Precipitants of progression in MS

1. Pregnancy
2. AF
3. Embolism
4. High-output states (e.g. anaemia)

Presenting features

Table 14.8 Potential presenting features of mitral stenosis

	Signs	Symptoms

Acute	Bi-basal crepitations – may extend apically
	Irregularly irregular pulse
	Unilateral hemiplegia, bi-temporal
	    hemianopia, dysphasia
		SOB
		Sense of impending doom
		Palpitations
		Arm/leg weakness, drooping of face,
		    slurring of speech
		Haemoptysis
		Chest pain

Chronic	Bi-basal crepitations – may extend apically Irregularly irregular pulse Tapping apex beat	Shortness of breath on exertion (SOBOE) Fatigue Hoarse voice Dysphagia Chronic plethora

---

Box 14.10   Pathophysiology of symptoms specific to mitral stenosis

1. Haemoptysis: alveolar capillary rupture, chronic bronchitis, bronchial vein rupture
2. Chest pain: usually occurs if cor pulmonale also present; can occur even with normal coronary arteries
3. Tapping apex beat: manifestation of S1 as a palpable beat
4. Chronic plethora: low cardiac output and severe pulmonary hypertension = chronic hypoxaemia causing cutaneous vasodilation)

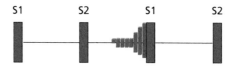

Figure 14.4 Auscultatory findings in mitral stenosis. Note the presence of presystolic potentiation due to atrial systole (increased amplitude of murmur in figure), which is only seen in sinus rhythm.

Table 14.9 Murmur characteristics of mitral stenosis

Location	Apex
Radiation	Axilla
Timing	Mid-diastolic
Pitch	Low
Manoeuvres	Rolled to left
	Breath held in end-expiration
Additional sounds	Loud S1: due to mitral valve closing following a greater excursion
	Loud S2: due to pulmonary hypertension
	Opening snap: sudden opening of stiffened mitral valve
Additional markers of severity	Length of murmur
	AF
	Loud S2
	RV heave
	Signs of decompensation (Chapter 11, Table 11.1)

Differentials

1. **Austin Flint murmur:** see Box 14.11
2. **Diastolic sounds:** S3, S4, pericardial rub
3. **Inflow obstruction:** left atrial myxoma, left atrial ball valve thrombus, H(O)CM
4. **Tricuspid stenosis:** see Section 14.8

See Chapter 6.

Box 14.11   Austin Flint murmur

- In patients with AR
- Blood falls back during early diastole hitting anterior leaflet of the mitral valve
- This narrows the mitral opening
- Functional mitral stenosis and a mid-diastolic murmur is generated

---

Key investigations
Bedside tests

Table 14.10 Bedside tests in patients with suspected MS

Test	Justification	Potential result
ABG	If patient is acutely SOB, crucial to outline severity using markers such as PaO_2, pH etc.	Low PaO_2 if MS becomes decompensated Exhaustion can cause hypercapnia and acidosis
Blood pressure	Hypotension could exacerbate lesion and cause a patient to decompensate	Systolic >135 mmHg
ECG	MS can induce non-specific ECG changes	See Box 14.12

Box 14.12   ECG findings in MS

1. **Prolonged P-wave** (P-mitrale): LA enlargement
2. **Peaked P-wave** (P-pulmonale): RA enlargement due to pulmonary hypertension
3. **Irregularly irregular QRS:** due to AF
4. **Right axis deviation:** RV hypertrophy due to pulmonary hypertension

Blood tests

Table 14.11 Blood tests in patients with suspected MS

Test	Justification	Potential result
Full blood count	Anaemia can precipitate a flow murmur/exacerbate existing murmurs	Low Hb defines anaemia Common in older patients
Thyroid function tests	Hyperthyroidism can precipitate a flow murmur/exacerbate existing murmurs	Hyperthyroid: TSH low
Urea and electrolytes	Renal function may dictate suitability of treatments	Renal disease: creatinine elevated
Glucose and cholesterol	Screen for underlying cardiovascular disease risk factors	Elevated if patient has undiagnosed diabetes or hypercholesterolaemia

Imaging

Table 14.12 Imaging modalities of use in patients with suspected MS

Test	Justification	Potential result
Chest X-ray	Look for evidence of end-organ damage Look for evidence of decompensation	Pulmonary oedema signs (see Box 11.5) Large left atrium – straightened left heart border and double shadow
Trans-thoracic echocardiogram	Assessment of severity of stenosis and presence of concomitant regurgitation Can be done at bedside if patient is acutely breathless	Area of the mitral valve orifice calculated
Transoesophageal echocardiogram	Accurate assessment of feasibility of repair	Valve leaflet and surrounding structures visualized

Special tests

Table 14.13 Special tests used to investigate MS

Test	Justification/comments	Potential result
Cardiac catheterization	Coronary artery disease may be managed surgically at time of valvular repair/replacement	Complete or partial occlusion of a major coronary artery

Management options

Conservative

1. Patient education regarding oral hygiene
2. Salt restriction if mild symptoms of pulmonary oedema develop
3. Surveillance with echo in asymptomatic patients

Medical

Medical therapies aim to manage complications arising from mitral regurgitation:

1. Consider long-term HF therapy as appropriate (Chapter 11)
2. If AF present, treat as appropriate (Chapter 13)

Invasive

Invasive therapy aims to repair or replace the affected valve. It is indicated in heavily calcified and rigid valves, or severe symptomatic disease (mitral valve area <1.5 cm^2).

Table 14.14 Invasive options for the management of mitral stenosis

	Balloon valvotomy/mitral valvuloplasty	Commissurotomy (very uncommon)	Mitral valve replacement (usual procedure)
Surgical approach	Non-surgical	Median sternotomy/left thoracotomy	Median sternotomy
Technique	Catheter via femoral vein	Can be either bypass or without bypass	Either tissue or mechanical valve
Advantages	Lower operative mortality	Gives option for those with calcification/regurgitation	Tissue – no warfarin Mechanical – long lasting
Disadvantages	Restricted to certain patients – no regurgitation or calcification	Higher operative mortality	Tissue – lasts 5–10 years Mechanical – need for anticoagulation

14.6 AORTIC STENOSIS (AS)

Pathophysiology

- **Progressive narrowing:** results in decreased flow across the valve
- **Stroke volume:** maintained by developing LV hypertrophy
- **Non-compliant LV:** results from progressive LV hypertrophy and increases end-diastolic pressures
- **Angina:** symptoms arise as high end-diastolic pressures reduce coronary artery perfusion
- **Syncope:** stenosis prevents an appropriate increase in cardiac output, combined with vasodilatation in skeletal muscle, results in decreased cerebral perfusion. Less commonly, syncope triggered by cardiac arrhythmias or complete heart block
- **Shortness of breath:** see Box 14.13

Box 14.13 Mechanism of shortness of breath in AS

1. High intramural pressure triggers baroreceptors
2. Results in bradycardia and inadequate cardiac output
3. Skeletal muscle vasodilation during exercise prevents adequate tissue oxygenation

Box 14.14   Potential (but uncommon) side effects of AS

1. GI bleeding:
   - Severe calcification of aortic valve may cause acquired von Willebrand syndrome
   - Large von Willebrand factor multimers are sheared (and activated) when passing across the tight calcified valve
2. Microangiopathic haemolytic anaemia (MAHA):
   - Red cells are sheared when passing across the tight calcified valve

Key data
Aetiology
1. **Degenerative:** calcification of the aortic valve
2. **Bicuspid aortic valve:** 1–2% of the general population
3. **Rheumatic heart disease:** chronic occurrence after acute rheumatic fever
4. **Supravalvular AS:** Williams syndrome or rubella

Prevalence
- 40 per 10^4
- 100–400 per 10^4 when >65 years

Mortality
Mortality is highly dependent on associated symptoms:

- Symptomatic angina – 50% mortality at 5 years
- Syncope – 50% mortality at 3 years
- SOB – 50% mortality at 2 years

Presenting features

Table 14.15 Potential presenting features of aortic stenosis

	Signs	Symptoms
Acute	Bi-basal crepitations – may extend apically Aortic dissection (see Box 14.15) Stroke: unilateral hemiplegia, bi-temporal hemianopia, dysphasia	Angina SOB Syncope Aortic dissection (see Box 14.15) Stroke: arm/leg weakness, drooping of face, slurring of speech
Chronic	Bi-basal crepitations – may extend apically Slow rising pulse Palpable systolic thrill Sustained heaving apex beat	Angina SOB Dizziness on standing PR bleeding/melena (angiodysplasia)

Box 14.15   Features of aortic dissection

1. Sudden, intense chest pain radiating to back and downwards migrating
2. Increased risk with bicuspid valves

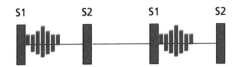

S1   S2   S1   S2

Figure 14.5 Auscultatory findings in aortic stenosis.

Table 14.16 Murmur characteristics of aortic stenosis

Location	Right sternal edge, second intercostal space
Radiation	Carotid arteries
Timing	Systolic – ejection
Pitch	Crescendo–decrescendo
Manoeuvres	Breath held in end-expiration
Additional sounds	Soft S1
	Soft S2: increasing calcification prevents valve from snapping shut
	S3: sign of fluid overload
	S4: increased ventricular wall stiffness due to hypertrophy
Additional markers of severity	Length of murmur
	Reversed split S2
	Narrow pulse pressure
	Signs of decompensation

Differentials
Most common
1. **Aortic sclerosis:** see Box 14.16
2. **Innocent murmur:** see Section 14.8
3. **Aortic regurgitation:** with a concomitant ejection systolic murmur due to increased flow
4. **Atrial septal defect:** see Chapter 18
5. **Pulmonary stenosis:** see Section 14.8

Dangerous
- **Coarctation of aorta:** see Chapter 18
- **Hypertrophic (obstructive) cardiomyopathy:** see Chapter 15

> **Box 14.16**   Aortic sclerosis
>
> 1. Thickening and calcification of one or more leaflets of the aortic valve
> 2. Increases turbulence of flow across the valve
> 3. Little/no obstruction of flow (c.f. aortic stenosis)

(See Audio Podcast 14.4 and 14.5 at **www.wiley.com/go/camm/cardiology**)

Key investigations
Bedside

Table 14.17 Bedside tests in patients with suspected AS

Test	Justification	Potential result
Arterial blood gas	If patient is acutely SOB, crucial to outline severity using markers such as PaO_2, pH etc.	Low PaO_2 if severe AS or AS becomes decompensated. Exhaustion can cause hypercapnia and acidosis
Blood pressure	Hypertension could exacerbate lesion and cause a patient to decompensate	Narrow pulse pressure is common in AS
ECG	AS can induce non-specific ECG changes	See Box 14.17

Box 14.17 ECG findings in AS

1. LVH with strain pattern
2. Bundle branch block (left or right)
3. First-degree heart block to third-degree heart block

Blood tests

Table 14.18 Blood tests in patients with suspected AS

Test	Justification	Potential result
Full blood count	Anaemia can precipitate a flow murmur/exacerbate existing murmurs	Low Hb defines anaemia Common in older patients
Thyroid function tests	Hyperthyroidism can precipitate a flow murmur/exacerbate existing murmurs	Hyperthyroid: TSH low
Urea and electrolytes	Renal function may dictate suitability of treatments	Renal disease: creatinine elevated
Glucose and cholesterol	Screen for underlying CVD risk factors	Elevated if patient has undiagnosed diabetes or hypercholesterolaemia

Imaging

Table 14.19 Imaging modalities of use in patients with suspected AS

Test	Justification	Potential result
Chest X-ray	Look for evidence of end-organ damage Look for evidence of decompensation	Pulmonary oedema signs (see Box 11.5) Calcification in valve or aortic root
Trans-thoracic echocardiogram	Assessment of severity of stenosis and presence of concomitant regurgitation Assess for bicuspid valve as underlying aetiology	Area of the through the aortic valve orifice calculated LVH may be present
Transoesophageal echocardiogram	Accurate assessment of feasibility of repair/replacement	Valve leaflet and surrounding structures visualized

Special tests

Table 14.20 Special tests used to investigate AS

Test	Justification/comments	Potential result
Cardiac catheterization	Coronary artery disease may be managed surgically at time of valvular repair/replacement	Accurate assessment of both coronary arteries and valve pressure gradients possible

Management options
Conservative
1. Patient education regarding oral hygiene
2. Surveillance with echo in asymptomatic patients

Medical
Medical therapies aim to manage complications arising from mitral regurgitation:

1. Beta-blockers reduce myocardial oxygen demand and reduce angina symptoms
2. Additional HF therapy as appropriate (see Chapter 11)
3. Avoid drugs which reduce afterload/systemic resistance in severe AS (e.g. ACE inhibitors, GTN)

Invasive
Invasive therapy aims to repair or replace the affected valve.

Box 14.18 Indications for invasive management in aortic stenosis

1. Severe AS:
   - Symptomatic
   - Undergoing CABG
2. Asymptomatic:
   - LVEF <50%
   - Abnormal exercise test related to AS

Table 14.21 Invasive options for the management of aortic stenosis

	Balloon valvuloplasty	TAVI (transaortic valve implant)	Aortic valve replacement
Surgical approach	Non-surgical	Non-surgical	Median sternotomy
Technique	Catheter via femoral vein	Catheter via transfemoral or transapical approach	Either tissue or prosthetic valve
Advantages	Gives option to those who are haemodynamically unstable	Gives option to those deemed unfit for valve replacement (according to EUROSCORE)	Tissue – no warfarin Prosthetic – long lasting
Disadvantages	Not definitive, bridge to TAVI or AVR	Centres need necessary expertise	Tissue – lasts 5–10 years Prosthetic – need for anticoagulation

14.7 AORTIC REGURGITATION (AR)

Pathophysiology
- **Incomplete ejection:** blood ejected from the LV during systole falls back during diastole
- **Ventricle dilatation:** increased stroke volume at end-diastole causes dilatation of the LV chamber

- **Hypertrophy:** LV hypertrophy may arise (late in the disease process)
- **Acute AR:** often catastrophic – ventricle has not had time to compensate and can lead to cardiogenic shock

---

Box 14.19 Eponymous signs in aortic regurgitation

1. **Watson's water hammer pulse:** collapsing radial pulse when arm is elevated
2. **Corrigan's pulse:** collapsing carotid pulse
3. **De Musset's sign:** head nodding in time with the heart beat
4. **Quincke's sign:** pulsation of the nail capillary bed
5. **Traube's sign:** systolic sound, 'pistol shot' heart over femoral artery
6. **Duroziez's sign:** compression of the femoral artery with stethoscope generates systolic and diastolic murmurs
7. **Muller's sign:** visible pulsation of the uvula

Box 14.20 Aortic regurgitation associated murmurs

1. **Ejection systolic murmur:** due to turbulent flow across aortic valve
2. **Austin Flint murmur:** see Box 14.11

Key data

Aetiology
1. **Hypertension**
2. **Infective endocarditis:** causes acute AR
3. **Aortic dissection:** proximal dissection (Stanford A) causes acute AR
4. **Aortic root disease:** ankylosing spondylitis or polycystic kidney disease
5. **Connective tissue disorders:** e.g. Marfan's
6. **Rheumatic heart disease:** chronic occurrence after acute rheumatic fever

Prevalence
- 0.5 per 10^4
- 10–20 per 10^4 when >65 years

Mortality
- 10-year survival of 50%
- Asymptomatic with EF >50% – 1% mortality at 5 years
- Symptomatic – 65% mortality at 5 years

Presenting features

Table 14.22 Potential presenting features of aortic regurgation

	Signs	Symptoms
Acute	Bi-basal crepitations – may extend apically	SOB Sense of impending doom
Chronic	Thrusting, displaced apex beat Eponymous signs (see Box 14.19)	SOBOE Angina Syncope

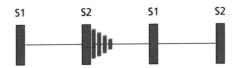

Figure 14.6 Auscultatory findings in aortic regurgitation.

Table 14.23 Murmur characteristics of aortic regurgitation

Location	Lower left sternal edge
Radiation	-
Timing	Early diastole
Pitch	High pitched
Manoeuvres	Leaning forward
	Breath held in end-expiration
Additional sounds	Ejection systolic murmur (ESM)
	Austin Flint murmur
	S3: sign of fluid overload
	S4: increased ventricular wall stiffness due to hypertrophy
Additional markers of severity	Low diastolic BP
	Wide pulse pressure
	Signs of decompensation

Differentials

1. Pulmonary regurgitation
2. Other diastolic noises, e.g. S3
3. Ruptured sinus of Valsalva aneurysm

Box 14.21   Valsalva aneurysm

- Aneurysm of the coronary sinus (normally right coronary sinus)
- Typically a congenital defect
- Other causes include: Ehlers–Danlos syndrome, atherosclerosis, syphilis

---

Key investigations
Bedside

Table 14.24 Bedside tests in patients with suspected AR

Test	Justification	Potential result
ABG	If patient is acutely SOB, crucial to outline severity using markers such as PaO_2, pH etc.	Low PaO_2 if AR becomes decompensated. Exhaustion can cause hypercapnia and acidosis
Blood pressure	AR often presents with characteristic blood pressure changes	AR: wide pulse pressure, low diastolic pressure
ECG	AR can induce non-specific ECG changes	See Box 14.22

Box 14.22 ECG findings in AR

1. LVH with strain pattern
2. Left axis deviation
3. Q-waves in lateral leads (due to prominent septal depolarization)

Blood tests

Table 14.25 Blood tests in patients with suspected AR

Test	Justification	Potential result
Full blood count	Anaemia can precipitate a flow murmur/exacerbate existing murmurs	Low haemoglobin defines anaemia
Thyroid function tests	Hyperthyroidism can precipitate a flow murmur/exacerbate existing murmurs	Hyperthyroid: low TSH
Urea and electrolytes	Renal function may dictate suitability of treatments	Renal disease: raised creatinine
Glucose and cholesterol	Screen for underlying CVD risk factors	High if patient has diabetes or hypercholesterolaemia

Imaging

Table 14.26 Imaging modalities of use in patients with suspected AR

Test	Justification	Potential result
Chest X-ray	Look for evidence of end-organ damage Look for evidence of decompensation	Pulmonary oedema signs (see Box 11.5) Cardiomegaly
Trans-thoracic echocardiogram	Assessment of severity of regurgitation and presence of concomitant stenosis	Area of the through the mitral valve orifice calculated

Special tests

Table 14.27 Special tests used to investigate AR

Test	Justification/comments	Potential result
Cardiac catheterization	Coronary artery disease may be managed surgically at time of valvular repair/replacement	Accurate assessment of both coronary arteries and valve pressure gradients possible

Management options
Conservative
- Patient education regarding oral hygiene
- Surveillance with echo in asymptomatic patients

Medical
Medical therapies aim to manage complications arising from aortic regurgitation:

- Consider long-term HF therapy as appropriate (see Chapter 11)
- Beta-blockers should be avoided as they prevent compensatory tachycardia, particularly in acute AR

Invasive
Invasive therapy aims to repair or replace the affected valve.

Box 14.23 Indications for invasive therapy in AR

1. Acute symptomatic AR
2. Severe AR + undergoing concomitant CABG/valve surgery
3. Asymptomatic + LVEF<50%/LVESD >50 mm

Table 14.28 Invasive options for the management of aortic regurgitation

	Aortic valve repair	Aortic valve/root replacement
Surgical approach	Median sternotomy	Median sternotomy
Technique	May include bicuspid aortic valve repair (through a smaller J incision) or repair of enlarged root	Either tissue or prosthetic valve
Advantages	Only in experienced centres	Tissue – no warfarin. Prosthetic – long lasting
Disadvantages	Restricted to certain patients	Tissue – lasts 5–10 years Prosthetic – need for anticoagulation

14.8 OTHER MURMURS TO BE AWARE OF

Hypertrophic (obstructive) cardiomyopathy (H(O)CM)
- HCM is discussed in detail in Chapter 15
- In approximately one third of cases, there is an element of obstruction of the outflow tract
- This can cause an audible ejection systolic murmur
- Murmur is louder when Valsalva manoeuvre performed (c.f. AS), which decreases LV filling, resulting in a narrower outlet during systole
- Patients can be young

Pulmonary and tricuspid valve disease
- Regurgitation:
  - Both are usually secondary lesions to pulmonary hypertension
  - Regurgitation more common than their stenotic counterparts
  - Murmur characteristics are similar to aortic and mitral regurgitation respectively
  - Pulmonary regurgitation is best heard at the second intercostal space on the left sternal edge
  - Tricuspid regurgitation is best heard over the left lower sternal edge; it rarely causes a pulsatile liver
  - 'Trivial TR' is commonly reported on echo and frequently found in healthy individuals
  - Signs and symptoms normally relate to the primary lesions (e.g. left-sided valvular disease), which are the root cause, rather than pulmonary or tricuspid lesions directly
- Pulmonary stenosis is normally a congenital lesion, often in conjunction with Fallot's tetralogy
- Tricuspid stenosis is normally secondary to endocarditis that has affected more than one valve; or rheumatic heart disease

Prosthetic heart valve murmur
- Associated median sternotomy/lateral thoracotomy scar
- Metal valve cause an audible click:
  a. First heart sound = mitral
  b. Second heart sound = aortic
- Tissue valve: often has normal heart sounds
- May be associated flow murmur:
  a. Aortic flow murmur = ejection systolic
  b. Mitral flow murmur = late diastolic
- Abnormal findings include regurgitant murmurs and muffling of mechanical heart sounds (suggesting failure of the valve)

Innocent murmur

- Develops as a result of increased blood flow over a valve (normally the aortic valve)
- Accentuated by high-output states (e.g. anaemia, pregnancy, after exercise)

Box 14.24 Characteristics of an innocent/flow murmur

1. Ejection or mid-systolic
2. Does not radiate
3. Heart sounds 1 and 2 are equal in intensity
4. No added heart sounds
5. Normal apex beat

(See Audio Podcast 14.6 and 14.7 at **www.wiley.com/go/camm/cardiology**)

14.9 KEY CLINICAL TRIALS

Key trial 14.1

Trial name: Long-term survival of patients undergoing mitral valve repair and replacement.
Participants: 47 279 patients >65 years old undergoing primary isolated mitral valve surgery.
Intervention: Mitral valve repair.
Control: Mitral valve replacement.
Outcome: Operative mortality for repair = 3.9%, operative mortality for replacement = 8.9%.
Reason for inclusion: In older patients with isolated mitral valve regurgitation, repair is more favourable than replacement.
Reference: Vassileva CM, Mishkel G, McNeely C, et al. Long-term survival of patients undergoing mitral valve repair and replacement. A longitudinal analysis of medicare fee-for-service beneficiaries. *Circulation.* 2013;127:1870-1876. http://circ.ahajournals.org/content/127/18/1870.

Key trial 14.2

Trial name: Re-interventions after percutaneous mitral commissurotomy during long-term follow-up, up to 20 years: the role of repeat percutaneous mitral commissurotomy.
Participants: 912 patients with good immediate results post percutaneous mitral commissurotomy (PMC); 20-year follow-up.
Intervention: Analysis of whether patients required further interventions, and effect on survival.
Control: N/A.
Outcome: 38% required subsequent interventions on the mitral valve. Median time was 117 months (repeat PMC) and 95 months (mitral surgery). Twenty-year survival was 38% for group without reintervention on mitral valve; 46% for those without surgery on mitral valve.
Reason for inclusion: This study shows that after successful PMC, reintervention is frequently needed (38%) but that almost half of patients remained free from surgery at 20 years.
Reference: Bouleti C, Lung B, Himbert D, et al. Reinterventions after percutaneous mitral commissurotomy during long-term follow-up, up to 20 years: the role of repeat percutaneous mitral commissurotomy. Eur Heart J. 2013;34:19231929. http://eurheartj.oxfordjournals.org.

Key trial 14.3

Trial name: PARTNER.
Participants: 358 high-risk AS patients deemed not suitable for aortic surgery.
Intervention: Transcatheter aortic valve implantation.
Control: Standard therapy – medical therapy, balloon aortic valvuloplasty (performed in 83.8%).
Outcome: At 1 year, rate of death was 30.7% with TAVI vs. 50.7% with standard therapy (p < 0.001). At 30 days, there was a higher rate of major strokes and vascular complications (5% vs. 1.1%, p = 0.06).
Reason for inclusion: This study shows that TAVI, in a certain subgroup of patients, is convincingly better for mortality and morbidity than standard therapy in the management of AS.

Reference: Leon MB, Smith CR, Mack M, et al. Transcatheter aortic-valve implantation for aortic stenosis in patients who cannot undergo surgery. N Engl J Med. 2010;363:1597-1607. http://www .nejm.org/doi/full/10.1056/NEJMoa1008232.

Key trial 14.4

Trial name: Early surgery versus conventional treatment in asymptomatic very severe aortic stenosis.
Participants: 197 asymptomatic patients with very severe aortic stenosis.
Intervention: Early surgery whilst patient was asymptomatic.
Control: Conventional treatment strategy – careful monitoring and surgery once symptoms had developed.
Outcome: All-cause mortality at 6 years: operated group = 2%, conventional group = 32%.
Reason for inclusion: In younger patients, early surgery was associated with significant benefits in all-cause mortality.
Reference: Kang DH, Park SJ, Rim JH, et al. Early surgery versus conventional treatment in asymptomatic very severe aortic stenosis. Circulation. 2010;121:1502-1509. http://circ.ahajournals.org/content/121/13/1502.

Key trial 14.5

Trial name: Is repair of aortic valve regurgitation a safe alternative to valve replacement?
Participants: 160 patients undergoing aortic valve repair.
Intervention: Aortic valve repair.
Control: N/A.
Outcome: At 4 years, mortality rate = 10%. Reoperation rate was 11% at 5 years.
Reason for inclusion: Aortic valve repair is a good option for selected patients, with low operative mortality and appears suitable particularly for young patients who wish to avoid chronic anticoagulation.
Reference: Minakata K, Schaff HV, Zehr KJ, et al. Is repair of aortic valve regurgitation a safe alternative to valve replacement? J Thorac Cardiovasc Surg. 2004;127:645-653. http://www .jtcvsonline.org/article/S0022-5223(03)01712-4/abstract.

GUIDELINES

European Society of Cardiology. Guidelines on the management of valvular heart disease. 2012. http:// www.escardio.org/guidelines-surveys/esc-guidelines/Pages/valvular-heart-disease.aspx

FURTHER READING

Prodromo J, D'Ancona G, Amaducci A, Pilato M. Aortic valve repair for aortic insufficiency: a review. J Cardiothorac Vasc Anesth. 2012;26(5):923–932. http://www.jcvaonline.com/article/S1053-0770(11)00534-9/abstract
A thorough discussion of the potential role aortic valve repair plays in the treatment of aortic regurgitation.
Rosenhek R, Zilberszac R, Schemper M, et al. Natural history of very severe aortic stenosis. Circulation. 2010;121(1):151–156.
An examination of the natural history of aortic stenosis over a period of 4 years.

www.wiley.com/go/camm/cardiology

For additional resources and to test your knowledge, visit the companion website at:

15 Cardiomyopathy

Anneline te Riele

University Medical Center Utrecht, the Netherlands

15.1 DEFINITION

A disorder of the myocardium in which the heart muscle is structurally and functionally abnormal, in the absence of another cause (e.g. hypertension, valvular disease).

15.2 UNDERLYING CONCEPTS

- **Ventricular dysfunction:** the key feature of cardiomyopathies. May be systolic, diastolic or combined
- **Compensatory mechanisms** (e.g. ventricular dilatation)**:** are in place to maintain cardiac output; but eventually, these compensatory mechanisms may fail, leading to heart failure
- **Systolic dysfunction:** a decrease in cardiac contractility, often estimated by ventricular ejection fraction
- **Diastolic dysfunction:** abnormal relaxation and filling pattern of the ventricle

15.3 CLINICAL TYPES

1. Hypertrophic cardiomyopathy (HCM): characterized by presence of increased ventricular wall thickness ($\geq$15 mm) in the absence of another cause
2. Dilated cardiomyopathy (DCM): characterized by ventricular systolic dysfunction and dilatation, in the absence of another cause
3. Restrictive cardiomyopathy (RCM): characterized by abnormal ventricular relaxation

Clinical Guide to Cardiology, First Edition. Edited by Christian F. Camm and A. John Camm.
© 2016 John Wiley & Sons, Ltd. Published 2016 by John Wiley & Sons, Ltd.
Companion website: www.wiley.com/go/camm/cardiology.

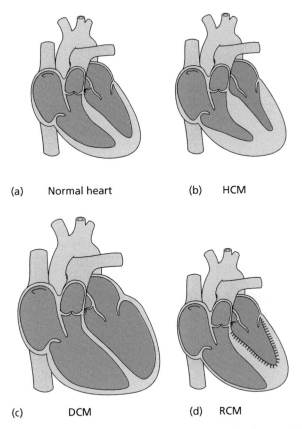

(a)   Normal heart   (b)   HCM

(c)   DCM   (d)   RCM

Figure 15.1 Clinical types of cardiomyopathy. (a) Normal heart. (b) HCM with the characteristically enlarged ventricular walls. (c) DCM characterized by enlarged ventricles which attempt to compensate for ventricular dysfunction. (d) RCM characterized by infiltration which stiffens the ventricular walls and causes diastolic dysfunction.

Table 15.1 Overview of differences between cardiomyopathies. DCM, dilated cardiomyopathy; HCM, hypertrophic cardiomyopathy; RCM: restrictive cardiomyopathy.

	HCM	DCM	RCM
Primary mechanism	Diastolic dysfunction	Systolic dysfunction	Diastolic dysfunction
Ventricular volume	↓	↑↑	↑
Ejection fraction	=/↑	↓↓	↓
Wall thickness	↑↑	↓	=/↑
Atrial size	↑	↑↑	↑
Congestive symptoms*	Rarely	Left-sided first, then right-sided	Common
Ventricular arrhythmias	Common, often during exercise	Common	Uncommon (except for sarcoidosis)
Atrial arrhythmias	Common	Common	Common
Conduction disturbances	Rarely	Occasional heart block	Occasional heart block

*Left-sided congestive symptoms: (exertional) dyspnoea, orthopnoea, paroxysmal nocturnal dyspnoea. Right-sided congestive symptoms: peripheral oedema, nausea, abdominal discomfort.

15.4 PRESENTATION

Although pathophysiology differs for each cardiomyopathy, all may present with heart failure and arrhythmias. Also, the approach to all patients is similar.

Table 15.2 Considerations in any patient with cardiomyopathy

History	Family history
	History of alcohol, chemotherapy or radiation therapy*
	Assessment of ability to perform routine activities
Physical examination	Comprehensive physical examination
	Assessment of volume status
Additional investigations	ECG
	Chest X-ray
	Blood tests: BNP, renal/liver function, troponin
	24-hour Holter monitoring
	Echocardiography +/- MRI

*These may inflict damage to the heart, leading to cardiomyopathy.

15.5 HYPERTROPHIC CARDIOMYOPATHY

Key data
Definition
A heart muscle disorder characterized by the presence of increased ventricular wall thickness ($\geq$15 mm) in the absence of another cause (e.g. hypertension, valve disease).

Subtypes
- **Obstructive:** LVOT obstruction due to severe septal hypertrophy; also known as HOCM (hypertrophic obstructive cardiomyopathy)
- **Non-obstructive:** no LVOT obstruction

Aetiology
1. Familial (70%):
   a. Sarcomeric protein mutations
   b. Metabolism disorders (e.g. Pompe, Anderson–Fabry)
2. Non-familial (30%):
   a. Idiopathic
   b. Obesity

Box 15.1   Sarcomeric protein mutations associated with HCM

1. Beta-myosin heavy chain
2. Myosin binding protein C
3. Cardiac troponin T

Incidence
- Unclear (many HCM cases go unnoticed)

Prevalence
- 20 per 10^4

Mortality
- 1% per year in diagnosed cases

Box 15.2   Factors associated with worse prognosis in HCM

1. Multiple pathogenic (sarcomere) mutations
2. Family history of sudden death
3. Severe ventricular hypertrophy (≥30 mm)
4. Severe LVOT obstruction (≥60 mmHg)
5. Extensive and diffuse delayed gadolinium enhancement on MRI
6. Abnormal blood pressure response to exercise
7. Previous (non-sustained) VT or VF
8. Decreased LV ejection fraction (<50%)

Outline of pathophysiology

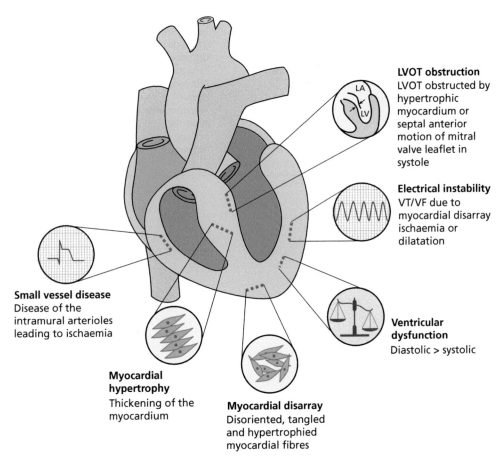

LVOT obstruction
LVOT obstructed by hypertrophic myocardium or septal anterior motion of mitral valve leaflet in systole

Electrical instability
VT/VF due to myocardial disarray ischaemia or dilatation

Ventricular dysfunction
Diastolic > systolic

Myocardial disarray
Disoriented, tangled and hypertrophied myocardial fibres

Myocardial hypertrophy
Thickening of the myocardium

Small vessel disease
Disease of the intramural arterioles leading to ischaemia

Figure 15.2 Pathophysiology of HCM.

Presenting features
1. **General findings/signs of congestion:**
   a. Dyspnoea
   b. Orthopnoea
   c. Peripheral oedema
   d. Raised JVP

2. **Cardiac findings:**
   a. Visible cardiac apex
   b. S4
   c. Pansystolic murmur – mitral valve regurgitation
   d. Systolic murmur beginning in mid-systole – LVOT obstruction
3. **Respiratory findings:**
   a. Bilateral crackles

Table 15.3 Presentation of hypertrophic cardiomyopathy

	Acute presentation	Chronic presentation
LVOT obstruction	Syncope Altered consciousness	Syncope Presyncope Dizzy spells (Transient) altered consciousness
Small vessel disease **Ventricular dysfunction**	Typical/atypical angina Dyspnoea Orthopnoea Peripheral oedema	Typical/atypical angina (Exertional) dyspnoea Orthopnoea Paroxysmal nocturnal dyspnoea Reduced exercise tolerance Fatigue Peripheral oedema
Electrical instability	Palpitations Syncope Sudden cardiac arrest Death	Palpitations Syncope Presyncope

Differentials
Most common
1. Athletic-induced hypertrophy
2. Hypertension-induced hypertrophy
3. Aortic stenosis
4. Ischaemic heart disease

Dangerous
1. Acute coronary syndrome
2. Congestive heart failure
3. Ventricular arrhythmia due to other causes

Key investigations
Bedside

Table 15.4 Bedside tests for suspected hypertrophic cardiomyopathy

Test	Justification	Potential result
ECG	LV hypertrophy causes characteristic changes	ECG changes outlined in Box 15.3
Blood pressure	Rule out hypertension-induced hypertrophy	Increased blood pressure suggests hypertensive cause

Box 15.3   ECG changes seen in HCM

1. High QRS voltage (e.g. Sokolow criteria: S in V_1 + R in V_5 or V_6 ≥35 mm)
2. Repolarization abnormalities (deep, negative T-waves, ST-segment depression)
3. Ventricular or atrial arrhythmias (e.g. ventricular tachycardia, atrial fibrillation)
4. May be normal (10% of HCM patients)

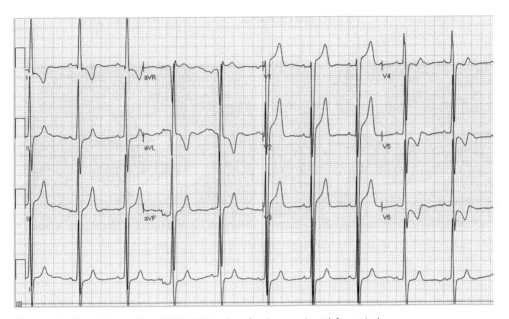

Figure 15.3 12-lead sinus rhythm ECG in HCM patient showing prominent left ventricular hypertrophy (Sokolow criteria).
Source: TP Mast, MD, and MJM Cramer, MD, University Medical Center Utrecht, the Netherlands.

Blood tests

Table 15.5 Blood tests for suspected hypertrophic cardiomyopathy

Test	Justification/comments	Potential result
Troponin	ACS is a common cause of arrhythmias	ACS – raised troponin
Urea and electrolytes	Rule out electrolyte abnormalities as arrhythmic cause	Hypokalaemia – common cause of ventricular arrhythmias
	Measure of renal function to assess forward heart failure	Heart failure – raised urea suggests renal dysfunction
BNP	Measure of heart failure	Heart failure – raised BNP (see Chapter 11)
Liver function tests	The liver may be affected in right-sided heart failure	Heart failure – total protein and albumin can be reduced in right-sided failure
Thyroid function tests	Potential endocrine cause of atrial fibrillation	Atrial fibrillation – may be raised if thyroid dysfunction is the underlying cause

Imaging

Table 15.6 Imaging modalities of use in suspected hypertrophic cardiomyopathy

Test	Justification/comments	Potential result
Chest X-ray	Assessment of cardiac size	Cardiac size likely to be normal, may be some atrial dilatation
Trans-thoracic echocardiogram	High sensitivity for detection	Increased ventricular wall thickness (Box 15.4)

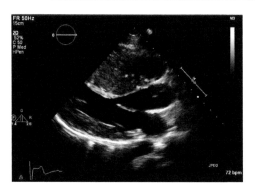 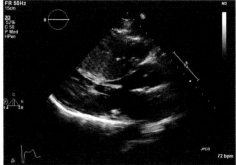

Figure 15.4 TTE in HCM. Parasternal long-axis TTE in HCM patient showing prominent septal hypertrophy (A and B), as well as septal anterior motion (anterior leaflet of mitral valve touching the septum in systole, B).
Source: TP Mast, MD, and MJM Cramer, MD, University Medical Center Utrecht, the Netherlands.

Box 15.4   Echocardiographic findings in HCM

1. Ventricular hypertrophy ≥15 mm (often septal > lateral wall)
2. LVOT gradient or septal anterior motion of mitral valve (mitral leaflet obstructs LVOT)
3. Abnormal diastolic function
4. Atrioventricular valve regurgitation
5. Atrial enlargement
6. Abnormal systolic function (severe cases)

Special tests

Table 15.7 Special tests used to investigate suspected hypertrophic cardiomyopathy

Test	Justification/comments	Expected result
Cardiac MRI	High sensitivity for detection	Increased ventricular wall thickness
Cardiac catheterization	Coronary artery disease can cause arrhythmias and heart failure	IHD – complete or partial occlusion of a major coronary artery
Exercise testing	LVOT may only be present with adrenergic drive	LVOT – drop in blood pressure/failure to increase during exercise testing (risk factor for sudden death)
	Arrhythmias may only present with adrenergic drive	Ventricular tachycardia (see Chapter 13)
24-hour Holter monitoring	Arrhythmias may only be detected during prolonged monitoring	Atrial fibrillation, ventricular tachycardia (see Chapter 13)

Management options
Conservative
1. Patients with moderate/severe HCM should not take part in competitive/vigorous exercise
2. Strictly manage cardiovascular risk factors

Medical
Medical therapy aims to reduce adrenergic drive and ventricular contraction. This can be accomplished by either:

1. Beta-blockers
2. Non-dihydropyridine calcium-channel blockers

Invasive
Invasive therapy aims to reduce septal hypertrophy and thus reduce the potential for LVOT obstruction or protect against sudden cardiac death:

1. Percutaneous alcohol septal ablation in obstructive HCM
2. Septal myectomy +/- mitral valvuloplasty
3. ICD in selected high-risk cases

Box 15.5   ICD indications in HCM

1. Unexplained syncope
2. Previous VT/VF
3. Non-sustained VT on Holter monitoring
4. Family history of sudden death
5. Severe LV hypertrophy (≥30 mm)
6. Abnormal blood pressure response to exercise

(See Audio Podcast 15.1 at **www.wiley.com/go/camm/cardiology**)

Heart transplantation can be considered in some individuals if other treatment options have failed.

Additional considerations
1. Heart failure: symptomatic improvement can be accomplished with loop diuretics. If heart failure is a major factor then full heart failure therapy should be considered (Chapter 11)
2. Atrial fibrillation: anticoagulation with vitamin K antagonists/novel oral anticoagulants should be considered in at-risk populations (Chapter 36)
3. Arrhythmias: in addition to beta-blockers or calcium-channel blockers, other therapies can be considered if ventricular/supraventricular arrhythmias are a substantial burden (Chapter 13)

(See Audio Podcast 15.2 at **www.wiley.com/go/camm/cardiology**)

15.6 DILATED CARDIOMYOPATHY

Key data
Definition
A heart muscle disorder characterized by left ventricular systolic dysfunction and left ventricular dilatation, in the absence of abnormal loading conditions (e.g. hypertension) or coronary artery disease.

Aetiology
1. Acquired (60%):
    a. Myocarditis
    b. Toxin exposure
    c. Tachycardiomyopathy

> **Box 15.6** Causes of DCM
>
> ABCCCD:
> - **A**lcohol abuse
> - Wet **b**eriberi
> - **C**oxsackie B virus
> - Chronic **c**ocaine use
> - **C**hagas disease
> - **D**oxorubicin toxicity (and other anthracyclines)

2. Familial (40%)

Incidence
- 0.5–1.0 per 10^4 per year

Prevalence
- 3–4 per 10^4

Mortality
- 5–8% per year

> **Box 15.7** Factors associated with poor prognosis in DCM
>
> 1. Male gender
> 2. Black race
> 3. Anaemia
> 4. LV ejection fraction <35%
> 5. NYHA functional class ≥II
> 6. Renal dysfunction
> 7. Broad QRS >120 ms
> 8. Persistent high left atrial pressure
> 9. Sustained ventricular arrhythmias

Outline of pathophysiology

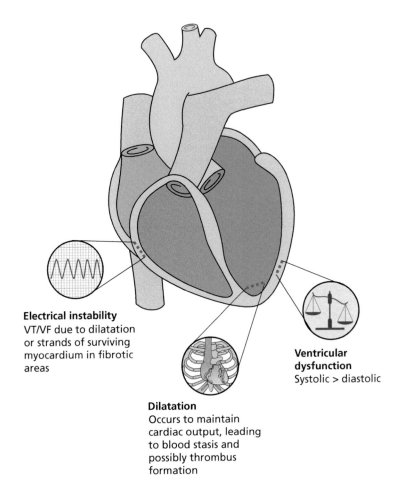

Electrical instability
VT/VF due to dilatation
or strands of surviving
myocardium in fibrotic
areas

**Ventricular
dysfunction**
Systolic > diastolic

Dilatation
Occurs to maintain
cardiac output, leading
to blood stasis and
possibly thrombus
formation

Figure 15.5 Pathophysiology of DCM.

Presenting features
1. **General findings:**
   a. Dyspnoea
   b. Orthopnoea
   c. Peripheral oedema
   d. Raised JVP
2. **Cardiac findings:**
   a. Cardiomegaly (lateral displacement of apex beat)
   b. S3
   c. Pansystolic murmur – atrioventricular valve regurgitation
3. **Respiratory findings:**
   a. Bilateral crackles

Table 15.8 Presenting features of dilated cardiomyopathy

	Acute presentation	Chronic presentation
Ventricular dysfunction	Dyspnoea Orthopnoea Peripheral oedema	(Exertional) dyspnoea Orthopnoea Paroxysmal nocturnal dyspnoea Reduced exercise tolerance Fatigue Peripheral oedema
(AV) Valve regurgitation	–	Dyspnoea Reduced exercise tolerance
Thromboembolism	Acute dyspnoea (right-sided embolus) Neurological symptoms (left-sided embolus)	–
Electrical instability	Palpitations Syncope Sudden cardiac arrest Death	Palpitations Syncope Presyncope

Differentials
Most common
1. Ischaemic cardiomyopathy
2. Valvular heart disease
3. Hypertrophic/restrictive cardiomyopathy

Dangerous
1. Congestive heart failure
2. Ventricular arrhythmia due to other causes
3. Acute coronary syndrome

Key investigations
Bedside

Table 15.9 Bedside tests for dilated cardiomyopathy

Test	Justification	Potential result
ECG	DCM causes characteristic changes	ECG changes outlined in Box 15.8
Blood pressure	Rule out hypertension-induced dilatation	Increased blood pressure suggests hypertensive cause

Box 15.8   ECG findings in DCM

1. Intraventricular conduction delay (e.g. LBBB)
2. Either increased voltage (enlarged ventricles) or reduced voltage (due to loss of muscle fibres/fibrosis)
3. P-mitrale – left atrial enlargement

Blood tests

Table 15.10 Blood tests for dilated cardiomyopathy

Test	Justification/comments	Potential result
Troponin	ACS is a common cause of arrhythmias	ACS – raised troponin
Urea and electrolytes	Rule out electrolyte abnormalities as arrhythmic cause	Hypokalaemia – common cause of ventricular arrhythmias
	Measure of renal function to assess forward heart failure	Heart failure – raised urea suggests renal dysfunction
BNP	Measure of heart failure	Heart failure – raised (see Chapter 11)
Liver function tests	The liver may be affected in right-sided heart failure	Heart failure – total protein and albumin can be reduced in right-sided failure
Thyroid function tests	Potential endocrine cause of atrial fibrillation	Atrial fibrillation – may be raised if thyroid dysfunction is the underlying cause
Haemoglobin	Anaemia is indicative of worse prognosis in DCM	Anaemia – decreased haemoglobin

Imaging

Table 15.11 Imaging modalities of use in dilated cardiomyopathy

Test	Justification/comments	Expected result
Chest X-ray	Assessment of cardiac size	Cardiomegaly/balloon appearance of the heart
Trans-thoracic echocardiogram	High sensitivity for detection	See Box 15.9

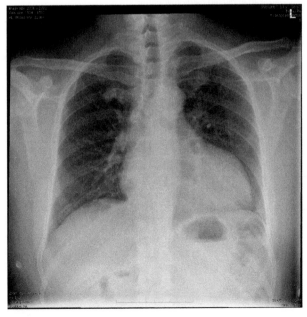

Figure 15.6 Chest X-ray in DCM patient showing enlarged heart with cardiothoracic ratio (CTR) >0.5.
Source: BK Velthuis, MD, University Medical Center Utrecht, the Netherlands.

Box 15.9 Echocardiographic findings in DCM

1. Dilated ventricle with reduced systolic function
2. Normal/decreased wall thickness
3. Atrial dilatation
4. Atrioventricular valve insufficiency
5. Intramural/apical thrombus

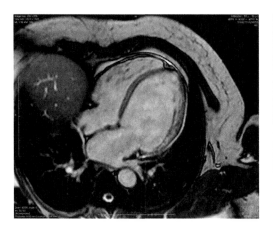 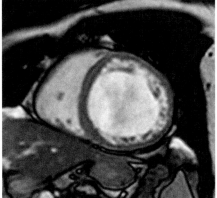

Figure 15.7 MRI IN DCM. Cardiac magnetic resonance imaging in DCM patient in the four-chamber (A) and short-axis (B) view showing an enlarged LV (end-diastolic volume 330 mL) with reduced wall thickness and reduced function (ejection fraction 28%).
Source: BK Velthuis, MD, University Medical Center Utrecht, the Netherlands.

Special tests

Table 15.12 Special tests undertaken in dilated cardiomyopathy

Test	Justification/comments	Expected result
Cardiac MRI	High sensitivity for detection	Dilated left ventricle with reduced systolic function
Cardiac catheterization	Coronary artery disease can cause of arrhythmias and heart failure	IHD – complete or partial occlusion of a major coronary artery
Exercise testing	Assessment of functional status	Decreased exercise tolerance suggests early heart failure
24-hour Holter monitoring	Arrhythmias may only present during prolonged monitoring	Atrial fibrillation, ventricular tachycardia (see Chapter 13)

Management options
Conservative
Encourage patient to abstain from toxin exposure (e.g. alcohol).

Medical

Medical therapy focuses on improving heart failure symptoms and prognosis. This is achieved primarily with:

1. ACE inhibitors/ARBs
2. Beta-blockers
3. Diuretic agents (e.g. loop or thiazide)
4. Anti-aldosterone agents

Invasive

Invasive therapy aims to improve heart failure symptoms and prevent sudden cardiac death:

1. Cardiac resynchronization therapy (CRT)
2. Implantable cardioverting defibrillator (ICD)
3. Heart transplantation

Box 15.10　CRT indications

1. QRS ≥130 ms, LBBB morphology
2. LV ejection fraction ≤35%
3. NYHA III despite adequate medical therapy

Box 15.11　ICD indications

1. Secondary prevention – prior VT/VF
2. Primary prevention – NYHA ≥II symptoms and LV ejection fraction ≤40%

Additional considerations

Additional considerations are the same as those in HCM (Section 15.5).

15.7 RESTRICTIVE CARDIOMYOPATHY

Key data
Definition
A heart muscle disorder characterized by abnormal ventricular relaxation, in the setting of normal systolic/diastolic volume and wall thickness.

Aetiology
1. Amyloidosis (familial/non-familial)
2. Sarcoidosis
3. Familial haemochromatosis
4. Scleroderma
5. Radiation damage

Incidence
Epidemiology figures are unclear for this condition: uncommon cardiomyopathy (approximately 5% of cardiomyopathies).

Prevalence
Epidemiology figures are unclear for this condition: uncommon cardiomyopathy (approximately 5% of cardiomyopathies).

Mortality
- 10–15% per year

Box 15.12   Factors associated with poor prognosis in RCM

1. Male gender
2. Age ≥70 years
3. Increased LV wall thickness
4. NYHA functional class ≥II
5. Left atrial diameter >60 mm

Outline of pathophysiology

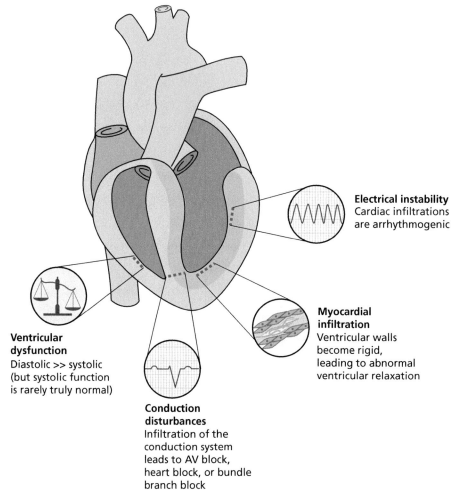

Electrical instability
Cardiac infiltrations
are arrhythmogenic

**Ventricular
dysfunction**
Diastolic >> systolic
(but systolic function
is rarely truly normal)

**Myocardial
infiltration**
Ventricular walls
become rigid,
leading to abnormal
ventricular relaxation

**Conduction
disturbances**
Infiltration of the
conduction system
leads to AV block,
heart block, or bundle
branch block

Figure 15.8 Pathophysiology of RCM.

Presenting features
1. **General findings:**
   a. Dyspnoea
   b. Orthopnoea
   c. Peripheral oedema
   d. Kussmaul's sign (paradoxical rise in JVP on inspiration)

2. **Cardiac findings:**
   a. Cardiomegaly (lateral displacement of visible heart beat)
   b. S3 and/or S4
   c. Pansystolic murmur – atrioventricular valve regurgitation
3. **Respiratory findings:**
   a. Bilateral crackles

Differentials
Most common
1. Constrictive pericarditis
2. Hypertrophic cardiomyopathy
3. Long-standing hypertension

Dangerous
1. Congestive heart failure due to other cardiomyopathy, or other causes
2. Ventricular arrhythmia due to other causes
3. Acute coronary syndrome
4. Hypertrophic obstructive cardiomyopathy

Key investigations
Bedside

Table 15.13 Bedside tests for RCM

Test	Justification	Expected result
ECG	RCM causes non-specific ECG changes	ECG changes outlined in Box 15.13
Blood pressure	Rule out hypertension-induced dilatation	Increased BP suggested hypertensive cause

---

Box 15.13   ECG Findings of RCM

1. Low-voltage QRS
2. Conduction disturbances (first-degree AV block, complete heart block, bundle branch block)

Blood tests

Table 15.14 Blood tests for RCM

Test	Justification/comments	Potential result
Troponin	ACS is a common cause of arrhythmias	ACS – raised troponin
Urea and electrolytes	Rule out electrolyte abnormalities as arrhythmic cause	Hypokalaemia – common cause of ventricular arrhythmias
	Measure of renal function to assess forward heart failure	Heart failure – raised urea suggests renal dysfunction
BNP	Measure of heart failure	Heart failure – raised (see Chapter 11)
Liver function tests	The liver may be affected in right-sided heart failure	Heart failure – total protein and albumin can be reduced in right-sided failure
Thyroid function tests	Potential endocrine cause of atrial fibrillation	Atrial fibrillation – may be raised if thyroid dysfunction is the underlying cause
Serum ACE	A non-specific marker of sarcoidosis	Sarcoidosis – raised

Imaging

Table 15.15 Imaging modalities of use in RCM

Test	Justification/comments	Expected result
Chest X-ray	Assessment of cardiac size	Cardiomegaly and atrial enlargement of the heart
Trans-thoracic echocardiogram	High sensitivity for detection	See Box 15.14

Box 15.14 Echocardiographic findings of RCM

1. Diastolic dysfunction
2. Systolic dysfunction
3. Increased wall thickness
4. Atrial enlargement
5. Atrioventricular valve regurgitation
6. Patchy intramural sparkling appearance with increased echodensity (amyloidosis)

Special

Table 15.16 Special tests for RCM

Test	Justification/comments	Expected result
Cardiac MRI	High sensitivity for detecting RCM	Granulomas, delayed gadolinium enhancement
Cardiac biopsy	May diagnose amyloidosis, sarcoidosis, haemochromatosis	Characteristic histological changes
Positron emission tomography (PET) scan	May diagnose sarcoidosis	Sarcoidosis – extracardiac granulomas
24-hour Holter monitoring	Arrhythmias may only be detected during prolonged monitoring	Atrial fibrillation, ventricular tachycardia (see Chapter 13)

Management options
RCM is very treatment resistant, and treatment options are limited.

Medical
Medical therapy focuses on improving heart failure symptoms and prognosis (see Chapter 11).

Invasive
Invasive therapy aims to overcome conduction blocks or reduce heart failure symptoms:

1. Dual-chamber pacemaker (in cases of conduction block)
2. Heart transplantation

Additional considerations
Additional considerations are the same as those in HCM (Section 15.5).

15.8 OTHER CARDIOMYOPATHIES

These additional cardiomyopathies are rare and unlikely to be encountered clinically. However, for completeness they are included here.

Non-compaction cardiomyopathy
The loose interwoven meshwork of myocardial fibres does not undergo compaction during embryogenesis, leading to regions of non-compacted myocardium. This results in heart failure (both diastolic and systolic dysfunction), systemic emboli and ventricular arrhythmias.

Arrhythmogenic (right ventricular) cardiomyopathy
Rare cardiomyopathy characterized by replacement of the myocardium with fibrofatty tissue, predominantly in the RV. Ventricular arrhythmias, sudden death and (right-sided) heart failure are characteristic features of the disease.

Takotsubo cardiomyopathy
Rare cardiomyopathy characterized by regional systolic dysfunction involving the LV apex and/or mid-ventricle ('transient apical ballooning syndrome'). Symptoms are often preceded by emotional or physical stress. LV function usually normalizes over a period of days to weeks and recurrence is rare.
(See Audio Podcast 15.3 at **www.wiley.com/go/camm/cardiology**)

GUIDELINES

European Society of Cardiology. Classification of the cardiomyopathies: a position statement from the European Society of Cardiology working group on myocardial and pericardial diseases. 2008. Eur Heart J. 2008;29:270–276.

American Heart Association. Contemporary definitions and classification of the cardiomyopathies. An American Heart Association Scientific Statement From the Council on Clinical Cardiology, Heart Failure and Transplantation Committee; Quality of Care and Outcomes Research and Functional Genomics and Translational Biology Interdisciplinary Working Groups; and Council on Epidemiology and Prevention. 2006. Circulation. 2006;113:1807–1816.

American College of Cardiology/American Heart Association. 2011 ACCF/AHA Guideline for the diagnosis and treatment of hypertrophic cardiomyopathy. 2011. JACC. 2011;58:e212–260.

FURTHER READING

Maron BJ, Maron MS. Hypertrophic cardiomyopathy. Lancet. 2013;381:242–255.
  Comprehensive review of HCM by two experts.
Jefferies JL, Towbin JA. Dilated cardiomyopathy. Lancet. 2010;375:752–762.
  Comprehensive review of DCM by two experts.
Dickstein K, Vardas PE, Auricchio A, et al. 2010 Focused update of ESC Guidelines on device therapy in heart failure: an update of the 2008 ESC Guidelines for the diagnosis and treatment of acute and chronic heart failure and the 2007 ESC Guidelines for cardiac and resynchronization therapy. Developed with the special contribution of the Heart Failure Association and the European Heart Rhythm Association. Eur Heart J. 2010;31:2677–2687.
  ESC guideline for ICD and CRT therapy in heart failure. Important for management decisions in end-stage cardiomyopathy associated with heart failure.

 For additional resources and to test your knowledge, visit the companion website at:

www.wiley.com/go/camm/cardiology

16 Hypertension

James Cranley

Papworth Hospital NHS Foundation Trust, Cambridge, UK

16.1 DEFINITION

Systemic arterial hypertension is defined as systolic blood pressure ≥140 mmHg and/or diastolic BP ≥90 mmHg.

16.2 UNDERLYING CONCEPTS

Defining hypertension
- **Normal distribution:** systemic arterial blood pressure has a positively skewed normal distribution and is continuously related to cardiovascular risk
- **Tipping point:** hypertension is defined as a blood pressure above which there is increased cardiovascular risk and treatment has a prognostic benefit

Pathophysiology
- **Volume:** pressure within the arterial tree is dependent both on the central blood volume and the volume of the arterial tree
- **Systemic resistance:** increased contraction of the arterial tree (primarily the arterioles) decreases its cross-sectional area, increasing resistance and elevating pressure. Resistance to flow is determined by Poiseuille's law (Box 16.1)

Box 16.1 Poiseuille's law

$$\Delta P = \frac{8\mu L Q}{\pi r^4}$$

- ΔP – pressure Loss
- L – length
- μ – dynamic viscosity
- Q – flow rate
- r – radius

- **Cardiac output:** high output increases the volume of blood passing through the arterial tree and can increase pressure as a result
- **Renal dysfunction:** regulation of volume and osmolality by the kidneys is required to maintain blood pressure; dysfunction can lead to fluid retention and increased pressure
- **Mean arterial pressure (MAP):** the mean arterial pressure is determined by the cardiac output and systemic vascular resistance

---

Clinical Guide to Cardiology, First Edition. Edited by Christian F. Camm and A. John Camm.
© 2016 John Wiley & Sons, Ltd. Published 2016 by John Wiley & Sons, Ltd.
Companion website: www.wiley.com/go/camm/cardiology.

Box 16.2   Mean arterial pressure

$MAP = (CO \times SVR) + CVP$

CVP can be approximated as 0 mmHg therefore the equation can be simplified:

$MAP = CO \times SVR$

In practice we do not use the CO and SVR to measure the MAP; instead we estimate it from the peak (systolic BP) and trough (diastolic BP) values:

$MAP = \frac{2}{3}$ Diastolic BP $+ \frac{1}{3}$ Systolic BP

- **Autoregulation:** the intrinsic ability of an organ to maintain a constant blood flow despite changes in perfusion pressure. This allows organ perfusion to remain stable despite fluctuations in BP (chronic hypertension causes a rightward shift in this relationship)

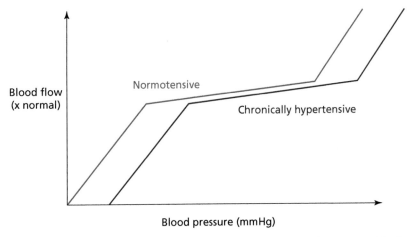

Figure 16.1 Autoregulation. Blood flow in an organ is maintained constant despite fluctuations in blood pressure through means of myogenic and metabolic mechanisms. In chronic hypertension there is a rightward shift in this relationship making them more vulnerable to hypoperfusion with lowering of blood pressure.

Major complications of hypertension
- **Atherosclerosis:** hypertension is a major risk factor for atherosclerosis-driven disease, including coronary/peripheral artery disease and cerebrovascular disease; hypertension increases risk of stroke seven fold
- **Aortic dissection:** the formation of a false lumen within the tunica media of the aorta

Box 16.3   Mechanisms by which hypertension increases the risk of aortic dissection

- **Direct:** high sheer stress promotes degeneration of the media (so-called 'cystic medial necrosis')
- **Indirect:** atherosclerotic disease affecting the vasa vasorum

- **Left ventricular pressure overload:** systemic arterial hypertension increases left ventricular afterload. Over time the pressure-overloaded left ventricle hypertrophies causing diastolic dysfunction; and eventually dilates, causing systolic dysfunction
- **Hypertensive nephropathy:** causing 10–30% of end-stage renal failure, this is characterized histologically by glomerular sclerosis

Box 16.4   Hypertensive nephropathy

- A direct result of hypertensive damage to the arterioles in the kidney
- Hypertension causes arteriole thickening through hyaline arteriolosclerosis
- Resulting ischaemia produces tubular atrophy and glomerular changes
- When advanced, results in renal failure

- **Hypertensive retinopathy:** as with arteries elsewhere, the retinal 'arteries' (histologically arterioles) become thickened and sclerotic ('arteriosclerosis'). Causes a series (see Box 16.5) of changes visible on fundoscopy and, rarely, decreased acuity

Box 16.5   Stages of hypertensive retinopathy

- **Grade 1:** tortuous arteries with thickened, shiny walls (silver wiring)
- **Grade 2:** thickened arteries compress the veins they cross anterior to (arteriovenous nipping)
- **Grade 3:** rupture of superficial precapillary arterioles or small veins (flame haemorrhages). Ischaemia in the nerve fibre layer causes axonal damage, leading to axoplasmic material deposition (cotton wool spots)
- **Grade 4 ('papilloedema'):** blurred optic disc, dilated veins with lack of venous pulsation, haemorrhages adjacent to disc

- **Hypertensive encephalopathy:** headache, confusion, seizures, eventually leading to reduced consciousness (focal neurological deficits are uncommon and suggest stroke)

Box 16.6   Hypertensive encephalopathy

- Occurs due to dilatation of cerebral arteries following failure of the normal cerebral arterial autoregulation
- Normally cerebral blood flow is kept constant by cerebral vasoconstriction in response to increases in blood pressure
  - Non-hypertension: flow is kept constant over a mean pressure of 60–120 mmHg
  - Hypertension: flow is constant over a mean pressure of 110–180 mmHg (due to arteriolar thickening)
- When blood pressure is raised above the upper limit of autoregulation, arterioles dilate
- Dilatation results in hyperperfusion and cerebral oedema

- **Ischaemic stroke:** hypertension is a major risk factor for ischaemic stroke. Note that stroke often presents with increased BP as a protective physiological mechanism, and caution should be used lowering blood pressure in the acute setting
- **Intracerebral haemorrhage:** haemorrhagic stroke accounts for 10–15% of strokes; hypertension increases the risk up to six fold

16.3 KEY DATA

Aetiology
- 'Essential'/primary (idiopathic) hypertension – 95%
- Secondary hypertension – 5%:
  - **a.** Renal: intrinsic renal disease (includes those presenting as nephritic syndrome)
  - **b.** Renovascular disease
  - **c.** Endocrine
  - **d.** Aortic coarctation
  - **e.** Pregnancy/eclampsia
  - **f.** Drugs

Box 16.7   Endocrine causes of secondary hypertension

1. Conn's syndrome
2. Cushing's syndrome
3. Acromegaly
4. Phaeochromocytoma
5. Hyperparathyroidism

Box 16.8   Drugs causing secondary hypertension

1. Steroids
2. Combined oral contraceptive pill
3. Monoamine oxidase inhibitors
4. NSAIDs
5. Cocaine
6. Nasal decongestants (e.g. ephedrine)

Incidence
- 78 per 10^4 per year

Prevalence

Table 16.1 Prevalence of hypertension within the population divided by age and gender

Age of patient (years)	Men	Women
45–54	33%	25%
≥75	66%	78%

Mortality
- 1.85 per 10^4 per year

16.4 CLINICAL TYPES

Primary vs. secondary hypertension
- **'Essential'/primary:** no identifiable cause, i.e. idiopathic
- **Secondary:** defined underlying cause such as renal or endocrine disease is found

Hypertensive emergency
- **Elevation:** a recent elevation in BP to very high levels, (e.g. systolic >180 mmHg and/or diastolic >100 mmHg) causing acute end-organ damage
- **Systems affected:** nervous, renal and cardiovascular systems
- **Prevalence:** only 1% of essential hypertensives develop hypertensive emergencies, but it is more prevalent in secondary hypertension. Therefore, it is important to look carefully for secondary causes of hypertension in those with hypertensive emergencies
- **Accelerated and malignant hypertension:** both are types of hypertensive emergency (these terms are out-dated and should be avoided since they are variably defined)
- **Treatment:** requires therapy to lower blood pressure within minutes to hours to prevent further end-organ damage

Box 16.9   Accelerated and malignant hypertension

1. Accelerated: a hypertensive emergency where there may be vascular damage on fundoscopic examination, (e.g. flame-shaped haemorrhages or soft exudates) but no papilloedema
2. Malignant: similar to accelerated HTN, but papilloedema is present on fundoscopy. Also defined as acute severe hypertension with encephalopathy

Note: these terms should be avoided due to inconsistent definitions

Hypertensive urgency
- **No damage:** recently and severely elevated blood pressure with no evidence of end-organ damage
- **Treatment:** no evidence suggests a benefit from rapidly reducing blood pressure in patients with hypertensive urgency. Aggressive therapy may harm the patient, resulting in cardiac, renal or cerebral hypoperfusion

16.5 PRESENTING FEATURES

On take (hypertensive emergencies)
Symptoms are common in acute and severely elevated blood pressure, in contrast to the insidious, asymptomatic presentation of chronic hypertension.

Table 16.2 Symptoms of hypertensive emergencies

System	Clinical features
Nervous system	Encephalopathy: headache, seizures, visual disturbance, focal neurological deficit, coma Haemorrhage: intracerebral haemorrhage, subarachnoid haemorrhage Retinopathy: fundoscopic changes
Cardiovascular (CV) system	Raised afterload: acute LV failure (causing pulmonary oedema), acute RV failure (secondary to LV failure) Coronary arteries: acute MI Cerebrovascular: ischaemic stroke Peripheral arteries: AAA rupture, acute aortic dissection Micro-angiopathic haemolytic anaemia (MAHA)
Renal system	Acute glomerulonephritis

Box 16.10   Most common hypertensive emergencies

1. Ischaemic stroke (24.5%)
2. Pulmonary oedema (22.5%)
3. Hypertensive encephalopathy (16.3%)
4. Congestive cardiac failure (12%)

(See Audio Podcast 16.1 at **www.wiley.com/go/camm/cardiology**)

In clinic (chronic hypertension)
- Features of chronically raised BP can be divided into those which are a consequence (i.e. features of end-organ damage) and those which are associated with secondary causes, if present
- Note that chronic hypertension is usually asymptomatic and presents differently to hypertensive emergencies. Patients may, however, exhibit symptoms and signs relating to end-organ damage, or (rarely) an underlying secondary cause

Table 16.3 Clinical features of chronic hypertensive end-organ damage

System	Clinical features
Nervous system	Headache Retinopathy: fundoscopic changes
CV system	Coronary arteries: angina, history of ACS, heart failure Cerebrovascular: TIA/stroke (weakness, sensory change, visual loss etc.) Peripheral arteries: history of/palpable AAA, claudication symptoms, bruits LVH-related: arrhythmia history (palpitations, syncope), exertional dyspnoea History of aortic dissection
Renal system	Nephropathy: frothy urine (proteinuria), haematuria, polyuria, malaise, itch

Table 16.4 Clinical features of secondary causes of hypertension (note that most hypertension is primary and will therefore not exhibit these features)

System	Cause	Clinical features
Renal causes	Polycystic kidney disease	FH of renal disease FH of sudden death (subarachnoid haemorrhage) Loin pains (cyst haemorrhage) Palpable enlarged kidneys
	Renal parenchymal disease	History of renal disease Recurrent urinary tract infection Haematuria/proteinuria Drug history (esp. nephrotoxins) Signs of systemic disease (e.g. SLE or systemic sclerosis)
	Renovascular disease	Renal bruits History of high CV risk/established CV disease (atheromatous) Young patient without risk factors (fibromuscular dysplasia)
Endocrine causes	Phaeochromocytoma	Episodes of headache Palpitations Pallor and diaphoresis
	Conn's disease	Episodes of muscle weakness Tetany (hypokalaemia)
	Cushing's syndrome	Truncal obesity Thin skin with bruises and striae Buffalo hump Proximal myopathy Acne
	Acromegaly	Large hands Frontal bossing Bitemporal hemianopia Macroglossia Prognathism Oily skin
	Hyperparathyroidism	Hypercalcaemia features – bone pain, polyuria, polydipsia, dehydration (nephrogenic diabetes insipidus), constipation, confusion, renal tract stones
Other causes	Drugs	Full DH (see Box 16.8)
	Pregnancy/eclampsia	Proteinuria Remember to ask about sexual history and last menstrual period
	Coarctation	Radio-radial or radio-femoral delay Weak femoral pulses Ejection systolic murmur

16.6 DIFFERENTIALS

There are no specific differentials for hypertension. Ensure that secondary conditions are fully considered.

16.7 KEY INVESTIGATIONS

Aims of investigations in hypertension

1. Assess end-organ damage
2. Assess for possible causes of secondary hypertension
3. Assess cardiovascular risk

The detail of investigation for secondary causes depends on the clinical context, for instance more investigation should be made in a young patient with very high blood pressure than in an older patient (in whom the cause is likely to be idiopathic).

Bedside tests

Table 16.5 Bedside tests of use in patients with hypertension

Test	Justification	Potential result
ECG	Examining for LV hypertrophy or signs of past/present ischaemia	LV hypertrophy: S-wave in V1 + R-wave in V5 or V6 $\geq$35 mm Past infarction: Q-waves Present ischaemia: T-wave or ST-segment changes
Urinalysis	May show end-organ damage or suggest a cause of secondary hypertension	End-organ damage: proteinuria Glomerulonephritis: proteinuria and haematuria
Urinary β-HCG	Pregnancy can be a cause of secondary hypertension	–
Ambulatory monitoring	Provides repeated blood pressure measurements outside of the clinical setting	See Table 16.9

Blood tests

Table 16.6 Blood tests of use in patients with hypertension

Test	Justification	Potential result
Urea and electrolytes	Renal profile may show end-organ damage Electrolyte derangement may suggest secondary hypertension	Renal failure: raised urea and creatinine Conn's syndrome: hypokalaemia and hypernatraemia
Random cortisol	Cushing's syndrome can be a cause of secondary hypertension	Cushing's: cannot be diagnosed with random cortisol but can be ruled out if within normal limits
Lipid profile	Cardiovascular risk profiling	Raised LDL and triglycerides increase cardiovascular risk
Glucose + HbA1c	Cardiovascular risk profiling	Raised glucose and HbA1c suggests diabetes
Calcium	Hyperparathyroidism may cause secondary hypertension	Hyperparathyroidism: hypercalcaemia

Imaging

In most cases imaging is not required, however, in some cases the modalities in Table 16.7 may be of use.

Table 16.7 Imaging modalities of use in patients with hypertension

Test	Justification	Potential result
Arterial ultrasound	Assess carotid, abdominal (renal) and peripheral arteries for stenosis (end-organ damage) – should be undertaken if indicated (e.g. bruits/claudication symptoms)	Stenosis
Renal ultrasound	To assess renal damage – should be undertaken if evidence of renal failure	Chronic disease: small kidney size Other causes of renal failure: obstruction, hydronephrosis, etc.
Renal MRI/CT angiogram	To assess renal arteries for stenosis, a potential cause of secondary hypertension	Renal artery stenosis: classically a 'string of beads' appearance in fibromuscular dysplasia

Special tests

Table 16.8 Special tests of use in patients with hypertension

Test	Justification	Potential result
Echocardiogram	To assess cardiac anatomy and function – indicated if signs of LV hypertrophy seen on ECG	Hypertrophy of the cardiac myocardium suggests long-standing hypertension
24-hour urinary metanephrines	Phaeochromocytoma is a rare cause of secondary hypertension	Phaeochromocytoma: raised urinary metanephrines

16.8 MANAGEMENT OPTIONS

Table 16.9 Diagnosis of hypertension based on clinic and home/ambulatory monitoring

		Home/ambulatory monitoring	
		Raised	Normal
Clinic measurement	Raised	Sustained hypertension	White coat hypertension
	Normal	Masked hypertension	Normotensive

Diagnosing hypertension

- **Grades:** hypertension is graded based on systolic and diastolic blood pressure. ESC grades (Table 16.10) correspond to NICE stages (Table 16.11)
- **Ambulation:** raised blood pressure in clinic should be further investigated using 24-hour ambulatory blood pressure monitoring (ABPM) to distinguish sustained hypertension from 'white coat' hypertension

Box 16.11   How to measure blood pressure

1. Allow patient to sit for 3–5 minutes before beginning
2. Take at least two BP measurements, in the sitting position, spaced 1–2 minutes apart
3. Consider the average BP if deemed appropriate
4. Take repeated measurements of BP to improve accuracy in patients with arrhythmias
5. Use an appropriate blood pressure cuff for the patient's arm size (the bladder of the cuff should fit around at least 80% of the arm, but not more than 100%).
6. Have the cuff at the heart level, whatever the position of the patient
7. Use phase I and V Korotkoff sounds to identify systolic and diastolic BP respectively
8. Measure lying and standing blood pressures in elderly patients (assess for orthostatic hypotension)

Table 16.10 ESC grades of hypertension (HTN) based on blood pressure (mmHg)

Category	Systolic BP		Diastolic BP
Optimal	<120	AND	<80
Normal	120–129	AND/OR	80–84
High–normal	130–139	AND/OR	85–89
Grade 1/mild HTN	140–159	AND/OR	90–99
Grade 2/moderate HTN	160–179	AND/OR	100–109
Grade 3/severe HTN	≥180	AND/OR	≥110

Table 16.11 NICE categorization of hypertension and corresponding management strategy (ABPM, ambulatory blood pressure monitoring; HBPM, home blood pressure monitoring)

Stage	Definition	Management overview
Stage 1	Clinic BP **140/90** mmHg or higher **and** ABPM/HBPM **135/85** mmHg or higher	Conservative management **and** drugs therapy only if CV risk high enough
Stage 2	Clinic BP **160/100** mmHg or higher **and** ABPM/HBPM **150/95** mmHg or higher	Conservative management **and** drug therapy
Stage 3	Clinic BP **180/110** mmHg or higher. No need for verification with ABPM/HBPM	Drug therapy immediately **and** Conservative management

When to treat hypertension
- Different organizations (NICE, ESC, AMA etc.) have slightly differing guidelines on treatment thresholds
- **CV risk:** the decision to treat depends on the overall cardiovascular risk of the patient, not BP alone
- **Calculation:** CV risk can be calculated 'exactly' or categorized using tables

Box 16.12   CV risk calculators

- Demographic (e.g. age, gender and ethnicity) and CV risk factors are used
- Entered into online algorithms (e.g. Q-risk, http://www.qrisk.org)
- Generate a 10-year CV mortality risk
- Patients categorized as low (0–10%), moderate (10–20%) and high (20–30%) and very high (>30%)

- **Conservative management:** should be undertaken in all patients with hypertension
- **Stage 1:** drug therapy should be undertaken if any of:
  a. End-organ damage
  b. Known cardiovascular disease

c. Known renal disease
d. Known diabetes mellitus
e. 10-year cardiovascular risk >20%
- **Stage 2/3:** drug treatment should be initiated in all patients in these categories
- **Clinical context:** when initiating therapy, particular attention should be given in the elderly and those with co-morbidities who may be more prone to adverse effects

Blood pressure goals
- **Aged <80 years:** <140/90 mmHg
- **Aged >80 years:** <150/90 mmHg
- **Diabetes with end-organ damage:** <130/80 mmHg
- **CKD + protein:creatinine ratio (PCR) >100 mg/mmol:** <130/80 mmHg

Treatment options

Box 16.13   Once a diagnosis of hypertension is made, the following should occur

1. Initiate of treatment
2. Investigate for end-organ damage
3. Investigate for secondary hypertension
4. Assess cardiovascular risk to guide further therapy
5. Optimize CV risk factors

Conservative
1. Salt restriction (5–6 g/day)
2. Moderate alcohol consumption (men: <21 units/week, women: <14 units/week)
3. Increased consumption of vegetables, fruits and low-fat dairy products
4. Weight reduction (BMI ≤25 kg/m^2)
5. Regular exercise (150 minutes of 'moderate dynamic exercise' per week)
6. Smoking cessation
7. Decrease consumption of caffeine-rich products

Medical
Therapy is divided into steps. If blood pressure does not reach appropriate levels incremental steps should be attempted.

Step 1:
- **<55 years:** ACEi/ARB (if ACEi not tolerated)
- **>55 years or Afro-Caribbean descent (any age):** calcium-channel blocker (CCB)
- If a CCB is not suitable or heart failure is present, offer a thiazide-like diuretic

Step 2:
- Offer a CCB in combination with ACEi/ARB
- If a CCB is not suitable/heart failure present, offer a thiazide-like diuretic
- **Afro-Caribbean descent:** consider ARB in preference to ACEi, in combination with a CCB

Step 3:
- Combination ACEi/ARB, CCB and a thiazide-like diuretic

Step 4:
- Consider seeking expert advice
- **K$^+$ ≤4.5 mmol/L:** consider low-dose (25 mg OD) spironolactone
- **K+ >4.5 mmol/L:** consider higher-dose thiazide-like diuretic
- **Diuretic not tolerated/contraindicated:** consider an alpha- or beta-blocker
- **Remains uncontrolled:** if blood pressure remains uncontrolled with optimal tolerated doses of four drugs, seek expert advice

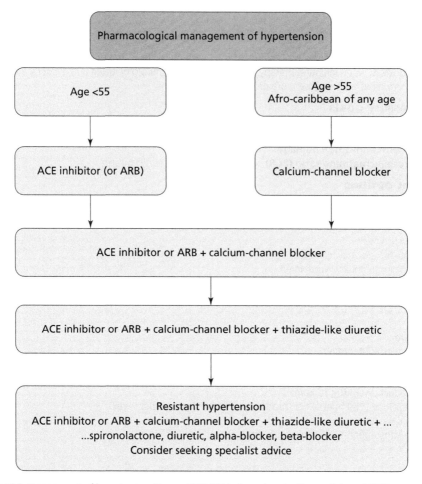

Figure 16.2 Management of hypertension. Source: NICE 2011. Reproduced with permission of NICE.

Lipid-lowering therapy:

- Initiating lipid lowering therapy should be based on overall CV risk, rather than cholesterol levels themselves (see Table 16.12)
- Target total cholesterol <4 mmol/L of which LDL should be <2 mmol/L
- Statins are recommended as first-line therapy

Table 16.12 General guidance for lipid lowering therapy

Prevention strategy	Indicated population
Primary prevention	10-year CV risk >20% All diabetics >40 years old All >75 years old
Secondary prevention	Anyone with previous atherosclerotic-driven disease (CAD, peripheral arterial disease (PAD) or CVD)

Invasive

Invasive management for hypertension is very rare, examples would include:

1. **Endocrine surgery:** Conn's, Cushing's disease, phaeochromocytoma
2. **Renal artery angioplasty:** for renovascular disease
3. **Renal denervation:** a catheter-based technique, evidence for this is inconclusive

---

Box 16.14   Managing hypertensive emergencies

- Severe (i.e. grade 3) hypertension is not uncommon in hospitalized patients
- Urgent management is only required in the presence of end-organ damage
- If no end-organ damage, oral therapy with outpatient follow-up is appropriate
- End-organ damage should prompt urgent senior input and lowering of blood pressure over minutes to hours
- Rapid lowering is best achieved by parenteral (usually IV) therapy
- The choice of therapy depends on the organ system damaged and is a senior lead decision

---

(See Audio Podcast 16.2, 16.3, 16.4 and 16.5 at **www.wiley.com/go/camm/cardiology**)

KEY CLINICAL TRIALS

Key trial 16.1

Trial name: ALLHAT, 2003.

Participants: 33 000 patients with grade 1 or 2 hypertension >55 years with at least one coronary artery disease risk factor.

Intervention: ACEi (lisinopril) or CCB (amlodipine).

Control: Thiazide diuretic (chlorthalidone).

Outcome: No difference in the primary end-point (fatal heart disease, non-fatal MI) but patients on the diuretic had a lower rate of heart failure (but higher serum glucose levels).

Reason for inclusion: Important trial showing that these three drugs were essentially as good as each other at preventing coronary events, with diuretics showing some promise in heart failure.

Reference: ALLHAT Officers and Coordinators for the ALLHAT Collaborative Research Group. Major outcomes in high-risk hypertensive patients randomized to angiotensin-converting enzyme inhibitor or calcium channel blocker vs diuretic: The Antihypertensive and Lipid-Lowering Treatment to Prevent Heart Attack Trial (ALLHAT). JAMA. 2002;288(23):2981–2997. doi:10.1001/jama.288.23.2981. http://jama.jamanetwork.com/article.aspx?articleid=195626.

Key trial 16.2

Trial name: ASCOT.

Participants: 19 000 patients with moderate/high-risk hypertension with at least three CV risk factors.

Intervention: Calcium-channel blocker (amlodipine) first, then adding in an ACEi (perindopril) as needed.

Control: Beta-blocker (atenolol) first, then adding in a thiazide diuretic (bendroflumethiazide) as needed.

Outcome: Intervention superior in preventing stroke, CV events, and all-cause mortality. Trial ended early (due to significant reduction in all-cause mortality), thus evidence for the primary end-point (non-fatal MI and fatal CAD) did not reach significance. Mean difference in BP-lowering effect between the groups was small (only 2.7 mmHg systolic).

Reason for inclusion: Large trial showing that ACEi and CCBs are a good combination. Contributed to the removal from guidelines of beta-blockers as first-, second- or third-line agents for hypertension.

Reference: Dahlöf B, et al. Prevention of cardiovascular events with an antihypertensive regimen of amlodipine adding perindopril as required versus atenolol adding bendroflumethiazide as required, in the Anglo-Scandinavian Cardiac Outcomes Trial-Blood Pressure Lowering Arm (ASCOT-BPLA): a multicentre randomised controlled trial. Lancet. 2005;366:895–906. http://www.thelancet.com/journals/lancet/article/PIIS0140-6736(05)67185-1/fulltext

Key trial 16.3

Trial name: ACCOMPLISH.

Participants: 11 000 high-risk hypertensive patients with age >60 years old, systolic blood pressure >160 mmHg or currently on antihypertensive therapy AND evidence of end-organ damage, but no previous cardiovascular events.

Intervention: Benazepril plus amlodipine.

Control: Benazepril plus hydrochlorothiazide.

Outcome: The composite primary end-point of cardiovascular events and cardiovascular death was significantly reduced in the amlodipine arm compared to hydrochlorothiazide. With respect to blood pressure, both drug combinations were equally effective, with a significant, but minimal difference in blood pressure.

Reason for inclusion: This trial partly explains why guidelines recommend ACEi and/or CCB as first-line, before adding in diuretics.

Reference: Jamerson K, et al. Benazepril plus amlodipine or hydrochlorothiazide for hypertension in high-risk patients. N Engl J Med. 2008;359:2417–2428. http://www.nejm.org/doi/full/10.1056/NEJMoa0806182

GUIDELINES

National Institute for Health and Clinical Excellence. CG127: Clinical management of primary hypertension in adults. 2011. http://www.nice.org.uk/guidance/CG127

European Society of Cardiology, European Society of Hypertension. 2013 ESH/ESC Guidelines for the management of arterial hypertension. 2013. http://www.escardio.org/guidelines-surveys/esc-guidelines/Pages/arterial-hypertension.aspx

FURTHER READING

Marik PE, Varon J. Hypertensive crises: challenges and management. Chest. 2007;132(5):1721. http://www.ncbi.nlm.nih.gov/pubmed/17565029
Excellent overview of the management of hypertensive emergencies

Krause T, et al. Management of hypertension: summary of NICE guidance. BMJ 2011;343:d4891.
Clear summary of management and assessment of chronic hypertension.

 For additional resources and to test your knowledge, visit the companion website at:

www.wiley.com/go/camm/cardiology

17 Pericardial Disease

Laura Ah-Kye

King's College Hospital NHS Foundation Trust, London, UK

17.1 DEFINITION

- **Pericarditis:** inflammation of the two-layered serofibrous sac surrounding the heart
- **Pericardial effusion:** increased fluid between the two layers of the sac surrounding the heart (pericardium)

17.2 UNDERLYING CONCEPTS

Anatomy
1. **Pericardium:** protects and restrains the heart. It consists of two layers:
   - Visceral pericardium: serous inner layer, adherent to the myocardium, which secretes pericardial fluid
   - Parietal pericardium: serofibrous outer layer, contiguous with the visceral pericardium
2. **Pericardial fluid:** separates the two layers
3. **Phrenic nerve:** innervates the parietal pericardium

(See Audio Podcast 17.1 at **www.wiley.com/go/camm/cardiology**)

Pathophysiology
1. **Inflammatory reaction:** involving the visceral and/or parietal pericardial layers. It may be divided into:
   - *Temporal:* acute, subacute or chronic
   - *Pathology:* fibrinous (dry), effusive, constrictive
2. **Pericardial effusion:** inflammatory response triggers production of cytokines and causes secretion of fluid from the visceral pericardium
3. **Cardiac tamponade:** occurs when fluid accumulation impedes diastolic filling, decreasing cardiac output
4. **Adhesive pericarditis:** presence of adhesions due to dense fibrous tissue between the pericardial layers, the pericardium and heart, or the pericardium and neighbouring structures
5. **Constrictive pericarditis:** fibrotic thickening of the pericardium due to chronic inflammation; a late complication of pericarditis

(See Audio Podcast 17.2 at **www.wiley.com/go/camm/cardiology**)

17.3 CLINICAL TYPES

Morphological classification
1. **Fibrinous:** pericarditis with a fibrinous (fibrin-containing) inflammatory exudate
2. **Effusive:** minimal inflammation with limited exudate; instead transudate (from the visceral pericardium) accumulates
3. **Purulent:** inflammation contains pus cells and microorganisms; seen in bacterial infections
4. **Granulomatous:** characterized by diffuse fibrin deposits associated with granulomatous reaction and large effusions; caused by tuberculosis, and rarely by fungal or parasitic infections
5. **Haemorrhagic:** bloody effusion; seen in acute MI, ventricular rupture and aortic dissection, cardiac procedures, drugs that alter clotting, tuberculosis and neoplasms

Clinical Guide to Cardiology, First Edition. Edited by Christian F. Camm and A. John Camm.
© 2016 John Wiley & Sons, Ltd. Published 2016 by John Wiley & Sons, Ltd.
Companion website: www.wiley.com/go/camm/cardiology.

Temporal classification

Table 17.1 Temporal classification of pericarditis

	Duration	Type
Acute	<6 weeks	Fibrinous
		Effusive
Subacute	6 weeks–6 months	Constrictive
		Effusive–constrictive
Chronic	>6 months	Constrictive
		Effusive
		Adhesive (non-constrictive)
Recurrent	N/A	Intermittent type (symptom-free intervals without therapy)
		Incessant type (relapse occurs with discontinuation of anti-inflammatory therapy)

17.4 ACUTE PERICARDITIS

Pathophysiology
- **Mechanism**: results from inflammation of the pericardial tissue
- **Types**: inflammation is either fibrinous (dry) or effusive
- **Pain**: a consequence of phrenic nerve innervation to the parietal pericardium

Key data
Aetiology
1. Idiopathic
2. Infectious
3. Immunological
4. Myocardial infarction
5. Metabolic disorders
6. Mediastinal radiotherapy
7. Neoplasm

Box 17.1　Common viral causes of acute pericarditis

1. Coxsackie B
2. Echo 8
3. Mumps
4. EBV
5. CMV
6. HIV
7. Parvo B1

Box 17.2　Common bacterial causes of acute pericarditis

1. Tuberculosis
2. Gram-positive:
   - *Staphylococcus aureus*
   - *Streptococcus*
   - *Pneumococcus*
3. Gram-negative:
   - *Neisseria meningitidis*
   - *Haemophilus influenzae*

Box 17.3   Immunological causes of acute pericarditis

1. SLE
2. Rheumatoid arthritis
3. Ankylosing spondylitis
4. Systemic sclerosis
5. Rheumatic fever
6. Post-myocardial infarction syndrome (Dressler's syndrome)

Box 17.4   Metabolic causes of pericarditis

1. Uraemia
2. Myxoedema
3. Hypercholesterolaemia

Incidence
- True incidence and prevalence of the disease are unknown
- 5% of chest pain presentations to emergency departments
- 0.1% of hospital admissions

Mortality
Mortality rate is dependent on the agent:

- Viral pericarditis is benign
- Mortality rate of bacterial pericarditis in treated patients is 40%
- Mortality rate approaches 85% for untreated tuberculous pericarditis

Box 17.5   Causes of mortality in bacterial pericarditis

1. Cardiac tamponade
2. Sepsis
3. Constriction

Presenting features
1. **Retrosternal chest pain:** see Table 17.2 (common)
2. **Pericardial friction rub:** see Box 17.6 (common)
3. **Fever:** often present due to inflammation
4. **Signs of effusion/tamponade:** see Section 17.5

Table 17.2 Differentiating features of pericarditis from common chest pain differentials

	Pericarditis	Myocardial infarction	Pulmonary embolism
Location	Retrosternal	Retrosternal	Variable
Character	Sharp	Crushing	Sharp
Onset	Sudden	Sudden	Sudden
Change with respiration	Increases with inspiration	No	May increase with inspiration
Positional	Worse when supine	No	No
Radiation	Jaw, neck, shoulder, arms	Jaw, neck, shoulder, arms	Shoulder
Duration	Hours to days	Minutes to hours	Hours to days
GTN response	No change	Improved	No change

Box 17.6   Features of a pericardial friction rub

1. **Auscultation:**
   - Comprised of three components timed with the heart beat
   - One systolic (between S1 and S2) rub: ventricular contraction
   - Two diastolic rubs: ventricular relaxation and atrial contraction
   - Not all components are audible in all patients
2. **Site**: widespread often loudest at left lower sternal border
3. **Position**: patient sitting forward
4. **Respiratory variation**: loudest during inspiration or forced expiration
5. **Sound characteristics**: high frequency, scratchy/grating/squeaking

Risk factors

1. **Male:** viral pericarditis has a 3:1 male:female ratio
2. **Age:** more commonly described in those aged 20–50 years
3. **Transmural MI:** see Box 17.7
4. **Cardiac surgery:** post-pericardiotomy syndrome, occurs in ≤20% of CABG cases after 1 month
5. **Neoplasm:** generally occurs due to metastasis and rarely from primary pericardial tumour
6. **Uraemia:** see Box 17.8

Box 17.7   Pericarditis as a result of transmural myocardial infarction

1. **'Early' (pericarditis epistenocardica):**
   - Local inflammation at the epicardial infarct border with direct exudation
   - Occurs in 5–20% of transmural infarcts
2. **'Delayed' (Dressler's syndrome):**
   - Presents 1 week to several months post infarction
   - 0.5–5% of infarcts
   - <0.5% in patients treated with thrombolytics
3. **Incidence:** infarct-related pericarditis has declined due to myocardial revascularization

Box 17.8   Pericarditis in renal failure

1. **Uraemic pericarditis:**
   - Reported in 6–10% of patients with renal failure
   - Due to azotaemia (blood urea nitrogen >21.4 mmol/L)
2. **Dialysis-associated pericarditis:**
   - Reported in up to 13% of patients receiving chronic haemodialysis

Differentials

Most common

1. Myocardial infarction or ischaemia
2. Pneumonia
3. Costochondritis

Uncommon but dangerous

1. Pneumothorax
2. Pulmonary embolism
3. Aortic dissection

Key investigations
Bedside tests

Table 17.3 Bedside tests of use in patients presenting with acute pericarditis

Test	Justification	Potential result
ECG	Pericarditis can lead to acute myocardial injury	Widespread saddle-shaped ST-segment elevation and PR depressions

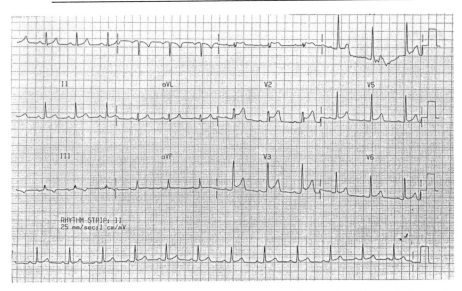

Figure 17.1 12-lead electrocardiogram from a patient with acute pericarditis showing widespread ST-segment elevation and PR-segment depression.

Blood tests

Table 17.4 Blood tests of use in patients presenting with acute pericarditis

Test	Justification	Potential result
FBC	Evidence of infection (WCC) Evidence of chronic disease (Hb)	Elevated WCC Decreased Hb
Serum troponin	Elevated levels reflect myocardial involvement	Elevated in 35–50% of patients with pericarditis (usually mild elevation) may suggest myo-pericarditis
ESR	Elevated levels are consistent with inflammatory state	Elevated
CRP	Elevated levels are consistent with inflammatory state	Elevated
Serum urea	Elevated levels of urea suggest a uraemic cause	Elevated in renal failure
Blood cultures	Evidence of infection	May be positive depending on aetiology
Viral serology	Evidence of infection	May be positive depending on aetiology
Auto-antibodies, complement level, rheumatoid factor	Evidence of autoimmune or inflammatory disease	May be positive depending on aetiology

Imaging

Table 17.5 Imaging modalities of use in patients with acute pericarditis

Test	Justification	Potential result
Trans-thoracic echocardiogram (TTE)	Indicated when pericardial effusions/cardiac tamponade suspected Also to differentiate from acute coronary syndrome	May show a pericardial effusion and absence of regional wall motion abnormalities
Chest X-ray	Concomitant lung pathology provides evidence of tuberculosis, fungal disease, pneumonia or neoplasm that may be related	Normal or water-bottle-shaped enlarged cardiac shadow

Special tests

Table 17.6 Special tests of use in patients with acute pericarditis

Test	Justification/comments	Potential result
Chest CT	May detect complications: effusion or constriction	Increased pericardial thickness, calcification, deformed ventricular contours, dilatation of the inferior vena cava and angulation of the ventricular septum
Cardiac MRI	Good sensitivity for detecting changes, constitution of pericardium and presence of pericardial fluid	Thickening of the pericardium with inflammation, evaluation of underlying myocardium, location of fluid
Pericardiocentesis/biopsy	Identification of the organism from pericardial fluid or pericardial biopsy	Dependent on aetiology

Management options

Treatment should be directed to a specific cause of pericarditis (Table 17.7).

Conservative

- **Exercise:** should be restricted for 4–6 weeks

Medical

Non-steroidal anti-inflammatory agents (NSAIDs) should be considered in all patients:

- **Duration:** 4 weeks; aiming to relieve chest pain and other inflammatory symptoms
- **Complications:** not prevented by NSAIDs (tamponade, constriction or recurrent pericarditis)
- **Ibuprofen:** 400 mg QDS; first-line medications – lower incidence of adverse reactions
- **Aspirin:** preferred in patients with a recent myocardial infarction (MI) – other NSAIDs impair scar formation; 2–4 g/day PO in three divided doses
- **Colchicine:** preferred in patients with recurrent pericarditis

Table 17.7 Treatments for various causes of acute pericarditis

Condition	Treatment
Viral/idiopathic	NSAIDs/aspirin
Bacterial/tuberculosis	Antibiotics + pericardiocentesis + NSAIDs
Acute myocardial infarction	Aspirin (avoid other NSAIDs)
Autoimmune	NSAIDs + corticosteroids
Uraemia	Dialysis (initiate or intensify)

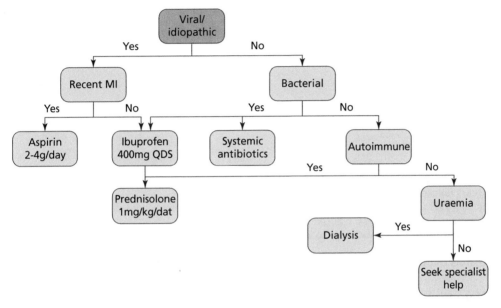

Figure 17.2 Flowchart of acute pericarditis management.

 (See Audio Podcast 17.3 at **www.wiley.com/go/camm/cardiology**)

17.5 CONSTRICTIVE PERICARDITIS

Constrictive pericarditis is a relatively rare, but disabling, consequence of chronic inflammation and fibrotic thickening of the pericardium. It leads to impaired ventricular filling, reducing stroke volume and cardiac output. Rhythm disturbance is common. Most cases occur within 3–12 months after the pericardial insult.

Pathophysiology
- **Granulation tissue**: may develop during pericardial healing or the resorption of a chronic effusion
- **Fibrosis**: develops due to ongoing inflammation increasing layer adherence and decreasing pericardial compliance
- **Ventricular filling**: decreases due to impaired ventricular dilatation against a stiffened pericardium
- **Venous congestion**: results from ventricular back pressure; causes fluid transudation from capillaries and resulting oedema

Key data
Aetiology
Can result from any cause of ongoing pericarditis, commonly:

1. Infection
2. Idiopathic
3. Previous cardiac surgery
4. Mediastinal radiotherapy
5. Chronic renal failure

Box 17.9 Infections that commonly result in constrictive pericarditis

1. Tuberculosis
2. Fungal (e.g. histoplasmosis)
3. Parasite (e.g. *Toxoplasma gondii*)

Incidence
• 9% of acute pericarditis cases

Mortality
• 30% at 5 years

Presenting features
1. **Heart failure signs and symptoms:** see Chapter 11
2. **Raised JVP:** rises with inspiration (Kussmaul's sign), and shows a prominent y descent
3. **Decreased apical impulse:** reduced by fibrotic pericardial layer
4. **Diastolic pericardial knock:** due to abrupt cessation of diastolic ventricular filling by the rigid pericardium
5. **History of pericardial disease or predisposing pericardial injury:** may predate clinical presentation by years

Differentials
1. Restrictive cardiomyopathy
2. Cardiac failure (from any other cause)
3. Cardiac tamponade
4. Right-sided valvular pathology
5. Pulmonary embolism
6. COPD

Key investigations
Bedside tests

Table 17.8 Bedside tests of use in patients presenting with constrictive pericarditis

Test	Justification	Potential result
ECG	Useful in any patient with cardiac features	Low QRS voltage Non-specific ST-segment or T-wave changes

Blood tests

Table 17.9 Blood tests of use in patients with constrictive pericarditis

Test	Justification	Potential result
FBC	Dilutional anaemia if CHF present Raised white cell count in infectious aetiology	Heart failure/chronic infection: low Hb Infection: raised WCC
Urea and electrolytes	Renal failure is a common cause of constrictive pericarditis	Raised creatinine/urea in renal failure
CRP	Raised in inflammatory conditions	Raised in constrictive pericarditis
Anti-nuclear antibodies	Systemic inflammatory conditions are common causes of constrictive pericarditis	Raised in systemic lupus erythematosus

Imaging

Table 17.10 Imaging modalities of use in patients with constrictive pericarditis

Test	Justification	Potential result
Chest X-ray	Fibrotic tissue often contains calcium	Pericardial calcifications Cardiac enlargement
TTE	Allows for direct visualization of the heart and surrounding vessels TOE allows measurement of the pericardial thickness	Pericardial thickening Prominent early diastolic filling with abrupt displacement of interventricular septum ('dip-plateau phenomenon') Systemic vein dilatation Decreased ventricular volume
CT/MRI	Accurate measurement of pericardial thickening Indication for surgery	Pericardial thickening (>2 mm) and/or calcification (Right) atrial enlargement Tube-like configuration of one or both ventricles Dilatation of the vena cava

Special tests

Table 17.11 Special tests of use in patients presenting with constrictive pericarditis

Test	Justification/comments	Potential result
Cardiac catheterization	Measurement of end-diastolic pressures	Elevated and equal LV/RV end-diastolic pressures (+/- 5 mmHg) Right ventricular systolic pressure <55 mmHg Mean pulmonary artery pressure >15 mmHg Right ventricular end-diastolic pressure >1/3 systolic pressure (narrow pulse pressure)
Coronary angiography	In all patients over 35 years and in patients with a history of mediastinal irradiation, regardless of the age	Irradiation is known to lead to constrictive pericarditis and coronary artery disease Prevalence of significant CAD among survivors is high and can be asymptomatic even in the presence of life-threatening CAD
Pericardial biopsy	Direct examination of the pericardium will provide definitive diagnosis if other tests inconclusive	Fibrotic thickening Chronic inflammation Granulomas Calcification

Management options

Medical
Treatment should be directed to a specific cause of pericarditis:

- **NSAIDs**: can be considered if there is a substantial inflammatory component (see Acute pericarditis, Section 17.4)
- **Steroids**: of some benefit if subacute constriction is present and fibrosis is yet to occur
- **Diuretics**: to alleviate congestive symptoms, however, rapid decrease in pre-load may reduce cardiac output

Interventional
- **Pericardiectomy:** the definitive treatment for permanent constriction
- **Cardiopulmonary bypass:** not recommended as bleeding risk is significantly increased following systemic heparinization
- **Mortality rate:** 6–12%

Box 17.10   Standard approach options for pericardiectomy

1. Antero-lateral thoracotomy (fifth intercostal space)
2. Median sternotomy

Box 17.11   Major complications of pericardiectomy

1. Acute perioperative cardiac insufficiency (intraprocedural myocardial damage)
2. Ventricular wall rupture
3. Excessive bleeding
4. Ventricular arrhythmias (myocardial irritation during procedure)

17.6 PERICARDIAL EFFUSION

Pathophysiology

Fluid content
- **Haemopericardium**: most commonly caused post intervention, also consider ventricular rupture post MI
- **Serous:** commonly congestive cardiac failure or uraemia
- **Serosanguinous:** caused by trauma or cardiopulmonary resuscitation
- **Chylous:** results from lymphatic obstruction or injury of the thoracic duct (rare)
- **Cholesterol:** seen in myxoedema (hypothyroidism)

Nature of effusion
- **Large effusions**: large effusions that develop slowly can be asymptomatic and not cause cardiac tamponade
- **Loculated effusions**: see Box 17.13
- **Cardiac tamponade:** accumulating effusion decreases diastolic filling, leading to low cardiac output, shock and death

---

Box 17.12   Common causes of large effusions

1. Neoplasm
2. Tuberculosis
3. Uraemic pericarditis
4. Myxoedema
5. Parasitoses

Box 17.13 Common causes of loculated effusions

1. Cardiac surgical interventions
2. Trauma
3. Purulent pericarditis

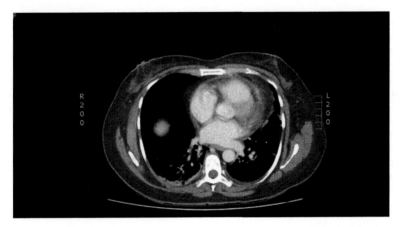

Figure 17.3 CT chest showing pericardial effusion.

(See Audio Podcast 17.4 at **www.wiley.com/go/camm/cardiology**)

Key data
Aetiology
Any cause of pericarditis can result in an infusion. Common causes include:

1. **Aortic dissection:** Stanford A type
2. **Infection:** e.g. tuberculosis
3. **Neoplasm:** especially lung or breast carcinoma
4. **Connective tissue disorders:** e.g. SLE
5. **Mediastinal radiotherapy**
6. **Cardiac intervention/surgery**

Incidence
True incidence and prevalence unknown. Incidence of iatrogenic effusions is, however, available:

- Trans-septal puncture: 1–3%
- Mitral valvuloplasty: 1–3%
- Pacemaker leads: 0.3–3.1%

Incidence of pericardial effusion in aortic dissection is 48% post-mortem and 17–45% in clinical series.

Mortality
Mortality in iatrogenic effusions:

- Trans-septal puncture <1%
- Mitral valvuloplasty <1%
- Pacemaker leads 0.1%

Aortic dissection is lethal if not operated.

Presenting features
Small, slowly accumulating effusions may be asymptomatic and have minimal clinical signs.

Box 17.14   The effect of effusions

- Although the size of the effusion is important in clinical effect, so is the speed of onset
- A slowly enlarging effusion may be asymptomatic even if large
- Small effusions may compromise a patient if they occur rapidly

1. **Symptoms from local compression:**
   - *Dyspnoea*: lung
   - *Dysphagia*: oesophagus
   - *Hoarseness*: recurrent laryngeal nerve
   - *Hiccups*: phrenic nerve
   - *Nausea*: diaphragm
   - *Ewart's sign*: large effusion compressing left lower lobe leading to apparent consolidation on clinical examination
2. **Signs of cardiac tamponade:**
   - *Beck's triad:* low BP, raised JVP, muffled HS
   - *Pulsus paradoxus:* pulse fades on inspiration due to a lowering of blood pressure
   - *Kussmaul's sign:* JVP rises on inspiration
   - *Unconsciousness*

Differentials
1. Restrictive cardiomyopathy
2. Acute pericarditis
3. Constrictive pericarditis

Key investigations
Bedside tests

Table 17.12 Bedside tests of use in patients presenting with a pericardial effusion

Test	Justification	Potential result
ECG	Useful in any patient with cardiac features	Low QRS and T-wave voltages PR-segment depression, ST-T changes, bundle branch block and electrical alternans (rarely seen in the absence of tamponade)

Blood tests

Table 17.13 Blood tests of use in patients presenting with a pericardial effusion

Test	Justification	Expected result
FBC	Dilutional anaemia if CHF present Raised white cell count in infectious aetiology	Low Hb Raised WCC may suggest bacterial pericardial effusion
Urea and electrolytes	Renal failure is a common cause of pericarditis	Raised creatinine/urea in renal failure and may suggest uraemic aetiology
CRP	Raised in inflammatory conditions	Raised in infective or inflammatory pericardial effusion
TSH	Hypothyroidism can cause pericardial effusions	Raised TSH in hypothyroidism
Anti-nuclear antibodies	Systemic inflammatory conditions are common causes of pericarditis	Raised in systemic lupus erythematosus
Blood cultures	When bacterial pericarditis and effusion is suspected	Positive blood culture in purulent pericardial effusion

Imaging

Table 17.14 Imaging modalities of use in patients presenting with a pericardial effusion

Test	Justification	Expected result
Chest X-ray	May show signs if a large pericardial effusion is present	Globular cardiomegaly with sharp margins ('water bottle' silhouette) Lucent line within the cardio-pericardial shadow (epicardial halo sign)
TTE	Preferred test to confirm the presence of a pericardial effusion	Separation of pericardial layers can be detected in echocardiography, when the pericardial fluid exceeds 15–35 mL
CT	To detect pericardial thickening or pericardial effusion	Rule out a constrictive pericarditis

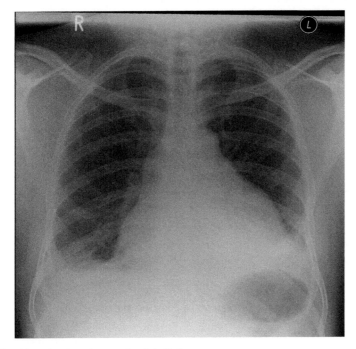

Figure 17.4 Chest X-ray showing a large pericardial effusion.

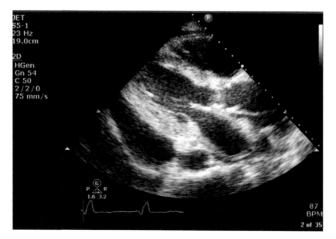

Figure 17.5 Trans-thoracic echocardiogram of a pericardial effusion.
Source: Fadi Jouhra, Kings College Hospital.

Special tests

Table 17.15 Special tests of use in patients presenting with a pericardial effusion

Test	Justification/comments	Expected result
Pericardiocentesis	Pericardial fluid and tissue analyses	Reveal the aetiology of the disease and permit further causative therapy
Pericardial biopsy	When fluid evaluation is non-diagnostic	Most useful when neoplastic or tuberculous effusions are suspected

Analysis of pericardial fluid

Diagnostic yield of fluid or tissue analysis is very low when performed for strictly diagnostic purposes without an obvious cause on initial evaluation.

Drainage is recommended in:

1. Tamponade
2. Large effusion (>20 mm) without evidence of tamponade that persists for 3 months
3. Suspected TB or bacterial pericarditis

Effusions are transudates or exudates. It is has been disputed whether classification is a useful biochemical characteristic as some studies suggest no difference in the absolute or relative LDH and protein contents among various causes of effusion.

Box 17.15   Criteria for defining an exudative pericardial effusion

- LDH >2000 U/L
- Total protein >30 g/L
- Fluid to serum LDH >0.6
- Fluid to serum protein >0.5

Box 17.16   Other analytical tests for pericardial fluid

1. Viral and bacterial culture
2. Viral PCR
3. Pericardial adenosine deaminase activity >667 nkat/L: tuberculous pericarditis
4. Pericardial interferon-gamma >200 pg/L: tuberculous pericarditis
5. Cytology: metastatic or primary malignancy

Management options
Treatment should be aimed at the underlying aetiology rather than the effusion itself wherever possible.

Medical
Small or resolving effusions can be treated with anti-inflammatory agents only (see Section 17.4).

Invasive
Pericardiocentesis indicated:

1. In haemodynamic compromise and cardiac tamponade
2. When there is no haemodynamic compromise and effusions >20 mm in diastole on echocardiography
3. For diagnostic purposes

Box 17.17   Contraindications to pericardiocentesis

1. **Absolute:**
   - Trauma
   - Ruptured ventricular aneurysm
   - Aortic dissection
2. **Relative:**
   - Uncorrected coagulopathy
   - Anticoagulant therapy
   - Thrombocytopenia
   - Small, posterior and loculated effusions

Surgical drainage indicated:

- In very large chronic effusions where alternative therapy (including pericardiocentesis) was not successful
- When pericardiocentesis is contraindicated

KEY CLINICAL TRIALS

Key Trial 17.1
Trial name: COPE.
Participants: 120 with first incidence of acute pericarditis.
Intervention: Aspirin 800 mg TDS for 7–10 days tapering over 3–4 weeks combined with colchicine for 3 months.
Control: Aspirin 800 mg TDS for 7–10 days tapering over 3–4 weeks.
Outcome: Colchicine was protective against recurrence – risk ratio 0.17 (95% CI 0.05–0.53, p = 0.003).
Reason for inclusion: Recurrent pericarditis is the most difficult complication of the disease, occurring in 15–50% of cases. The optimal management for preventing recurrences has not been established.
Reference: Imazio M, et al. Colchicine in addition to conventional therapy for acute pericarditis: results of the COlchicine for acute PEricarditis (COPE) trial. Circulation. 2005;112:2012–2016.
http://circ.ahajournals.org/content/112/13/2012.full.pdf+html

GUIDELINES

European Society of Cardiology. Guidelines on the diagnosis and management of pericardial diseases. 2004. http://www.ncbi.nlm.nih.gov/pubmed/15120056/

FURTHER READING

Lange RA, Hillis LD. Clinical practice: acute pericarditis. N Engl J Med. 2004;351:2195–2202. http://www.nejm.org/doi/full/10.1056/NEJMcp041997.
A comprehensive review of acute pericarditis published in the New England Journal of Medicine.
Shabetai R. Pericardial effusion: haemodynamic spectrum. Heart. 2004;90:255–256.
Description and explanation of haemodynamic abnormalities caused by effusive pericarditis and cardiac tamponade.

 For additional resources and to test your knowledge, visit the companion website at:

www.wiley.com/go/camm/cardiology

18 Congenital Heart Disease

Rahul K. Mukherjee

King's College Hospital NHS Foundation Trust, London, UK

18.1 DEFINITION

A cardiac or great vessel abnormality present at birth that may present from birth onwards.

18.2 UNDERLYING CONCEPTS

Acyanotic

Definition: conditions in which there is no increase in deoxygenated blood entering the systemic circulation.

- **Pathology:** mainly consist of either left-to-right shunts or obstructive lesions
- **Shunts:** left-to-right shunts cause oxygenated blood to enter the right heart due to lower pressures and resistance
- **Obstruction:** significant narrowing of a valve or blood vessel creates a pressure gradient which is necessary to create flow across a stenotic site

---

Box 18.1   Subtypes of acyanotic congenital heart disease

1. Left-to-right shunts:
    a. Atrial septal defect (ASD)
    b. Ventricular septal defect (VSD)
    c. Patent ductus arteriosus (PDA)
    d. Patent foramen ovale (PFO)
2. Obstructive lesions:
    a. Coarctation of the aorta
    b. Pulmonary stenosis

Cyanotic

- **Definition:** conditions in which deoxygenated blood bypasses the lungs and enters the systemic circulation
- **Cyanosis:** blue discoloration of the skin develops as less oxygenated blood is delivered to the tissues
- **Pathophysiology:** structural defect which promotes right-to-left shunting

---

Box 18.2   Subtypes of cyanotic congenital heart disease

1. Fallot's tetralogy
2. Transposition of the great arteries
3. Eisenmenger's syndrome

Clinical Guide to Cardiology, First Edition. Edited by Christian F. Camm and A. John Camm.
© 2016 John Wiley & Sons, Ltd. Published 2016 by John Wiley & Sons, Ltd.
Companion website: www.wiley.com/go/camm/cardiology.

18.3 ATRIAL SEPTAL DEFECT

Definition
Incomplete separation of the atria allowing flow between the chambers.

Pathophysiology and anatomy
- **Septum primum:** the initial outgrowth of tissue growing into the atrial cavity
- **Septum secundum:** a semi-lunar growth of tissue from the upper wall of the atria which develops on the right side of the septum primum
- **Cardiac septation:** abnormalities during development result in excessive resorption of the septum primum or in deficient growth of the septum secundum
- **Shunting:** the degree of left-to-right shunting depends on the defect size and the filling properties of the ventricles

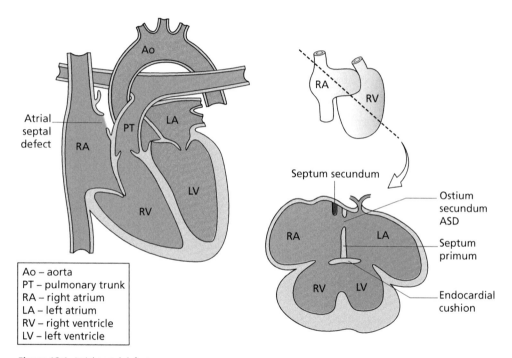

Ao – aorta
PT – pulmonary trunk
RA – right atrium
LA – left atrium
RV – right ventricle
LV – left ventricle

Figure 18.1 Atrial septal defect.

Key data
Aetiology
Syndromes associated with the development of ASDs or atrioventricular septal defects (AVSDs) include:

1. Holt–Oram syndrome: absent radial bone in arm, ASD and first-degree heart block
2. Down's syndrome: trisomy of chromosome 21
3. Noonan syndrome: autosomal dominant disorder consisting of pulmonary stenosis, septal defects, cardiomyopathy, learning difficulties and short stature
4. Alagille syndrome: autosomal dominant disorder causing a variety of defects in the heart, kidneys and liver
5. Patau syndrome: trisomy of chromosome 13

Box 18.3 Maternal risk factors in the development of ASDs

1. Use of beta-blockers
2. Alcohol
3. Smoking
4. Advanced maternal age
5. Pre-pregnancy obesity

Incidence
- 6 per 10^4 live births

Mortality
- 20% of ASDs will close spontaneously in the first year of life
- 30% of patients may develop dyspnoea by the third decade
- 10% develop supraventricular tachycardias (SVTs) and right heart failure by age 40 years
- 25% lifetime risk of mortality ascribed to unrepaired ASDs

Clinical types
1. **Ostium secundum ASD:** (70%) at site of foramen ovale
2. **Ostium primum ASD:** (15%) at the anterior and inferior aspect of the septum with mitral and tricuspid valve involvement
3. **Sinus venosus ASD:** (14%) posterior to the fossa ovalis and below the entrance of the superior vena cava (SVC) into the right atrium
4. **Coronary sinus ASD:** (1%) defect involves the coronary sinus

Presenting features

Table 18.1 Auscultatory findings in atrial septal defects

Location	Upper left sternal edge
Radiation	Back
Timing	Systolic
Pitch	Ejection
Manoeuvres	Increases on inspiration
Additional sounds	Wide fixed splitting of S2 (no change with breathing) Ejection click
Additional markers of severity	Signs of Eisenmenger's syndrome (RV heave, cyanosis, clubbing, raised JVP, peripheral oedema)

Table 18.2 Presenting features of atrial septal defect

	Acute presentation	Chronic presentation
Neurological (stroke) – due to paradoxical embolism	Limb weakness Speech and visual disturbances Facial droop	Residual weakness
Ventricular (right) dysfunction	Dyspnoea Peripheral oedema	(Exertional) dyspnoea Orthopnoea/paroxysmal nocturnal dyspnoea Fatigue Peripheral oedema Raised JVP Clubbing Cyanosis
Electrical instability	Palpitations (AF or atrial flutter) Syncope	Palpitations Syncope Pre-syncope

Differentials
Differentials of an ejection systolic murmur in a child
1. Pulmonary stenosis
2. Aortic stenosis
3. Innocent flow murmur

Differentials of splitting of the second heart sound
1. Physiological splitting (inspiration)
2. Pathological splitting during inspiration:
   - Right bundle branch block
   - Pulmonary stenosis
3. Fixed splitting of S2 (there is a split S2 but splitting does not vary with inspiration):
   - Atrial septal defect
4. Reversed splitting (increased splitting of S2 during expiration):
   - Left bundle branch block
   - Aortic stenosis

Not to miss
- Infective endocarditis: should be considered in all patients with a potentially new murmur

Key investigations
Suspicion of an ASD is normally investigated by ECG and TTE. Other investigations listed below should only be considered if required by the clinical picture.

Bedside

Table 18.3 Bedside tests in patients with suspected atrial septal defects

Test	Justification	Expected result
ABG	Patients with ASD may be breathless due to pulmonary hypertension	Type 1 respiratory failure if pulmonary hypertension present
ECG	ASDs are associated with non-specific ECG changes	See Box 18.4
Blood pressure	Hypertension can worsen left-to-right shunts due to increased afterload	Normal or high

Box 18.4   ECG findings in atrial septal defects

1. RBBB (often incomplete)
2. Left axis deviation (ostium primum defects)
3. Right axis deviation (ostium secundum defects)
4. Inverted P-waves in inferior leads (sinus venosus defects)
5. Right ventricular hypertrophy
6. Right atrial hypertrophy (P pulmonale)

Blood tests

Table 18.4 Blood tests in a patient with suspected atrial septal defect

Test	Justification	Expected result
FBC	Higher risk of endocarditis in structural heart disease (although risk is minimal in isolated ASD); polycythaemia if the patient develops Eisenmenger's syndrome	Raised WCC in endocarditis; raised haemoglobin if Eisenmenger's present
CRP	Higher risk of endocarditis in structural heart disease (although risk is minimal in isolated ASD)	Raised CRP in endocarditis
Blood cultures	To identify organism if suspecting endocarditis (consider in any new murmur)	Positive blood cultures in endocarditis

Imaging

Table 18.5 Imaging modalities used in the diagnosis of an atrial septal defect

Test	Justification	Potential result
Chest X-ray	Identify features of pulmonary hypertension	Prominent pulmonary arteries with increased pulmonary vascular markings. Double right heart border due to enlarged left atrium
Trans-thoracic echocardiogram	To determine the location and direction of shunt	Flow visualized through incomplete atrial septum

Special tests

Table 18.6 Special tests to be considered when investigating an atrial septal defect

Test	Justification	Expected result
Cardiac catheterization	To determine the severity of pulmonary hypertension and cardiac output	Decreased blood oxygen saturation in the right/left heart which helps assess the magnitude of the shunt

Management options
Conservative
Reassurance and cardiac surveillance; consider with small defects (<5 mm) and normal PA pressures.

Medical

Diuretics for congestive symptoms. If pulmonary hypertension develops consider:

- Calcium-channel blockers (e.g. nifedipine)
- Endothelin-receptor antagonists (e.g. bosentan)
- Prostacyclin analogues (e.g. epoprostenol/treprostenil)

Invasive

- ASD closure (percutaneous or surgical)

Box 18.5   Indications for ASD closure. Source: European Society of Cardiology Guidelines for the management of grown-up congenital heart disease (2010)

1. Patients with a significant shunt (>10 mm) and/or signs of RV volume overload
2. Development of a paradoxical embolism
3. Patients with significant pulmonary vascular resistance but <2/3 of systemic vascular resistance
4. Should not be undertaken if patient has developed Eisenmenger's physiology

---

18.4 VENTRICULAR SEPTAL DEFECT

Definition

A defect in the tissue wall separating the left and right ventricles.

Pathophysiology and anatomy

- **Septal components:** the majority of the septum is thick and muscular (muscular septum) whilst the upper/posterior part is thin and fibrous (membranous septum)
- **Embryology:** at 4–8 weeks of gestation, the single ventricular chamber divides. The septum is formed from the membranous portion of the interventricular septum, the endocardial cushions and bulbus cordis (proximal part of the truncus arteriosus)
- **Failure of septation:** results in a defect in the interventricular septum allowing communication between the systemic and pulmonary circulations

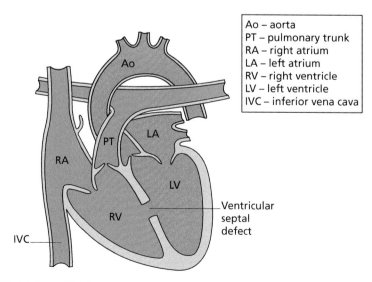

Ao – aorta
PT – pulmonary trunk
RA – right atrium
LA – left atrium
RV – right ventricle
LV – left ventricle
IVC – inferior vena cava

Figure 18.2 Ventricular septal defect.

Key data
Aetiology
VSDs can be both congenital and acquired.
  Congenital causes include:

1. Di George syndrome (22q11 deletion)
2. Down's syndrome: trisomy of chromosome 21
3. Edward's syndrome: trisomy of chromosome 18
4. Patau syndrome: trisomy of chromosome 13
5. Wolf–Hirschhorn syndrome (4p deletion): causes a number of craniofacial abnormalities, neurological and congenital heart defects

  Acquired (unlikely in children) causes include:

1. Myocardial infarction
2. Iatrogenic (e.g. septal puncture during RV pacing)

Box 18.6   Maternal risk factors for VSD development

1. Diabetes mellitus
2. Alcohol consumption (fetal alcohol syndrome)
3. Phenylketonuria

Incidence
• 4 per 10^4 live births

Mortality
• **Small defects:** excellent survival
• **Large defects:** if unrepaired, can result in the development of complications and early mortality
• **Repaired defects:** associated with a 3% operative mortality rate, survival after repair is excellent

Clinical types
1. **Perimembranous VSD:** (80%) occur in the membranous septum and lie in the LV outflow tract just below the aortic valve
2. **Supra-cristal VSD:** (5–8%) lie beneath the pulmonary valve and communicate with the RV outflow tract above the crista supraventricularis
3. **Muscular (trabecular) VSD:** (5–20%) occur in the muscular septum
4. **Posterior VSD:** (8–10%) lie posterior to the septal leaflet of the tricuspid valve

---

Box 18.7   Gerbode defect

Perimembranous ventricular septal defect associated with left ventricle–right atrial defect

---

Presenting features

Table 18.7 Auscultatory findings in ventricular septal defects

Location	Lower left sternal edge
Radiation	Throughout the praecordium
Timing	Pansystolic
Pitch	Harsh
Manoeuvres	Intensifies upon expiration
Additional markers of severity	Signs of Eisenmenger's syndrome (RV heave, cyanosis, clubbing, raised JVP, peripheral oedema, absence of a murmur)

Table 18.8 Presenting features of ventricular septal defects

	Acute presentation	Chronic presentation
Infective endocarditis	Dyspnoea Fevers Lethargy Malaise	
Ventricular dysfunction	Dyspnoea Orthopnoea Peripheral oedema	(Exertional) dyspnoea Orthopnoea Paroxysmal nocturnal dyspnoea Reduced exercise tolerance Fatigue Peripheral oedema
Electrical instability	Palpitations Syncope Sudden cardiac death (ventricular arrhythmias)	Palpitations Syncope Pre-syncope

(See Audio Podcast 18.1 at **www.wiley.com/go/camm/cardiology**)

Differentials
Differentials of a pansystolic murmur in a child:

1. Tricuspid regurgitation
2. Mitral regurgitation
3. Patent ductus arteriosus (continuous murmur, see Section 18.6)

Not to miss
• **Infective endocarditis:** should be considered in all patients with a potentially new murmur

Key investigations
Bedside

Table 18.9 Bedside tests in patients with suspected ventricular septal defects

Test	Justification	Potential result
ABG	Patients with VSD may be breathless due to pulmonary hypertension	Type 1 respiratory failure if pulmonary hypertension present
ECG	VSDs are associated with non-specific ECG changes	LVH due to volume overload. Patients who develop Eisenmenger's due to equalization of pressures may have RVH
24-hour Holter monitoring	VSDs may be associated with heart rhythm disturbances	Ventricular arrhythmias

Blood tests

Table 18.10 Blood tests in a patient with suspected ventricular septal defect

Test	Justification	Potential result
FBC	Higher risk of endocarditis in structural heart disease Polycythaemia may occur in Eisenmenger's physiology	Raised WCC in endocarditis; Raised haemoglobin if development of Eisenmenger's physiology
CRP	Higher risk of endocarditis in structural heart disease	Raised CRP in endocarditis
Blood cultures	To identify organism if suspecting endocarditis (consider in any new murmur)	Positive blood cultures in endocarditis

Imaging

Table 18.11 Imaging modalities used in the diagnosis of an ventricular septal defect

Test	Justification	Potential result
Chest X-ray	Identify features of pulmonary hypertension	Prominent pulmonary arteries with increased pulmonary vascular markings. Double right heart border due to enlarged left atrium. Larger defects may be associated with cardiomegaly
Trans-thoracic echocardiogram	To determine the location, size and direction of shunt. Assess ventricular function	Flow visualized through incomplete ventricular septum. If repaired, may see residual shunt

Special tests

Table 18.12 Special tests to be considered when investigating a ventricular septal defect

Test	Justification	Potential result
Cardiac catheterization	To determine the severity of pulmonary hypertension and cardiac output. Make an assessment of the reversibility of pulmonary hypertension	Decreased blood oxygen saturations in the right/left heart

Management options
Conservative
Reassurance (if small defect and normal PA pressures).

Medical
Diuretics for congestive symptoms. If pulmonary hypertension develops consider:

- Calcium-channel blockers (e.g. nifedipine)
- Endothelin-receptor antagonists (e.g. bosentan)
- Prostacyclin analogues (e.g. epoprostenol/treprostenil)

Invasive
- VSD closure (percutaneous or surgical)

Box 18.8   Indications for VSD closure. Source: European Society of Cardiology Guidelines for the management of grown-up congenital heart disease (2010)

1. Symptoms due to left-to-right shunting through the VSD without severe pulmonary vascular disease
2. Asymptomatic patients with evidence of LV volume overload
3. History of endocarditis
4. VSD-associated aortic valve cusp prolapse
5. Pulmonary hypertension when there is still net left-to-right shunt
6. Should not be undertaken if patient has developed Eisenmenger's physiology

18.5 COARCTATION OF THE AORTA

Definition
Narrowing of the aorta where the ductus arteriosus inserts.

Pathophysiology and anatomy
- **Afterload:** obstruction decreases blood flow to the lower torso and limbs leading to increased afterload of the left ventricle
- **Blood pressure:** increased in the aorta and arterial branches proximal to the coarctation site (arms) and decreased distally (limbs)
- **Collaterals:** collateral circulation develops over time in the internal mammary, subclavian, intercostal and spinal arteries

Key data
Aetiology
The underlying cause of coarctation is unknown but there are a number of associated conditions:

1. Bicuspid aortic valve (50–85% of cases)
2. Turner syndrome (35% of cases have coarctation)
3. Berry aneurysms
4. Mitral valve abnormalities
5. VSD
6. Patent ductus arteriosus
7. Tricuspid atresia
8. Aortic arch hypoplasia
9. Hypoplastic left heart syndrome

Incidence
- 4 per 10^4 live births

Mortality
- Following surgical correction, a 15% mortality rate is seen at 20 years

Box 18.9   Causes of death in patients with aortic coarctation

1. Coronary artery disease
2. Ventricular arrhythmia
3. Heart failure
4. Stroke
5. Ruptured aortic aneurysm

Clinical types
1. **Infantile type (preductal):** proximal to the origin of the left subclavian artery
2. **Adult type (post/juxtaductal):** distal to the origin of the left subclavian artery

Presenting features

Table 18.13 Auscultatory findings with coarctation of the aorta

Location	Aortic area
Radiation	To the back
Timing	Ejection systolic murmur
Pitch	Constant
Additional sounds	Ejection click
	Bruits heard over collaterals in the anterior axilla, scapula and left sternal border
Additional markers of severity	Hypoplastic limbs

Table 18.14 Presenting features in coarctation of the aorta

	Acute presentation	Chronic presentation
Infective endocarditis	Dyspnoea Fevers Lethargy Malaise	
Large/small vessel disease	Tearing chest pain radiating to the back following recent repair (e.g. due to aortic dissection or aortic aneurysm rupture)	Hypertension of unknown cause (especially in a young patient)
Morphological changes	–	Hypoplastic limbs (due to reduced distal perfusion)

Differentials
Most common
1. Aortic stenosis
2. Aortic sclerosis
3. Pulmonary stenosis

Dangerous
- Aortic aneurysm rupture

Not to miss
1. Turner syndrome
2. Aortic arch hypoplasia

Key investigations
Bedside

Table 18.15 Bedside tests in patients with suspected coarctation of the aorta

Test	Justification	Potential result
Blood pressure in both arms	Coarctation may lead to a differential BP depending on site of stenosis	Difference in BP in both arms
ECG	Increased afterload may result in left ventricular hypertrophy	LVH, biphasic P-waves

Blood tests

Table 18.16 Blood tests in a patient with suspected coarctation of the aorta

Test	Justification	Potential result
FBC	Higher risk of endocarditis in structural heart disease. Needed preoperatively to check haemoglobin	Raised WCC in endocarditis. Needed preoperatively to check haemoglobin
CRP	Higher risk of endocarditis in structural heart disease	Raised CRP in endocarditis
Urea & electrolytes	Reduced perfusion distally may result in abnormal renal function Co-existent hypertension due to coarctation may also result in hypertensive nephropathy	Deranged renal function (due to either effects of coarctation or hypertensive nephropathy)
Group and save/cross-match	Needed preoperatively or prior to percutaneous intervention	Results as per individual

Imaging

Table 18.17 Imaging modalities used in the diagnosis of coarctation of the aorta

Test	Justification	Potential result
Chest X-ray	To assess aortic knuckle, demonstrate presence of collaterals	Rib notching, prominent aortic knuckle, pulmonary congestion, cardiomegaly
Trans-thoracic echocardiogram	Occasionally coarctation may be seen on two-dimensional echo May be used to assess the presence of associated cardiac defects, e.g. bicuspid aortic valve	Presence of bicuspid aortic valve

Special tests

Table 18.18 Special tests to be considered when investigating coarctation of the aorta

Test	Justification	Potential result
Right and left heart catheterization	To measure peak–peak gradient across the stenotic lesion	Increased peak—peak gradient
Aortic angiography	Demonstrate presence of collaterals	Collateral circulation involving the internal mammary, subclavian, intercostal and spinal arteries
Magnetic resonance imaging	Determine involvement of adjacent vessels Monitor for the presence of aneurysms and re-stenosis	May demonstrate involvement of other major arteries

Management options
Conservative
• Surveillance

Medical
Anti-hypertensive medications in patients with hypertension associated with coarctation:

1. ACE inhibitors
2. Calcium-channel blockers
3. Diuretics

Invasive
1. Catheter-based intervention – balloon angioplasty with stent insertion
2. Surgical repair – resection of coarctation segment with end-to-end anastomosis of the aorta
3. Patch aortoplasty
4. Left subclavian flap angioplasty

Box 18.10   Indications for invasive intervention in coarctation of the aorta

1. Pressure difference >20 mmHg between upper and lower limbs
2. Hypertensive patients with >50% aortic narrowing relative to the aortic diameter at the diaphragm
3. Pathological blood pressure response during exercise
4. Significant left ventricular hypertrophy

18.6 OTHER FORMS OF CONGENITAL HEART DISEASE

Patent ductus arteriosus
- Derived from the sixth aortic arch, it connects the proximal left pulmonary artery with the descending aorta
- Allows blood to bypass the unexpanded lungs and enter the aorta for oxygenation from the placenta
- After birth, increased pO_2 causes abrupt muscle contraction leading to closure
- In some the ductus remains open, causing left-to-right shunt
- With a large PDA, LV volumes must increase to supply both cardiac output and the left-to-right shunt
- 80 cases per 10^4 live births
- Untreated, 60% mortality at 60 years
- Presents with continuous murmur throughout systole and diastole

Fallot's tetralogy
- Cyanotic condition which presents with children squatting to improve pulmonary circulation (by increasing systemic resistance)
- Four defining components:
  - Ventricular septal defect
  - Pulmonary stenosis
  - Right ventricular outflow tract obstruction
  - Over-riding aortic arch
- Initial symptoms are dependent on the severity of right ventricular hypertrophy
- 3 cases per 10^4 live births
- Untreated, 25% mortality at 1 year

Box 18.11   Syndromes associated with Fallot's tetralogy

1. Di George syndrome (22q11 deletion)
2. Alagille syndrome
3. Fetal alcohol syndrome
4. Maternal phenylketonuria

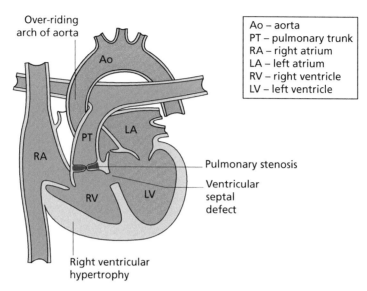

Over-riding
arch of aorta

Ao

Ao – aorta
PT – pulmonary trunk
RA – right atrium
LA – left atrium
RV – right ventricle
LV – left ventricle

LA

PT

RA

Pulmonary stenosis

Ventricular
septal
defect

RV   LV

Right ventricular
hypertrophy

Figure 18.3 Diagram of Fallot's tetralogy.

Transposition of the great arteries

- The aorta arises from the right ventricle and the pulmonary artery from the left ventricle
- Deoxygenated systemic venous blood is recirculated via the abnormal aortic connection back to the systemic circulation, bypassing the lungs
- Incompatible with life unless there is mixing of oxygenated and deoxygenated blood via a shunt
- 2–3 cases per 10^4 live births
- Untreated, 90% mortality at 1 year

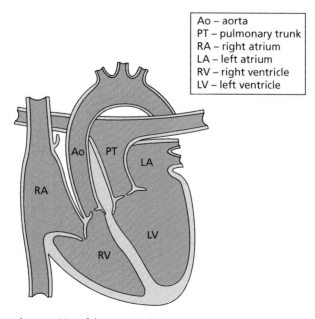

Ao – aorta
PT – pulmonary trunk
RA – right atrium
LA – left atrium
RV – right ventricle
LV – left ventricle

Ao PT

LA

RA

LV

RV

Figure 18.4 Diagram of transposition of the great arteries.

Box 18.12   Causes of Eisenmenger's syndrome

1. Atrial septal defect
2. Atrioventricular septal defect
3. Ventricular septal defect
4. Patent ductus arteriosus
5. Aortopulmonary window

Box 18.13   Eisenmenger's syndrome

1. Occurs in patients with long-standing left-to-right shunts
2. Increased pulmonary blood flow leads to pulmonary vasculature remodelling and pulmonary hypertension
3. Pulmonary hypertension results in shunt reversal
4. Development of cyanosis and right heart failure

 (See Audio Podcast 18.2 and 18.3 at **www.wiley.com/go/camm/cardiology**)

KEY CLINICAL TRIALS

Key trial 18.1

Trial name: PC Trial.
Participants: Patent foramen ovale and confirmed thromboembolic event.
Intervention: Percutaneous closure with Amplatzer PFO occluder.
Control: Medical therapy.
Outcome: No reduction in risk of embolic events/death.
Reason for inclusion: Negative outcome in a large clinical trial using a percutaneous intervention to treat PFOs in patients with a confirmed complication of PFO.
Reference: Meier B, Kalesan B, Mattle HP, et al. Percutaneous closure of patent foramen ovale in cryptogenic embolism. N Engl J Med. 2013;368(12):1083–1091.

Key trial 18.2

Trial name: BREATHE-5.
Participants: WHO class III Eisenmenger's syndrome (heart failure classification – not the same as NYHA classification).
Intervention: Bosentan therapy (endothelin-receptor antagonist).
Control: Placebo.
Outcome: Intervention improved exercise capacity and haemodynamics.
Reason for inclusion: Clear benefits observed with a medical therapy in Eisenmenger's syndrome.
Reference: Galie N, Beghetti M, Gatzoulis MA, et al. Bosentan therapy in patients with Eisenmenger syndrome: a multicenter, double-blind, randomised, placebo-controlled study. Circulation. 2006;114: 48–54.

Key trial 18.3

Trial name: Surgical treatment for secundum ASD trial.
Participants: >40 years old with an ostium secundum ASD.
Intervention: Surgical closure of ASD.
Control: Medical therapy.
Outcome: Surgical closure is superior in decreasing cardiovascular events and overall mortality.
Reason for inclusion: Demonstrated clear benefits in undertaking surgical closure of ASDs.
Reference: Attie F, Rosas M, Granados N, et al. Surgical treatment for secundum atrial septal defects in patients ≥40 years old. A randomized clinical trial. J Am Coll Cardiol. 2001;38(7):2035–2042.

GUIDELINES

American College of Cardiology and American Heart Association. Guidelines for the Management of Adults with Congenital Heart Disease. 2008. http://circ.ahajournals.org/content/118/23/e714

European Society of Cardiology. Guidelines for the management of grown-up congenital heart disease. 2010. http://eurheartj.oxfordjournals.org/content/31/23/2915.full.pdf

FURTHER READING

Briggs LE, Kakarla J, Wessels A. The pathogenesis of atrial and atrioventricular septal defects with special emphasis on the role of dorsal mesenchymal protrusion. Differentiation. 2012;84:117–130.
Excellent explanations of the embryological abnormalities resulting in the development of atrial septal defects.

Therrien, J and Webb, G. Clinical update on adults with congenital heart disease. Lancet. 2003;362:1305–1313.
Good coverage of a range of congenital heart defects – targeted at a general audience.

Penny, DJ and Wesley Vick, G. Ventricular septal defect. Lancet. 2011;377:1103–1112.
Recent clinical update on the pathophysiology and management of VSDs.

Rosenthal, E. Coarctation of the aorta from fetus to adult: curable condition or lifelong disease process? Heart. 2005;91(11):1495–1502.
Good review on coarctation of the aorta.

 For additional resources and to test your knowledge, visit the companion website at:

www.wiley.com/go/camm/cardiology

PART 4
Imaging

19 Electrocardiogram

Christian F. Camm
John Radcliffe Hospital, Oxford, UK

19.1 DEFINITION

An interpretation of the electrical activity of the heart through the use of cutaneous electrodes which can be recorded in real-time.

19.2 OUTLINE OF PROCEDURE

• 10 electrodes are placed on the skin in predefined positions

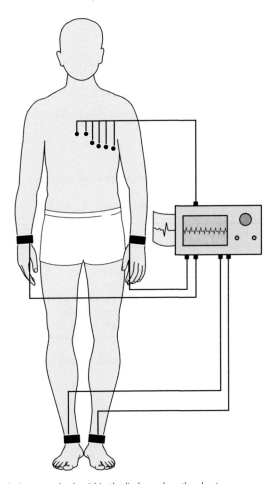

Figure 19.1 Image of lead placement both within the limbs and on the chest.

Clinical Guide to Cardiology, First Edition. Edited by Christian F. Camm and A. John Camm.
© 2016 John Wiley & Sons, Ltd. Published 2016 by John Wiley & Sons, Ltd.
Companion website: www.wiley.com/go/camm/cardiology.

- Electrodes are connected to wires which feed into the ECG device
- Multiple electrodes are combined in different patterns to generate 'leads'

Box 19.1   Definition of terms

- Electrode: physical wire and skin contact which detects the electrical activity of the heart
- Lead: a combination of electrodes which generate the electrical image

19.3 INDICATIONS

An ECG is not recommended as a general screening tool in patients without risk factors for cardiac disease or suggestive symptoms. The following symptoms would indicate the need for an ECG:

1. Palpitations
2. Chest pain
3. Murmur
4. Syncope/collapse
5. Breathlessness
6. Peripheral oedema
7. Heart failure
8. Irregular pulse

19.4 PERI-PROCEDURAL MANAGEMENT

There are no specific peri-procedural management concerns. The ECG is a non-invasive investigation.

19.5 KEY FEATURES

Leads

- Leads are generated by combining the signals from two or more electrodes

Table 19.1 Generation of ECG limb leads from electrodes (LL, left leg)

Lead	Positive pole	Negative pole	Axis
I	Left arm	Right arm	0°
II	Left leg	Right arm	60°
III	Left leg	Left arm	120°
aVL	Left arm	Left leg + right arm	30°
aVR	Right arm	Left leg + left arm	150°
aVF	Left leg	Left arm + right arm	90°

- Chest leads (V1–V6) are generated by using the corresponding chest lead as the positive pole
- Chest lead negative pole is Wilson's central terminal

Box 19.2   Wilson's central terminal

- A composite pole made from the signals of multiple electrodes
- Used as the negative pole for V1–V6

$$V_W = \frac{1}{3}(RA + LA + LL)$$

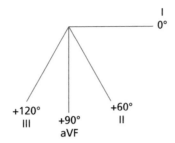

Figure 19.2 Direction of ECG limb leads.

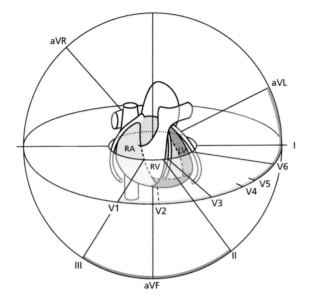

Figure 19.3 The view each lead provides of the heart. Note the two separate axes (coronal and axial).

Waves

Waves are defined deflections (positive or negative) from the isoelectric and can be either normal or pathological.

Table 19.2 Non-pathological waves that may be seen when interpreting an ECG

Wave	Representation	Normal dimensions
P	Atrial depolarization	<120 ms duration <2.5 mm amplitude
QRS	Ventricular depolarization	<120 ms duration
T	Ventricular repolarization	<160 ms duration
U	Interventricular septal repolarization	N/A

(See Audio Podcast 19.1 at **www.wiley.com/go/camm/cardiology**)

Table 19.3 Pathological waves that may be seen when interpreting an ECG

Wave	Representation	Location
J/Osborne	Hypothermia/hypercalcaemia	QRS-ST junction
Delta	Accessory electrical conduction pathway	Prior to QRS complex
Epsilon	Arrhythmogenic right ventricular dysplasia	End of QRS complex

Box 19.3   Q-waves

- Small (<1 mm): may represent septal depolarization; often seen in chest leads
- Large (>1 mm): represent previous myocardial infarction (full-thickness)

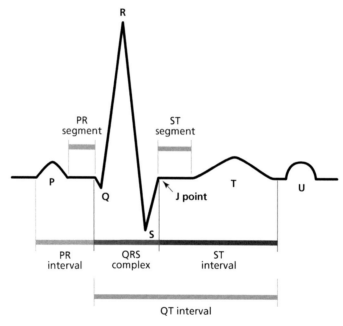

Figure 19.4   ECG waves and segments.

Segments and intervals
- **Segment:** the period of time between the end of one wave and the beginning of another
- **Interval:** a period of time including a segment and at least one wave

Table 19.4 Segments and Intervals that may be seen when interpreting an ECG

Segment/interval	Representation	Normal dimension
PR interval	Time taken for electrical impulse to travel from the SAN, through the AV node to the ventricles	120–200 ms
PR segment	Time from the end of atrial activation to the start of ventricular activation	50–120 ms
ST segment	Period when the ventricles are depolarized	80–100 ms
QT interval	Duration between ventricular depolarization and repolarization	Dependent on heart rate (see Box 19.4)

Box 19.4   How to calculate the corrected QT interval

Bazzett's formula is easier, however, Fridericia is more accurate.

$$QT/\sqrt{RR} \qquad QT/\sqrt[3]{RR}$$

$$\text{Bazzett} \qquad\qquad \text{Fridericia}$$

19.6 INTERPRETATION

Sequence of interpretation
The sequence provided here should be used when interpreting any ECG. It covers all the major aspects and prevents elements being missed.

Clinical details

Table 19.5 Important clinical details to be considered when assessing an ECG

Item	Importance
Demographic information	Age and gender may predispose to certain ECG findings
Presenting symptoms	Symptoms will give clues as to potential findings:
	• Palpitations: rhythm abnormalities
	• Chest pain: ischaemic changes
	• Syncope: rhythm abnormalities/hypertrophy

Technical aspects
- Vertical dimension represents voltage (10 mm = 1 mV)
- Horizontal dimension represents time (5 mm = 200 ms)

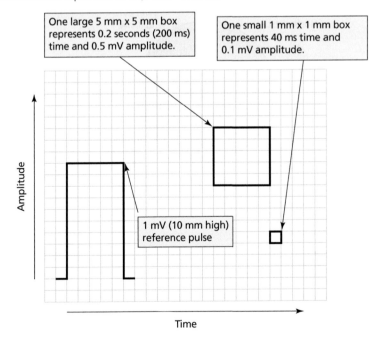

One large 5 mm x 5 mm box represents 0.2 seconds (200 ms) time and 0.5 mV amplitude.

One small 1 mm x 1 mm box represents 40 ms time and 0.1 mV amplitude.

1 mV (10 mm high) reference pulse

Amplitude

Time

Figure 19.5 ECG graph paper detailing the technical aspects of an ECG.

Rate

The ventricular rate can be calculated using one of two common methods.

Table 19.6 Methods of calculating ventricular rate on an ECG

Method	Explanation	Advantages
RR interval	Take the number of large squares on ECG paper in 1 minute (300) and divide by the number of squares between two sequential R waves	Fast
R-wave count	A 12-lead ECG strip takes 10 seconds. Multiply the number of RR intervals on the strip by 6	Slower, but takes into account variability in rhythm throughout the trace

Rhythm

- Rhythm is concerned with the regularly of the ventricular depolarization
- Should be defined as regular, regularly irregular, or irregularly irregular

Box 19.5   How to assess regularity of rhythm

1. Place piece of paper against ECG trace
2. Mark on paper the location of several R-waves
3. Shift paper along, if marks continue to line up the rhythm is regular

Axis

- Represents the overall direction of ventricular depolarization
- Normally between −30° and +90°
- Usually calculated by the ECG machine and displayed on the print-out
- Cardiac axis can be assessed by using the net depolarization of leads I, II and aVF

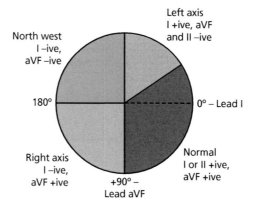

Figure 19.6 Axis of overall ventricular depolarization.

Box 19.6   Causes of left axis deviation

1. Left ventricular hypertrophy
2. Left anterior fascicular block
3. Inferior myocardial infarction
4. Wolff–Parkinson–White syndrome (right-sided accessory pathway)
5. Ostium primum ASD
6. Normal variant

Box 19.7   Causes of right axis deviation

1. Normal variant (children/thin adults)
2. Right ventricular hypertrophy
3. Chronic lung disease
4. Anterolateral myocardial infarction
5. Left posterior fascicular block
6. Pulmonary embolus
7. Wolff–Parkinson–White syndrome (left-sided accessory pathway)

P/PR:	102/148 ms
QRS:	88 ms
QT/QTc:	454/473 ms
P/QRS/T axis:	72/61/88 deg
Heart rate:	71 BPM

Figure 19.7 Standard information found on most ECG print outs. Axis of the atrial (P) and ventricular (QRS) depolarization are displayed as the fourth item on the list.

Waves and segments
P-waves:

- Best seen in lead II
- Should precede each QRS complex

Box 19.8   P-wave abnormalities

- P-mitrale – elongation of the P-wave (>120 ms) due to left atrial enlargement
- P-pulmonale – increased amplitude of the P-wave (>2.5 mm) due to right atrial enlargement

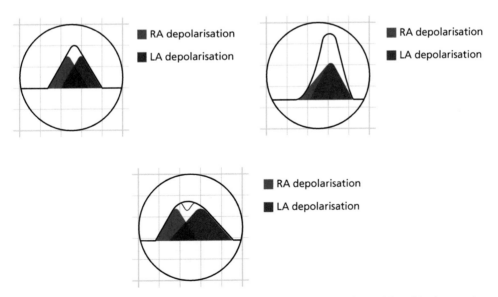

Figure 19.8 P-wave morphology. (A) Normal morphology. (B) 'Pulmonale' P-wave due to right atrial enlargement. (C) 'Mitrale' P-wave due to left atrial enlargement.

PR interval:
- Should have a consistent duration
- Shortening (<120 ms) suggests an accessory pathway bypassing the AV node
- Elongation (>200 ms) suggests impaired AV conduction

QRS complex:
- Normally consistent amplitude within leads
- Elongation (>120 ms) suggests delayed conduction within the His bundle or Purkinje fibres

Box 19.9 Causes of QRS complexes >120 ms

1. Left bundle branch block
2. Right bundle branch block
3. Ventricular origin
4. Idiopathic ventricular conduction delay
5. Hyperkalaemia
6. Ventricular paced rhythm
7. Ventricular pre-excitation (WPW pattern)

- Increased amplitude suggests ventricular hypertrophy or abnormal ventricular conduction

Box 19.10 Left ventricular hypertrophy

- Increased muscle bulk of left ventricle increases amplitude of depolarization (QRS complex)
- V1 (looking away from left ventricle) has an increased negative depolarization (S-wave)
- V6 (looking towards the left ventricle) has an increased positive depolarization (R-wave)
- If S-wave depth in V1 and R-wave height in V6 combined are >35 mm this suggests LVH

ST segment:
- Should be isoelectric, elevation/depression suggests pathology
- Myocardial ischaemia/infarction is a common cause of deviation, the location of these changes relates to the vascular territory
- Pathological deviation usually presents in contiguous leads (see Table 19.7)

Box 19.11 Causes of ST elevation

1. Infarction
2. Pericarditis
3. Bundle branch block
4. LV aneurysm
5. Brugada syndrome
6. Benign early repolarization

Table 19.7 Coronary arteries supplying specific ECG leads

Leads	Location	Vascular supply
II, III, aVF	Inferior	Right coronary artery
V1, V2	Septal	Left coronary artery
V3, V4	Anterior	Left anterior descending artery
V5, V6, I	Lateral	Left circumflex artery

T-wave:

- Should be positive in most leads
- Normally negative in aVR and V1 (occasionally V2)

Box 19.12 Causes of T-wave inversion

1. Ischaemia
2. Infarction
3. Bundle branch block
4. Pulmonary embolism
5. Digoxin use
6. Hypokalaemia
7. Cardiomyopathy
8. Normal variant
9. Left ventricular hypertrophy

Common ECG patterns
Sinus rhythm

Table 19.8 The typical features of an ECG showing (normal) sinus rhythm

Item	Detail
Rate	60–100 bpm
Rhythm	Regular
Axis	Normal
P-waves	Present
PR interval	120–200 ms
QRS complex	Narrow (<100 ms), normal amplitude
ST segment	Isoelectric
T-waves	Normal morphology

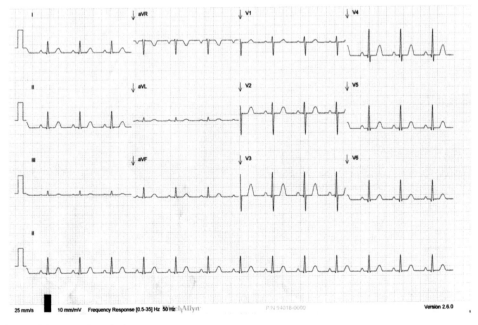

25 mm/s   10 mm/mV   Frequency Response [0.5-35] Hz 50 Hz WelchAllyn   P/N 94018-0000   Version 2.6.0

Figure 19.9 ECG – sinus rhythm.

- Sinus rhythm: any rhythm that is initiated at the sinoatrial node
- Normal sinus rhythm: a rhythm initiated at the sinoatrial node and where all components are within normal parameters

Sinus arrhythmia

Table 19.9 The typical features of an ECG showing sinus arrhythmia

Item	Detail
Rate	60–100 bpm
Rhythm	Regularly irregular (with breathing)
Axis	Normal
P-waves	Present
PR interval	120–200 ms
QRS complex	Narrow (<100 ms), normal amplitude
ST segment	Isoelectric
T-waves	Normal morphology

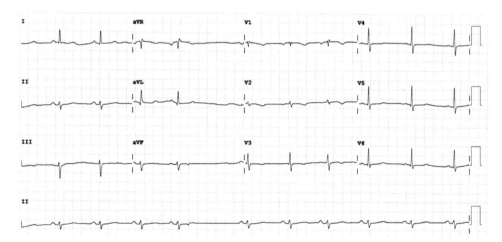

Figure 19.10 ECG – sinus arrhythmia.

Box 19.14   Physiology of respiratory sinus arrhythmia

- Inhalation decreases vagal tone, increasing heart rate
- Exhalation increases vagal tone, decreasing heart rate

Atrial fibrillation

Table 19.10 The typical features of an ECG showing atrial fibrillation

Item	Detail
Rate	Variable
Rhythm	Irregularly irregular
Axis	Normal
P-waves	Absent
PR interval	N/A
QRS complex	Narrow, normal amplitude
ST segment	Isoelectric
T-waves	Normal morphology

See Figure 13.2.

Supraventricular tachycardia

Table 19.11 The typical features of an ECG showing supraventricular tachycardia

Item	Detail
Rate	>100 bpm
Rhythm	Regular
Axis	Normal
P-waves	Often absent
PR interval	N/A
QRS complex	Narrow, normal amplitude
ST segment	Isoelectric
T-waves	Normal morphology

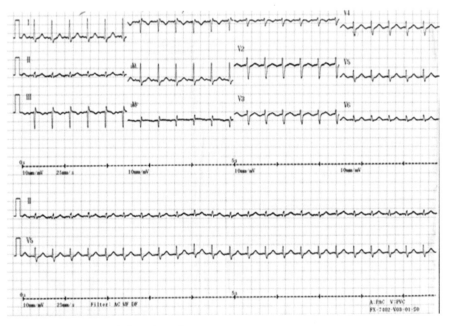

Figure 19.11 ECG – supraventricular tachycardia.

Infarction

Table 19.12 The typical features of an ECG showing infarction

Item	Detail
Rate	60–100 bpm
Rhythm	Regular
Axis	Variable
P-waves	Present
PR interval	120–200 ms
QRS complex	Narrow, normal amplitude
ST segment	Positive or negative deflection >1 mm in limb leads >2 mm in chest leads
T-waves	Variable – inverted, hyperacute

See Figure 2.3.

Left bundle branch block

Table 19.13 The typical features of an ECG showing left bundle branch block

Item	Detail
Rate	60–100 bpm
Rhythm	Regular
Axis	Normal/left
P-waves	Present
PR interval	120–200 ms
QRS complex	>120 ms V1 – W morphology V6 – M morphology
ST segment	Isoelectric
T-waves	Variable – inverted

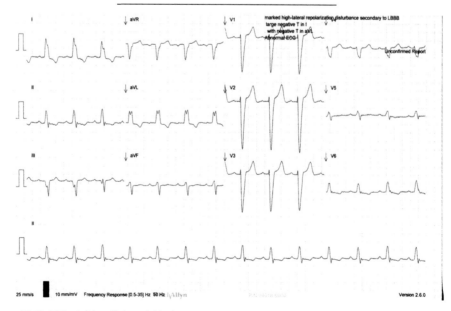

Figure 19.12 ECG – left bundle branch block.

Right bundle branch block

Table 19.14 The typical features of an ECG showing right bundle branch block

Item	Detail
Rate	60–100 bpm
Rhythm	Regular
Axis	Normal/right
P-waves	Present
PR interval	120–200 ms
QRS complex	>120 ms
	V1 – M morphology
	V6 – W morphology
ST segment	Isoelectric
T-waves	Variable – inverted

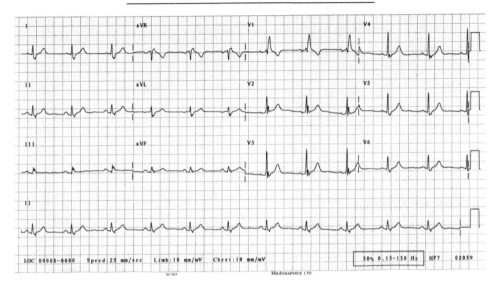

Figure 19.13 ECG – right bundle branch block.

Ventricular tachycardia

Table 19.15 The typical features of an ECG showing ventricular tachycardia

Item	Detail
Rate	>100 bpm
Rhythm	Regular
Axis	Variable
P-waves	Absent
PR interval	N/A
QRS complex	Widened (>120 ms)
ST segment	Variable
T-waves	Variable – often not seen

See Figure 13.6.

Ventricular fibrillation

This rhythm is characterized by a lack of distinct QRS complexes and should immediately trigger a cardiac arrest call.

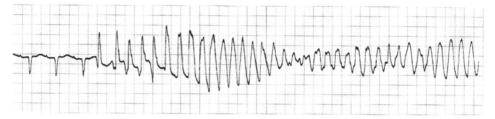

Figure 19.14 ECG – polymorphic ventricular tachycardia (torsades de pointes).

19.7 POTENTIAL COMPLICATIONS

The ECG is generally regarded as a safe procedure with no known serious complications.

Most common
• Skin sensitivity to electrodes

Dangerous
Nil

GUIDELINES

Society for Cardiological Science and Technology. Recording a standard 12-lead electrocardiogram, an approved methodology. 2010.
   http://www.scst.org.uk/resources/consensus_guideline_for_recording_a_12_lead_ecg_Rev_072010b.pdf

FURTHER READING

Corrado D, et al. Recommendations for interpretation of 12-lead electrocardiogram in the athlete. Eur Heart J. 2009;31(2):243–259.
   Extensive athletic training leads to cardiac remodelling which can appear pathological if not interpreted correctly. This review explores this challenge.
Moyer VA, et al. Screening for coronary heart disease with electrocardiography: U.S. Preventive Services Task Force recommendation statement. Ann Intern Med. 2012;157(7):512–518.
   This statement of recommendation discusses the balance of evidence for using ECGs to screen for coronary heart disease.

 For additional resources and to test your knowledge, visit the companion website at:

www.wiley.com/go/camm/cardiology

20 Transoesophageal Echocardiogram

Stephanie Hicks
King's College Hospital NHS Foundation Trust, London, UK

20.1 DEFINITION

A diagnostic ultrasound device passed via the mouth into the oesophagus, to the level of the heart, which is used to construct images of the heart chambers, valves and surrounding structures.

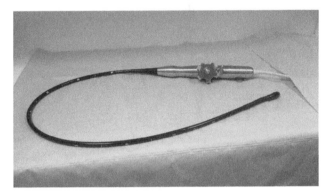

Figure 20.1 TOE probe.

20.2 OUTLINE OF PROCEDURE

Table 20.1 Transoesophageal echo procedure

Patient positioning	Left lateral position
Average procedure length	20–25 minutes
Performing clinician	Cardiologist
Other clinicians required	Anaesthetist (if performed in theatre)
Location	Varied (cardiac procedure suite, intensive care unit, theatre)
Medication given	Local anaesthetic spray (to numb back of mouth)
	Short-acting benzodiazepine (e.g. midazolam, procedural sedation)
Other equipment	Mouth guard (to protect teeth)
Procedural process	Ultrasound probe passed into the mouth and down the oesophagus
	The probe is manipulated along its course by the performing clinician in order to image important structures (listed below)
	Ultrasound images are displayed in real time to guide the operator as the procedure takes place
Structures imaged	Left and right ventricles
	Left and right atria
	Cardiac valves
	Interatrial septum
	Left atrial appendage
	Aorta (up to level of upper abdomen)

Clinical Guide to Cardiology, First Edition. Edited by Christian F. Camm and A. John Camm.
© 2016 John Wiley & Sons, Ltd. Published 2016 by John Wiley & Sons, Ltd.
Companion website: www.wiley.com/go/camm/cardiology.

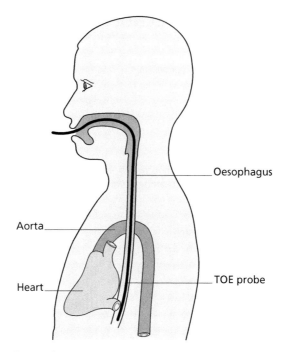

Oesophagus

Aorta

Heart

TOE probe

Figure 20.2 Positioning of TOE probe.

20.3 INDICATIONS

- Used in the evaluation of cardiac and aortic structure and function
- Limited to situations where findings will alter management and TTE is non-diagnostic

Some of the main indications for its use include:

1. Suspected infective endocarditis/identification of vegetations on cardiac valves
2. Identification of embolic source (see Box 20.1)
3. Identification of septal defects
4. Evaluation of prosthetic heart valve function
5. Suspected aortic dissection
6. Intraoperatively (see Box 20.2)
7. Preoperative assessment prior to cardiac intervention (e.g. transcatheter valve implantation)
8. Guidance of transcatheter procedures (e.g. septal defect closure)
9. Critically ill patients in an ITU setting (see Box 20.3)

Box 20.1   Intracardiac sources of embolism

1. Left atrial thrombus
2. Atrial tumours
3. Paravalvular abscesses
4. Left ventricular apex or aneurysm
5. Foramen ovale/atrial septal defect
6. Atrial septal aneurysm

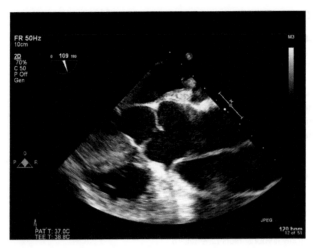

Figure 20.3 TOE image of an aortic dissection.

Box 20.2 Intraoperative indications for TOE

1. Valvular replacement surgery
2. Thoracic aortic surgical procedures
3. Coronary artery bypass graft surgery
4. Non-cardiac surgery where the patient has known or suspected cardiovascular pathology that may affect outcome

Box 20.3 Indications for TOE in ITU patients

1. Persistent unexplained hypoxaemia
2. Persistent unexplained hypotension
3. Evaluation of suspected complication of myocardial infarction (e.g acute mitral regurgitation, free wall rupture/tamponade or right ventricular involvement)

Box 20.4 Absolute contraindications to TOE

1. Perforated viscus
2. Oesophageal stricture
3. Oesophageal tumour
4. Oesophageal perforation/laceration
5. Oesophageal diverticulum
6. Active upper GI bleed

Box 20.5 Relative contraindications to TOE

1. History of GI surgery
2. Recent upper GI bleed
3. Barrett's oesophagus
4. History of dysphagia
5. Severe cervical arthritis
6. Symptomatic hiatus hernia
7. Oesophageal varices
8. Coagulopathy, thrombocytopenia
9. Active oesophagitis/peptic ulcer disease

(See Audio Podcast 20.1 at **www.wiley.com/go/camm/cardiology**)

20.4 PERI-PROCEDURAL MANAGEMENT

Prior to procedure
- **Blood tests:** none as routine (INR if on warfarin)
- **Imaging:** TTE (for elective/non-emergency patients)
- **Fasting:** 6 hours prior to procedure (4 hours for clear fluids)
- **Cannula:** yes (for IV sedation)
- **Nursing requirement:** no routine nursing escort required
- **LMWH:** can be continued prior to TOE
- **Other considerations:** dentures removed (can be damaged)

Box 20.6   Who to call when you are struggling to cannulate the patient

1. A fellow F1/F2
2. Your immediate senior (e.g. SHO, SpR)
3. Vascular access nurse
4. On-call anaesthetist (only if your seniors have failed)

Post procedure
- **Recovery:** transferred to recovery area until sedation has worn off
- **Monitoring:** routine observations (heart rate, blood pressure and oxygen saturations)
- **Blood tests:** no routine blood tests required
- **Patient advice:** cannot drive or operate heavy machinery for 24 hours; avoid food and drink for 2 hours after procedure; will need chaperone to accompany home

20.5 INTERPRETATION

As a junior doctor, you would not be expected to interpret ultrasound images from a TOE. A written report should be provided by the performing physician (see Figure 20.4).
   Key findings to look out for are as follows.

Left ventricle
- **Size:** dilatation or hypertrophy
- **Systolic function:** ejection fraction value (normal = 50–65%), description of wall motion abnormalities (sign of previous infarction)

Right ventricle
- **Size:** should be two thirds of the size of the left ventricle
- **Pressure:** right ventricular systolic pressure (RVSP) is a guide to the presence of pulmonary hypertension (normal range = 15–30 mmHg)

Atria
- **Size:** LA dilatation can be associated with AF
- **Septal flow:** colour Doppler can show atrial septum flow (evidence of ASD)

Valves
- **Stenosis:** indicated by raised mean gradient across the valve and a reduced valve area
- **Regurgitation:** can be determined by the presence of a regurgitant fraction on colour Doppler
- **Vegetations:** often described as 'mobile echogenic nodules' situated on valves

Aorta
- **Aortic root:** increased size can suggest an aortic root aneurysm
- **False lumen:** indicative of aortic dissection

Pericardium

- **Effusion:** presence of effusion and any associated respiratory variation or raised tricuspid inflow (indicators of tamponade)
- **Thickness:** pericardial thickening of ≥3 mm indicative of constrictive pericarditis

---

Interpretation Summary

A two-dimensional transthoracic echocardiogram was performed. Patient tachycardic during the study. Heart rate 110–115 bpm.

The left ventricle is normal in size. There is normal left ventricular wall thickness. The left ventricle is hyperdynamic.

Small pericardial effusion. Size approximately 5 mm posteriorly, 8–10 mm laterally and behind the right heart. No significant respiratory variation on transmitral and tricuspid inflows. No obvious RV diastolic collapse. IVC is normal in size with >50% collapse.

There is trace tricuspid regurgitation. RVSP estimated at 27–32 mmHg assuming RAP is 5–10 mmHg.

Left Ventricle

The left ventricle is normal in size. There is normal left ventricular wall thickness. The left ventricle is hyperdynamic. No regional wall motion abnormalities noted.

Right Ventricle

The right ventricle is normal in size and function.

Atria

The left atrial size is normal. Right atrial size is normal. No obvious atrial septum flow/shunt seen using colour Doppler.

Mitral Valve

The mitral valve is normal in structure and function. There is trace mitral regurgitation.

Tricuspid Valve

The tricuspid valve leaflets are thin and pliable. There is trace tricuspid regurgitation. RVSP estimated at 27–32 mmHg assuming RAP is 5–10 mmHg.

Aortic Valve

The aortic valve is trileaflet. The aortic valve opens well. No aortic regurgitation is present.

Pulmonic Valve

The pulmonic valve is normal in structure and function. Trace pulmonic valvular regurgitation.

Great Vessels

The aortic root is nromal size.

Pericardium/Pleural

Small pericardial effusion. Size approximately 5 mm posteriorly, 8–10 mm laterally and behind the right heart. No significant respiratory variation on transmitral and tricuspid inflows.

Figure 20.4 Copy of a TOE report.

20.6 POTENTIAL COMPLICATIONS

Most common

1. Lip injury (13%)
2. Voice hoarseness (12%)
3. Dysphagia (1.8%)
4. Minor pharyngeal bleeding (0.2%)

Dangerous

1. Bronchospasm (0.07%)
2. Cardiovascular complications, e.g. dysrhythmias (0.06–0.3%)
3. Oesophageal perforation (0.01–0.04%)
4. Death (<0.01%)

Box 20.7   Symptoms of bronchospasm

1. Shortness of breath
2. Chest tightness
3. Wheeze

(See Audio Podcast 20.2 at **www.wiley.com/go/camm/cardiology**)

GUIDELINES

European Society of Cardiology. Recommendations for transoesophageal echocardiography: update 2010. 2010. http://www.escardio.org/communities/EACVI/publications/Documents/eae-tee-recommendations-up2010.pdf

FURTHER READING

Hilberath JN, Oakes DA, Shernan SK, et al. Safety of transesophageal echocardiography. J Am Soc Echocardiogr. 2010;23:1115–1127.
   Outlines the key complications associated with TOE.
Evangelista A & Gonzalez-Alujas MT. Echocardiography in infective endocarditis. Heart. 2004;90(6):614–617.
   Comparison of the sensitivity of TOE compared to TTE in detecting characteristic findings in infective endocarditis, as well as outlining the role of TOE in the diagnosis of infective endocarditis.
Hahn RT, Abraham T, Adams MS, et al. Guidelines for performing a comprehensive transoesophageal echocardiographic examination: recommendations from the American Society of Echocardiography and the Society of Cardiovascular Anesthesiologists. J Am Soc Echocardiogr. 2013;26:921–964.
   Outlines the key indications for use of TOE.

 For additional resources and to test your knowledge, visit the companion website at:

www.wiley.com/go/camm/cardiology

21 Trans-Thoracic Echocardiogram

Fritz-Patrick Jahns

King's College Hospital NHS Foundation Trust, London, UK

21.1 DEFINITION

A trans-thoracic echocardiogram (TTE) is a non-invasive diagnostic imaging procedure, which uses high-frequency ultrasound waves to view the heart.

21.2 OUTLINE OF PROCEDURE

Table 21.1 Procedure of trans-thoracic echocardiography

Patient positioning	Left lateral position with the left arm behind their head (may need to move during the examination)
Average procedure length	20–30 minutes
Performing clinician	Cardiologist or cardiac sonographer/technician
Other clinicians required	None
Location	Usually cardiac diagnostic department or bedside (may also be used in satellite locations, e.g. A&E, theatres, etc.)
Medication given	None
Other equipment	Electrocardiogram (ECG) recorded throughout
Structures imaged	Atria and ventricles – most importantly the left ventricle (LV)
	Cardiac valves – most commonly aortic and mitral valves
	Pericardium/pericardial sac
	Cardiac wall thickness and muscle contractions – e.g. evidence of hypertrophy/regional wall abnormalities
	Ascending aorta
	Intracardiac masses (if any)

Clinical Guide to Cardiology, First Edition. Edited by Christian F. Camm and A. John Camm.
© 2016 John Wiley & Sons, Ltd. Published 2016 by John Wiley & Sons, Ltd.
Companion website: www.wiley.com/go/camm/cardiology.

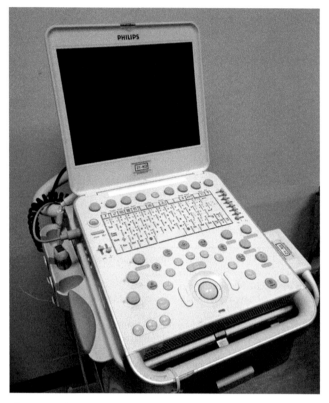

Figure 21.1 Echocardiogram machine.

(See Audio Podcast 21.1 at **www.wiley.com/go/camm/cardiology**)

21.3 INDICATIONS

Used for diagnosis of cardiac pathologies, assessment/surveillance of known pathologies, and in guiding some therapeutic techniques.

Assessment/diagnosis of valvular pathology
- New murmurs
- Suspected infective endocarditis (although has limited diagnostic capability when compared to a transoesophageal echocardiogram (TOE))
- Assessment of prosthetic valves
- Surveillance of known valvular pathology, e.g. progression of aortic stenosis

Suspected/known structural cardiac disease (diagnosis and/or surveillance)
- Ischaemic heart disease
- Cardiomyopathy
- Cardiac masses
- Septal defects

Diagnosis of pericardial disease
- Pericarditis
- Pericardial effusion

Procedural guidance
- Pericardiocentesis
- Ablation
- Therapeutic septal perforation
- Placement of devices (e.g. septal and left atrial appendage occlusion)

Risk assessment/stratification
- Risk of thromboembolism in atrial fibrillation (AF)
- Preoperatively in patients with known ischaemic heart disease/new murmur
- Stress echocardiogram to evaluate myocardial ischaemia

Box 21.1   Major causes of technical difficulty in performing a TTE

1. Patients with chronic lung disease
2. Patients with a large body habitus
3. Patients who have undergone recent cardiac surgery

Box 21.2   Imaging limitations of a TTE (also indications for a TOE)

1. **Structures:** poor imaging of small or remote cardiac elements (e.g. aorta, left atrial appendage, coronary arteries)
2. **Pathology:** lower sensitivity for certain findings (e.g. left atrial appendage thrombus)
3. **Attenuation:** increased compared to TOE (i.e. comparatively poor image quality)

(See Audio Podcast 21.2 and 21.3 at **www.wiley.com/go/camm/cardiology**)

21.4 PERI-PROCEDURAL MANAGEMENT

Prior to procedure
- **Blood tests:** none as routine
- **Imaging:** none as routine
- **Fasting:** not required prior to procedure
- **Cannula:** not normally required; may be needed if used for procedural guidance or for stress echocardiography
- **Nursing requirement:** not normally required; may be needed if unwell/haemodynamically unstable
- **LMWH:** can be continued (as with all medications) prior to TTE
- **Other considerations:** loose clothing/hospital gown should be worn to ensure appropriate exposure

Post procedure
- **Recovery:** none as routine; can be discharged when needed
- **Monitoring:** none as routine
- **Blood tests:** none as routine
- **Antibiotics:** none as routine
- **Patient advice:** patient can return to normal activities immediately post procedure

21.5 INTERPRETATION

A written report should be provided by the performing physician/technician (see Figure 21.5). Important findings include the following:

Left ventricle
- **Size:** may be small, dilated or hypertrophied
- **Intraventricular masses:** e.g. ventricular thrombus
- **Systolic function:** ejection fraction value (normally 55–65%), description of wall motion abnormalities (e.g. akinesis/hypokinesis)

Right ventricle
- Similar information as for the left ventricle
- **Size:** most useful information; often quantified in comparison to the left ventricle (the RV is normally two thirds the size of the LV)

Atria
- **Size:** normal/dilated (often in conjunction with diastolic dysfunction)
- **Septal defects:** e.g. aneurysmal septum (best seen with spectral Doppler echocardiography)

Valvular function (mainly aortic and mitral)
- **Stenosis/regurgitations:** reported as mild, moderate or severe using gradients and valve surface areas
- **Vegetation:** e.g. in infective endocarditis

Pericardium
- **Pericardial sac:** effusions/tamponade, pericardial thickening (pericarditis)

Box 21.3   Main TTE imaging modes

1. Two-dimensional (2D) imaging
2. Three-dimensional (3D) imaging
3. M-mode imaging
4. Doppler imaging

Box 21.4   Major TTE imaging views

1. **Parasternal long-axis:** assess the LV (size, function, wall thickness), LA, and mitral and aortic valves
2. **Parasternal short-axis:** assess the LV at various levels (including various regional walls), the RV and outflow tract, the tricuspid and pulmonary valves and the pulmonary arteries
3. **Apical (two-chamber or four-chamber):** assess the LV, RV, LA and RA (all together in four-chamber views) and the pericardium
4. **Subcostal:** assess the LV and RV, as well as the atrial and ventricular septa
5. **Suprasternal:** used to assess the aorta and various branches (i.e. left subclavian and common carotid)

Images from different views are often used in conjunction in the diagnosis of cardiac disease

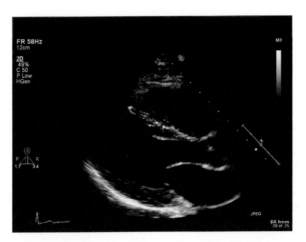

Figure 21.2 Parasternal long-axis view (TTE) showing the left ventricle (LV), left atrium (LA), and right ventricle (RV). The mitral and aortic valves are also seen.

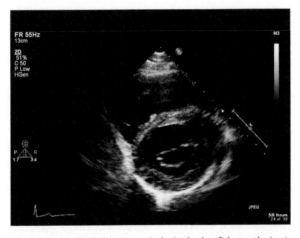

Figure 21.3 Parasternal short-axis view (TTE) showing typical mitral valve 'fish mouth view'.

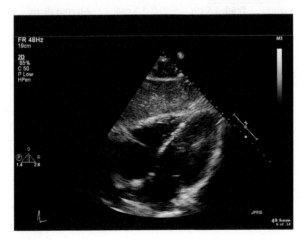

Figure 21.4 Sub-costal view. Showing the left (LA) and right (RA) atria and the left (LV) and right (RV) ventricles.

Adult Transthoracic Echocardiogram Report	
Name:	**Study Date:**
MRN:	**Patient Location:**
DOB: (dd/MM/yyyy)	**Gender:**
Age:	**Ethnicity:**
Reason For Study:	
History:	

Interpretation Summary

A two-dimensional transthoracic echocardiogram with M-mode and Doppler was performed.

The left ventricle is normal in size. Proximal septal thickening is noted. Left ventricular systolic function is normal. The right ventricle is normal in size and function.

Bi-atrial dilatation.

There is mild to moderate mitral regurgitation. There is mild to moderate tricuspid regurgitation.

Severe valvular aortic stenosis. Moderate aortic regurgitation.

Right ventricular systolic pressure is estimated at 33 mmHg + RAP 5–10 mmHg.

Left Ventricle

The left ventricle is normal in size. Proximal septal thickening is noted. Left ventricular systolic function is nromal. Ejection Fraction => 55%.

Right Ventricle

The right ventricle is normal in size and function.

Atria

The left atrium is moderately dilated. The right atrium is mild to moderately dilated.

Mitral Valve

There is mild mitral leaflet thickening. There is mild mitral annular calcification. There is mild to moderate mitral regurgitation.

Tricuspid Valve

The tricuspid valve leaflets are thickened and/or calcified, but open well. There is mild to moderate tricuspid regurgitation. Right ventricular systolic pressure is estimated at 33 mmHg + RAP 5–10 mmHg.

Aortic Valve

The aortic valve is severely calcified. Severe valvular aortic stenosis. Moderate aortic regurgitation.

Pulmonic Valve

The pulmonic valve is not well seen, but is grossly normal. Mild pulmonic valvular regurgitation.

MMode/2D Measurements & Calculations

LVIDd: 4.5 cm   (3.9–5.3 cm)   **IVSd:** 1.1 cm   (0.8–1.1 cm)   **Ao root diam:** 3.1 cm   (2.0–3.8 cm)

LVPWd: 0.79 cm   (0.5–1.1 cm)   **AVA(V,D):** 0.70 cm^2

EDV (Teich): 91.2 ml   **Ao root area:** 7.5 cm^2 **LVOT Area:** 2.7 cm^2 **LA Area:** 33.1 cm^2

RA Area: 26.6 cm^2 **TAPSE:** 1.9 cm

Doppler Measurements & Calculations

MVE max vel: 154 cm/sec   **Ao max PG (faully):** 81 mmHg   **AIP1/2t:** 740 msec   **LV V1 max PG:** 5 mmHg

Ao V2 mean: 319 cm/sec   **LV V1 mean PG:** 2 mmHg

Ao mean PG (fully): 42 mmHg   **LV V1 max:** 120 cm/sec

Ao V2 VTI: 94 cm   **LV V1 mean:** 76 cm/sec

LV V1 VT1: 24 cm

SV (LVOT): 67 ml   **TR max vel:** 289 cm/sec   **AV peak vel:** 495 cm/sec   **DSI:** 0.24

TR max PG: 33 mmHg

E/E'_Lat: 17

AVA(I,D): 0.71 cm^2

Figure 21.5 Sample TTE report.

21.6 POTENTIAL COMPLICATIONS

Most common
• Mild chest discomfort during manipulation of the transducer

Dangerous
None

GUIDELINES

The British Society of Echocardiography Education Committee. A minimum dataset for a standard transthoracic
echocardiogram. 2012. http://cdn1.cache.twofourdigital.net/u/bsecho/media/71250/tte_ds_sept_2012.pdf

 For additional resources and to test your knowledge, visit the companion website at:

www.wiley.com/go/camm/cardiology

22 Cardiac MRI

Kristopher Bennett
Whipps Cross Hospital, London, UK

22.1 DEFINITION

A non-invasive three-dimensional imaging technique using high-intensity magnetic fields and radio waves for assessment of the structure and function of the cardiovascular system.

22.2 OUTLINE OF PROCEDURE

Table 22.1 Outline of procedure of cardiac MRI

Patient positioning	Supine
Average procedure length	60 minutes
Performing clinician	Radiographer
Other clinicians required	Radiologist/cardiologist for image interpretation
Location	Radiology department
Medication given	Contrast agents (e.g. gadolinium chelates)
	Stress agents (e.g. adenosine or dipyridamole)
	Sedative agents (if claustrophobia/anxiety)
Other equipment	None
Structures imaged	Cardiac MRI can image most cardiovascular structures but it is particularly useful for imaging the following:
	Left and right ventricles
	Left and right atria
	Cardiac valves and associated structures
	Coronary arteries
	Pericardium
	Great vessels

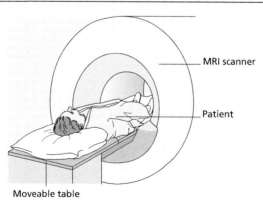

Figure 22.1 Line drawing of a typical MRI scanner.

(See Audio Podcast 22.1 at **www.wiley.com/go/camm/cardiology**)

Clinical Guide to Cardiology, First Edition. Edited by Christian F. Camm and A. John Camm.
© 2016 John Wiley & Sons, Ltd. Published 2016 by John Wiley & Sons, Ltd.
Companion website: www.wiley.com/go/camm/cardiology.

Procedure
1. The patient lies supine on the table
2. ECG monitoring is applied if required (voltage-gated imaging)
3. Technician remotely controls the movement of the table through the scanner
4. Technician initiates drug administration and communicates remotely
5. Images are processed and analysed by a radiologist/cardiologist

22.3 INDICATIONS

Cardiac MRI has a wide range of clinical applications:

1. Defining cardiac structure (see Box 22.1)
2. Quantifying left/right ventricular function
3. Assessing myocardial viability (including scars)
4. Quantifying blood flow (e.g. valvular disease, shunts)
5. Coronary artery MR angiography
6. Avoidance of other tests (e.g. poor echo windows, avoiding invasive tests)

Box 22.1 Common structural indications for cardiac MRI

1. Congenital heart disease (prior to and post surgery)
2. Aortic disease (especially aneurysm, dissection and intramural thrombus)
3. Constrictive pericarditis or pericardial masses
4. Differentiating cardiac neoplasm and thrombus
5. PFO

22.4 PERI-PROCEDURAL MANAGEMENT

Prior to procedure
1. **Blood tests:** U&E to define renal function if contrast planned (GFR <30 mL/min/1.73m^2 is a relative contraindication to gadolinium contrast agents)
2. **Imaging:** none as routine
3. **Fasting:** not routinely required
4. **Cannula:** yes – minimum 20 gauge
5. **Nursing requirement:** no routine nursing escort required
6. **LMWH:** can be continued prior to MRI
7. **Other considerations:** exclude pregnancy in women of child-bearing age; ask about absolute contraindications (see Box 22.2)

Post procedure
- **Recovery:** none as routine
- **Monitoring:** none as routine; assessment of pacemaker or ICD if present
- **Blood tests:** no routine blood tests required
- **Antibiotics:** none as standard
- **Patient advice:** none (patient can return to normal routine immediately unless sedation given)

Box 22.2   Foreign body contraindications to cardiac MRI

1. Electromechanical implants:
- Pacemakers/ICDs*
- Pacing wires*
- Hydrocephalus shunts
- Cochlear implants

2. Ferromagnetic implants and metals:
- Cerebral aneurysm clips
- Swan–Ganz catheter
- Metallic foreign bodies particularly in eyes or critical area (e.g. shrapnel)

* Some newer pacemakers and wires are MRI compatible.

Box 22.3   Generally safe for cardiac MRI

1. Cardiac:
- Sternal wires
- Coronary stents
- Heart valves and annuloplasty rings
- Epicardial wires

2. Orthopaedic implants*

3. Dental implants

4. Contraceptive devices

*Some advocate allowing 6 weeks for the implant to embed firmly in tissue before scanning.

Box 22.4   Relative contraindications for cardiac MRI

- Acutely deteriorating patients
- Claustrophobia
- Pregnancy

(See Audio Podcast 22.2 at **www.wiley.com/go/camm/cardiology**)

22.5 INTERPRETATION

The key findings to look out for depend upon the indication.

Defining cardiac anatomy

- **Pericardium:** haemorrhagic and non-haemorrhagic pericardial effusions can be differentiated, pericardial masses (e.g. cysts, lipomas or metastatic deposits) may be seen, pericardial thickening (>3 mm) is suggestive of constrictive pericarditis
- **Cardiac mass:** tumours, thrombi and vegetations can be differentiated
- **Aorta:** a false lumen and intimal flap are indicative of aortic dissection and dilatation is suggestive of aneurysm
- **Interatrial septum:** atrial septal defects and patent foramen ovale can be identified
- **Myocardium:** specific cardiomyopathies can be identified by morphology and tissue appearances, hyper-enhancing areas of inflammation suggest myocarditis

Quantifying left/right ventricular function

- **Size:** dilatation or hypertrophy
- **Systolic function:** ejection fraction value, regional wall motion abnormalities (suggestive of infarcted myocardium)

Assessing myocardial viability
- **Normal myocardium:** appears dark (low signal intensity) due to rapid contrast washout
- **Viable myocardium:** stunned/hibernating myocardium appears dark (rapid contrast washout) but with associated regional wall motion abnormality
- **Non-viable myocardium:** fibrosis, scar and acute infarcts appear bright (high signal intensity or delayed hyper-enhancement) due to delayed contrast washout

Quantifying blood flow
- **Valvular stenosis:** a reduced valve area, the presence (and velocity) of a stenotic jet and a raised mean pressure gradient
- **Valvular regurgitation:** indicated by regurgitant jets which can be measured to calculate a regurgitation fraction

Coronary artery MR angiography
- **Coronary artery disease:** regional wall motion abnormalities (stress testing), perfusion defects (perfusion imaging)
- **Anomalous coronary arteries:** anomalous origins of the left main and right coronary arteries

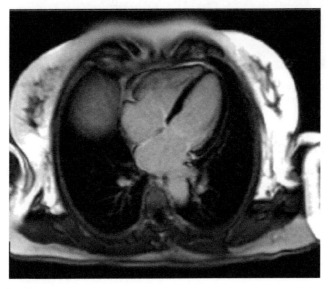

Figure 22.2 Normal cardiac MRI.
Source: Reproduced with permission from Dr Michael Papadakis, Lecturer in Cardiology, St. George's University of London.

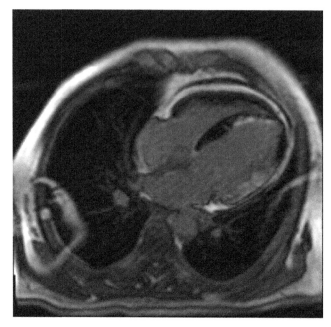

Figure 22.3 Delayed gadolinium hyper-enhancement.
Source: Reproduced with permission from Dr Michael Papadakis, Lecturer in Cardiology, St. George's University of London.

22.6 POTENTIAL COMPLICATIONS

Provided contraindications are excluded, cardiac MRI is a safe, non-invasive test with no ionizing radiation and minimal potential side effects. Most of the potential complications are due to contrast or stress agents administered during the procedure.

Most common
1. Claustrophobia (2–3%)
2. Adverse reactions to gadolinium contrast agents:
  • Headache, nausea, dizziness or altered taste (1–2%)
  • Urticarial rash or other allergic response (0.5%)

Dangerous
1. Anaphylaxis to gadolinium contrast agents (<0.001%)
2. Nephrogenic systemic fibrosis
  • No reported cases with eGFR >60 mL/min/1.73m^2
  • 1–7% with eGFR <30 mL/min/1.73m^2

Box 22.5   Nephrogenic systemic fibrosis

• This is a rare but serious complication of gadolinium-based contrast agents (not reported when eGFR >60 mL/min/1.73m^2)
• Patients with CKD (especially those on dialysis) and AKI are at particular risk
• The latent period between exposure and disease onset is usually 2–4 weeks
• It typically manifests as symmetrical, bilateral fibrotic papules, plaques or nodules; usually first appearing on the distal lower limbs before spreading proximally
• Systemic involvement may cause fibrosis of lung, pleura, myocardium, pericardium and muscles leading to contractures

KEY CLINICAL TRIALS

Key trial 22.1

Trial name: MR-IMPACT II.

Participants: 533 patients scheduled for X-ray coronary angiography (CXA) or single-photon emission computed tomography (SPECT).

Intervention: Cardiac MRI performed within 4 weeks of SPECT and CXA.

Control: All patients received CXA within 4 weeks of cardiac MRI as the reference standard for coronary artery disease (CAD).

Outcome: Sensitivity for detecting CAD was superior for cardiac MRI compared to SPECT but specificity was inferior. No severe adverse events related to cardiac MRI were reported.

Reason for inclusion: Cardiac MRI is emerging as an alternative to SPECT in CAD. This trial demonstrates cardiac MRI is a safe alternative to SPECT for detecting CAD.

Reference: Schwitter J, et al. MR-IMPACT II: Magnetic Resonance Imaging for Myocardial Perfusion Assessment in Coronary artery disease Trial: perfusion-cardiac magnetic resonance vs. single-photon emission computed tomography for the detection of coronary artery disease: a comparative multicentre, multivendor trial. Eur Heart J. 2013;34(10):775–781. http://circ.ahajournals.org/content/121/5/692.extract

Key trial 22.2

Trial name: CE-MARC.

Participants: 752 patients with suspected angina pectoris and at least one cardiovascular risk factor.

Intervention: Cardiac MRI compared to SPECT and x-ray angiography for diagnostic accuracy of ischaemic heart disease.

Control: X-ray angiography was used as the reference standard for coronary artery disease.

Outcome: Cardiac MRI showed superior sensitivity and negative predictive value over SPECT for detecting coronary artery disease with comparable specificity and positive predictive value.

Reason for inclusion: CE-MARC is the largest, prospective, real world evaluation of cardiac MRI and has established cardiac MRI's high diagnostic accuracy in coronary heart disease and its superiority over SPECT.

Reference: Greenwood JP, Maredia N, Younger JF, et al. Cardiovascular magnetic resonance and single-photon emission computed tomography for diagnosis of coronary heart disease (CE-MARC): a prospective trial. The Lancet. 2012;379(9814):453–460. http://www.ncbi.nlm.nih.gov/pubmed/22196944

GUIDELINES

European Society of Cardiology. Cardiovascular magnetic resonance pocket guide. 2013. http://www.escardio.org/communities/EACVI/publications/Pages/cmr-pocket-guide.aspx

FURTHER READING

American College of Radiology. ACR Manual on Contrast Media. 2013. Available online at: http://www.acr.org/~/media/ACR/Documents/PDF/QualitySafety/Resources/Contrast%20Manual/2013_Contrast_Media.pdf (accessed 25/02/14)

This online manual published by the American College of Radiology provides guidelines on the safe use of imaging contrast media, such as gadolinium for cardiac MRI. This will be useful for clinicians for determining the suitability of patients for cardiac MRI.

Petersen SE, et al. On behalf of the Education Committee of the European Association of Cardiovascular Imaging Association (EACVI). Update of the European Association of Cardiovascular Imaging (EACVI) Core Syllabus for the European Cardiovascular Magnetic Resonance Certification Exam. Eur Heart J Cardiovasc Imaging. 2014;15(7):728–729. http://www.ncbi.nlm.nih.gov/pubmed/24855220

A detailed review of the key areas of knowledge for those interested in cardiac MRI.

For additional resources and to test your knowledge, visit the companion website at:

www.wiley.com/go/camm/cardiology

23 Cardiac CT

Madeline Moore

King's College Hospital NHS Foundation Trust, London, UK

23.1 DEFINITION

Multi-detector row computed tomography (MDCT) is a diagnostic imaging tool that uses X-ray beams in multiple directions creating image slices that can be used to reconstruct two-dimensional (2D) and three-dimensional (3D) radiographic images of the heart and surrounding structures.

23.2 OUTLINE OF PROCEDURE

Table 23.1 Procedure for cardiac CT

Patient positioning	Supine
Average procedure length	20 minutes
Performing clinician	Radiographer
Other clinician required	Cardiologist to administer drugs
	Radiologist/Cardiologist to interpret images
Location	CT suite
Medication given	Iodine-based intravenous contrast to opacify the blood vessels (essential for angiogram only)
	Beta-blocker/CCB to slow the heart rate: aim <65 bpm
	Sublingual GTN may be given to dilate coronary vessels
	Benzodiazepine may be given as a sedative if anxious
Other equipment	Nil
Structures imaged	Left and right atria
	Left and right ventricles
	Cardiac valves
	Great vessels
	Coronary arteries
	Thorax

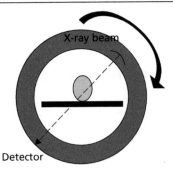

Figure 23.1 Multi-detector CT uses multiple rows (often ≥ 64) of detectors opposite the X-ray beams. The more detectors present the faster the speed of image acquisition. The ring is known as the gantry. This rotates around the patient as the patient passes through the ring at a set speed.

23.3 INDICATIONS

MDCT coronary angiogram
- Suspected coronary artery disease particularly in low- to intermediate-risk patients
- Coronary artery anomalies: evaluates malignant or non-malignant anomalous vessels
- Assessment of bypass grafts: evaluates patency, occlusions, aneurysms, pseudoaneurysms
- Cardiac surgery patient: as part of a pre-assessment
- Stents: re-stenosis assessment in selected patients
- Left ventricular function and myocardial perfusion
- Non-cardiac findings

Coronary artery calcium score
- Diagnosis of coronary artery disease (CAD) in low- to intermediate-risk patients
- Risk stratification

Box 23.1   Contraindications for CT coronary angiogram

1. Acute renal failure
2. Congestive cardiac failure (severe)
3. Pyrexia of unknown origin or acute infection
4. Allergy to contrast
5. Pregnancy
6. Hyperthyroidism (iodine-based contrast)

Box 23.2   Use of CT angiography in stent assessment

1. Re-stenosis assessment is only useful in selected patients
2. Accuracy is dependent on stent type, diameter and location
3. A stent <3 mm diameter unlikely to be measurable
4. CT artefacts known as 'blooming' severely impair the visualization of small stents

---

Box 23.3   Use of cardiac CT in patients with previous CABG

1. Re-operation has a high operative mortality and morbidity
2. Mediastinal anatomy may have been altered, e.g. adhesions
3. Assessment of pre-existing grafts and mediastinal anatomy can modify surgical approach
4. Angiogram is important for preoperative assessment to decrease operative morbidity

---

23.4 PERI-PROCEDURAL MANAGEMENT

Prior to procedure
- **Blood tests:** renal function for those with renal impairment; contrast is nephrotoxic
- **Imaging:** intra-procedural ECG ('gated ECG') is used simultaneously with the CT to achieve minimal motion artefacts
- **Fasting:** not required
- **Cannula:** minimum 20 gauge, for IV contrast, beta-blocker and sedation
- **LMWH:** continue as normal
- **Other considerations:**
  - Beta-blocker 2 days prior to procedure or intra-procedurally
  - Patient will need to hold their breath for approximately 10–30 seconds during the procedure for optimal images
  - Patient should be able to elevate their arms whilst going through the scanner

Post procedure
- **Recovery:** few hours rest if sedative or beta-blocker used; IV fluids with N-acetylcysteine (NAC) if known renal impairment
- **Monitoring:** vital observations
- **Blood tests:** renal function the following day
- **Patient advice:** can return to normal activities post procedure

23.5 INTERPRETATION
- A written report should be provided by the performing physician or radiologist
- During a CT angiogram calcium scoring is calculated simultaneously, however a calcium score can be calculated without the need for contrast

CT contrast coronary angiogram
Coronary artery system
- The presence and extent of coronary artery occlusion

Other cardiac findings
- Presence of valvular calcification
- Appearance of cardiac chambers
- Pericardial thickening and presence of effusion

Pulmonary images
- Presence of focal or diffuse abnormalities in the lungs
- Presence of pleural effusions

Box 23.4   Non-cardiac findings

1. All anatomy scanned should be reviewed
2. About 60% of all CT coronary angiograms show non-cardiac findings
3. 20% of these findings require follow-up

Calcium scoring
A score (e.g. Agatston score) is calculated based on the density and area of calcification in a given coronary artery. A total score is created by summing these individual scores.

Table 23.2 Coronary artery calcium scores and their meaning

Score	Interpretation
0	No calcified plaques
1–99	Mild plaque burden
100–399	Moderate burden
>400	Severe burden

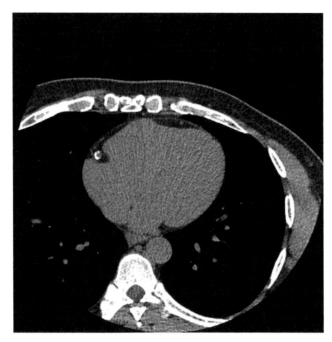

Figure 23.2 Axial slice of a cardiac CT for calcium scoring demonstrating a calcified plaque in the right mid stem of the RCA. The Agastson score was 115 for this vessel.

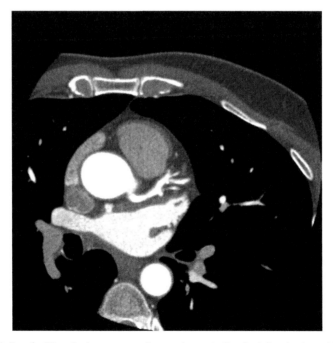

Figure 23.3 Axial slice of a CT contrast coronary angiogram demonstrating the left main stem which is unobstructed.

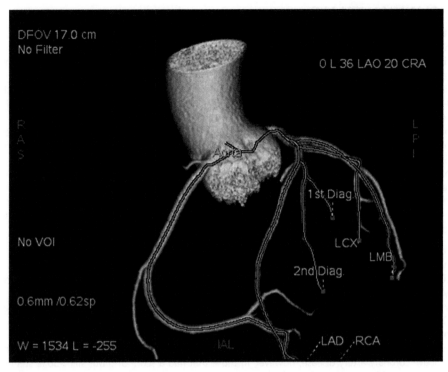

DFOV 17.0 cm
No Filter

0 L 36 LAO 20 CRA

R
A
S

L
P
I

1st Diag.

No VOI

LCX
LMB

2nd Diag.

0.6mm /0.62sp

W = 1534 L = -255

IAL

LAD RCA

Aorta

Figure 23.4 CT contrast coronary angiogram is used to create a 3D reconstruction of the coronary arteries to allow detailed views of the anatomy.

(See Audio Podcast 23.1 at **www.wiley.com/go/camm/cardiology**)

23.6 POTENTIAL COMPLICATIONS

1. Contrast nephropathy 3.7% (in patient with a pre-existing creatinine >200 μmol/L)
2. Contrast allergy (0.6%)

Box 23.5   Common signs/symptoms of iodine contrast allergy

1. Itching
2. Generalized rash or urticaria
3. Nausea and/or vomiting
4. Headache
5. Wheeze
6. Swelling or the lips or tongue
7. Acute bronchospasm
8. Anaphylaxis

It is important to note that MDCT has a high radiation dose. CT coronary angiogram has three times the radiation dose of a conventional coronary angiogram.

KEY CLINICAL TRIALS

Key trial 23.1

Trial name: ROMICAT.

Participants: Observational cohort study of 369 patients who suffered acute chest pain with normal initial troponin and non-ischaemic ECG.

Intervention: 64-slice coronary CT angiography performed to detect coronary plaque and stenosis. End-points included ACS during hospitalization and major adverse cardiac events (MACE) during the 6 month follow up.

Outcome: 50% of the patients with low to intermediate chance of ACS who suffered with acute chest pain did not have CAD on the CT and did not have ACS. Sensitivity and negative predictive value for ACS were 100% and 100% in the absence of CAD.

Reason for inclusion: Demonstrates the clinical application of CT angiography.

Reference: Hoffmann U, et al. Coronary computed tomography angiography for early triage of patients with acute chest pain – The Rule Out Myocardial Infarction Using Computer Assisted Tomography (ROMICAT) Trial. J Am Coll Cardiol. 2009;53(18):1642–1650. http://www.ncbi.nlm.nih.gov/pmc/articles/PMC2747766/

Key trial 23.2

Trial name: CONFIRM.

Participants: 10 000 symptomatic patients having undergone both coronary CT angiogram and coronary artery calcification (CAC) scoring.

Intervention: The study assessed the prevalence and severity of coronary artery disease as determined by CAC and CT angiography.

Outcome: 84% of patients with a CAC score 0 had no coronary artery disease demonstrated on a coronary CT angiogram. End-point events occurred in 0.8% of patients with a CAC score of 0 and no obstructive coronary artery disease, however, in those that had a score of 0 but still >50% stenosis on the coronary CT angiogram, 3.9% had an event.

Reason for inclusion: This study demonstrated that despite having a CAC score of 0 obstructive CAD can occur and this is associated with cardiovascular events. CAC scoring does not add prognostic value if a coronary CT angiogram has already been performed.

Reference: Villines TC, et al. Prevalence and severity of coronary artery disease and adverse events among symptomatic patients with coronary artery calcification scores of zero undergoing coronary computed tomography angiography: results from the CONFIRM (Coronary CT Angiography Evaluation for Clinical Outcomes: An International Multicenter) registry. J Am Coll Cardiol. 2011;58(24):2533–2540. http://www.ncbi.nlm.nih.gov/pubmed/22079127?dopt=Abstract.

GUIDELINES

National Institute for Health and Care Excellence (NICE). CG95: Chest pain of recent onset. 2010. http://www.nice.org.uk/guidance/CG95

European Society of Cardiology. ESC Guidelines on the management of stable coronary artery disease. 2012. http://eurheartj.oxfordjournals.org/content/34/38/2949.full.pdf

American College of Cardiology. Expert Consensus document on coronary computed tomographic angiography: a report of the American college of cardiology foundation task force on expert consensus documents. 2010. http://circ.ahajournals.org/content/121/22/2509.full.pdf

FURTHER READING

Schoenhagen P, Hachamovitch R, Achenbach S. Coronary CT angiography and comparative effectiveness research. J Am Coll Cardiol Img. 2011;4(5):492–495. doi:10.1016/j.jcmg.2011.02.013
Reviews coronary CT angiography research.

Hou ZH et al. Prognostic value of coronary CT angiography and calcium score for major adverse cardiac events in outpatients. JACC Cardiovascular Imaging. 2012;5(10):990–999 doi: 10.1016/j.jcmg.2012.06.006.
Evaluates the prognostic value of calcium scoring and CT angiography for major cardiac events.

Moscariello A, et al. Coronary CT angiography versus conventional cardiac angiography for therapeutic decision making in patients with high likelihood of coronary artery disease. Radiology. 2012;265(2):385–392 doi: 10.1148/radiol.12112426. Epub 2012 Aug 8

Coronary CT angiography versus conventional cardiac angiography for therapeutic decision making in patients with high likelihood of coronary artery disease.

 For additional resources and to test your knowledge, visit the companion website at:

www.wiley.com/go/camm/cardiology

24 Cardiac Catheterization

Fritz-Patrick Jahns

King's College Hospital NHS Foundation Trust, London, UK

24.1 DEFINITION

Cardiac catheterization is an invasive imaging procedure that allows real-time evaluation of various cardiac structures and cardiac function, as well as haemodynamic monitoring of intracardiac volumes and pressures and evaluation of coronary blood supply.

24.2 OUTLINE OF PROCEDURE

Table 24.1 Procedure for cardiac catheterization

Patient positioning	Supine
Average procedure length	30–60 minutes
Performing clinician	Interventional cardiologist
Other clinicians required	Specialist nurse Technicians (e.g. radiographer, cardiac physiologists)
Location	Cardiac catheter suite
Medication given	Sedation (as required) – commonly midazolam or fentanyl Local anaesthetic – commonly lidocaine Contrast agents Verapamil/lidocaine/adenosine (for rhythm control) GTN (relief of vasospasm and chest pain) Papaverine (for prevention or relief of vasospasm) Heparin
Other equipment	Vascular access needle (2–5 cm long, 18–21 gauge) Guide wire (usually 30–50 cm long) Cardiac catheters Cardiac monitoring equipment Fluoroscopy Vascular sealing material Splint (used by some to prevent excessive movement of puncture site)
Structures imaged	Right heart chambers and valves Left heart chambers and valves Coronary arteries Aorta Pulmonary artery

---

Box 24.1   Common cardiac catheters

1. Pigtail catheter
2. Pulmonary artery catheter
3. Judkins catheter

Clinical Guide to Cardiology, First Edition. Edited by Christian F. Camm and A. John Camm.
© 2016 John Wiley & Sons, Ltd. Published 2016 by John Wiley & Sons, Ltd.
Companion website: www.wiley.com/go/camm/cardiology.

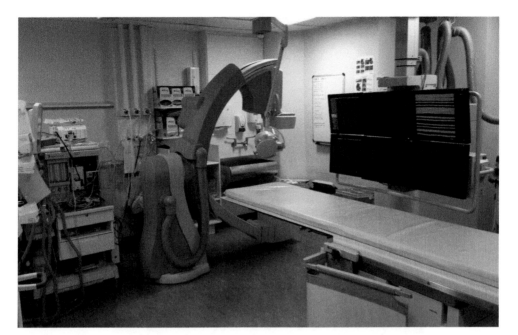

Figure 24.1 Cardiac catheterization suite.

The procedure

1. Preparation: site thoroughly cleaned (and shaved as necessary) and fully exposed with optimal patient positioning

2. Vascular access: either into central vein, or central/peripheral artery via one of two methods

---

Box 24.2   Methods of vascular access

1. Cut-down method: insertion of a catheter through an incision into the blood vessel under direct visualization

2. Percutaneous method: insertion of the catheter via a guide wire inserted through a hollow needle punctured through the skin into the blood vessel

---

3. Guide wire: (in percutaneous vascular access) inserted through the needle and left within the vessel

4. Guiding catheter: inserted either over guide wire (in percutaneous vascular access) or directly into the vessel (in cut-down vascular access) and advanced into heart chambers

5. Contrast medium: injected to image cardiac chambers, vessels and/or coronary arteries

6. Balloon catheter: advanced across the valve into the pulmonary artery and inflated – used to equalize left- and right-sided pressures

7. Withdrawal: catheter is withdrawn and pressure applied to area of access

8. Further imaging (as necessary)

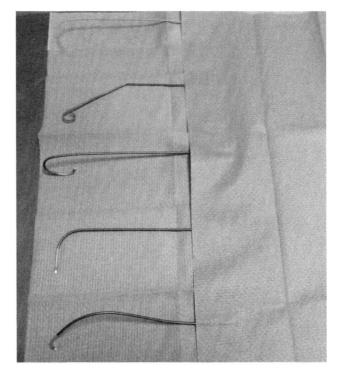

Figure 24.2 Sample cardiac catheters.

Table 24.2 Outline of left vs. right heart catheterization

	Left	Right
Access point	Peripheral artery (e.g. radial, femoral)	Central vein (e.g. internal jugular, femoral)
Structures visualized	Aorta, coronary arteries, left atrium and ventricle, aortic and mitral valves	Right atrium and ventricle, tricuspid and pulmonary valves, pulmonary arteries
Common diagnostic/ therapeutic use	Coronary angiogram +/− stenting Diagnostic imaging +/− biopsy Preoperative assessment Ventriculography Aortography	Haemodynamic measurements Diagnostic imaging +/− biopsy

24.3 INDICATIONS

- **Chambers:** to assess output and pressures in the various cardiac chambers
- **Valves:** to assess size, structure and function
- **Pulmonary disease:** pulmonary resistance and pulmonary artery pressures may be measured
- **Coronary arteries:** to assess flow, extent of disease and anatomy, and determine the need for intervention (e.g. angioplasty or surgery)
- **Congenital heart disease:** diagnose the lesion and determine the severity (e.g. septal defects, PDA)
- **Diagnostic biopsies:** pre- and post-transplant, cardiomyopathy, myocarditis and sarcoid
- **Heart failure:** evaluate myocardial contractility and degree of heart failure
- **Aorta:** to assess the vessel size and structure
- **Imaging mechanisms:** e.g. intravascular ultrasound (IVUS) and fractional flow reserve (FFR)

Box 24.3   Four main subtypes of cardiac catheterization

1. Left heart catheterization
2. Right heart catheterization
3. Ventriculography
4. Coronary angiogram (see Chapter 26)

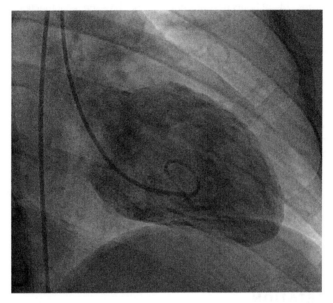

Figure 24.3 Fluoroscopic imaging: left ventriculogram.

(See Audio Podcast 24.1 and 24.2 at **www.wiley.com/go/camm/cardiology**)

24.4 PERI-PROCEDURAL MANAGEMENT

Prior to procedure

- **Blood tests:**
  - ○ *Urea and electrolytes*: to assess risk of contrast nephropathy
  - ○ *Clotting*: to assess risk of bleeding peri-procedure
- **Investigations:**
  - ○ Baseline ECG
  - ○ Baseline CXR: useful for comparison in suspected adverse events
- **Fasting:** 6 hours prior to the procedure
- **Cannula:** minimum 20 gauge (for fluid therapy or sedation)
- **Nursing requirement:** not normally required; may be needed if unwell/haemodynamically unstable
- **LMWH:**
  - ○ Prophylactic dose – hold for 12 hours prior to procedure
  - ○ Therapeutic dose – hold 24 hours prior to procedure
- **Warfarin:** often held prior to procedure (with an aim of INR <1.6), however varies
- **Other considerations:**
  - ○ Most other medications can be continued
  - ○ Confirm allergy status (especially iodine)
  - ○ Loose clothing/hospital gown should be worn
  - ○ Ensure the area of catheter insertion is clean and shaved if necessary

Post procedure
- **Recovery:** often required for a few hours especially in cases where sedation was used. *Firm pressure* required over the puncture site (especially with femoral access), particularly when the patient sneezes/coughs to avoid risks of bleeding; in some cases, a collagen sealing material is used
- **Monitoring:**
  - Cardiac monitoring often required for 1–2 hours post procedure
  - Routine observations (heart rate, blood pressure and oxygen saturations)
- **Blood tests:**
  - *Urea and electrolytes:* 24–48 hours post procedure if poor baseline renal function
  - *Clotting:* may be required if patient's anticoagulation therapy was altered
- **Antibiotics:** none as routine
- **Patient advice:** the patient should remain in bed, supine for 4–6 hours

Patient advice
- **Home:** will need to be accompanied if an outpatient procedure, particularly if sedatives used
- **Dressings:** remove entry site dressing 1 day post procedure, keep area clean and dry
- **Showering:** not for 24 hours – increased risk of bleeding
- **Driving:** can be resumed after 24 hours if no intervention performed
- **Activity:** no heavy lifting or strenuous activity for the first 2 weeks
- **Metformin:** restart after 48 hours (unless pre-existing renal failure)

Box 24.4   Discharge instructions for patients post procedure (day case)

1. Arrange for transportation home – do NOT drive yourself
2. If bleeding occurs, apply firm pressure to the site and notify a health professional
3. Do NOT attempt any heavy lifting or strenuous activities for 2 weeks post procedure
4. You may resume a normal diet and take regular medications

24.5 INTERPRETATION

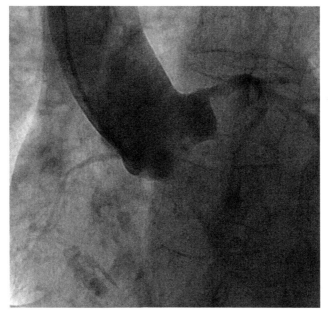

Figure 24.4 Fluoroscopic imaging: aortogram.

A written report should be provided by the performing clinician, describing the structures visualized, measurements taken and actions performed (if any).

Left heart
- **Function:** including size, volume, wall motion, contractility, presence or absence of defects (e.g. VSD)
- **Volumes and pressures:** e.g. LV end-diastolic/end-systolic volume, LV end-diastolic pressure
- **Valves:** function, size, presence/absence of defect in the mitral and aortic valves

Right heart
- **Right ventricle:** structure and function
- **Pulmonary:** arterial and wedge pressure
- **Valves:** function, size, presence/absence of defects in the tricuspid and pulmonary
- **Haemodynamics:** monitoring of central venous oxygen saturation and pressure

Coronary arteries
- **Disease severity:** presence/absence and extent
- **Interventions:** e.g. angioplasty

24.6 POTENTIAL COMPLICATIONS

General complications
1. Damage to vascular entry point (0.5–1.5%), e.g. haematoma/bleeding and infection
2. Reactions to contrast agents: mild nausea/hot flushes, vomiting, anaphylaxis
3. Contrast nephropathy
4. Vasovagal reaction
5. Cardiac tamponade
6. Air embolism
7. Transient arrhythmias

Box 24.5   Transient arrhythmia with cardiac catheterization

1. Often transient
2. Supraventricular/ventricular tachycardia/fibrillation
3. Due to direct mechanical stimulation of the nodes or chamber walls during the procedure

---

Right heart catheterization
1. Pulmonary haemorrhage/infarction due to rupture of the pulmonary artery on balloon inflation
2. Pneumothorax (if neck/chest veins are used)

Left heart catheterization
1. Stroke
2. Myocardial infarction
3. Acute coronary dissection
4. Peripheral vascular complications
5. Pseudoaneurysm
6. Death (0.1%)

GUIDELINES

American College of Cardiology Foundation, American Heart Association. ACCF/SCAI/AATS/AHA/ASE/ASNC/HFSA/ HRS/SCCM/SCCT/SCMR/STS 2012 Appropriate Use Criteria for Diagnostic Catheterization American College of Cardiology Foundation Appropriate Use Criteria Task Force. 2012. http://content.onlinejacc.org/cgi/content/full/ j.jacc.2012.03.003v1

FURTHER READING

Moore RK, et al. Spectral analysis, death and coronary anatomy following cardiac catheterization. Int J Cardiol. 2005;118(1):4–9.
Risks and data associated with cardiac catheterization.
McDaniel MC, et al. Contemporary clinical applications of coronary intravascular ultrasound. J Am Coll Cardiol Intv. 2011:4(11):1155–1167.
Recent evaluation of the evidence surrounding the use of IVUS.

 For additional resources and to test your knowledge, visit the companion website at:

www.wiley.com/go/camm/cardiology

PART 5
Interventional Therapies

25 Pacemakers and Implantable Cardiac Defibrillators

Lucy Carpenter ·
Barts Health NHS Trust, London, UK

25.1 DEFINITION

Pacemaker
An artificial device that provides electrical stimulation to maintain a normal rate of cardiac depolarization and contraction.

Implantable cardiac defibrillator (ICD)
An artificial device that provides electrical stimulation to restore a normal cardiac rhythm and prevent sudden cardiac death when ventricular arrhythmias are detected.

25.2 OUTLINE OF DEVICES

Permanent pacemakers
Single-chamber pacemaker
- Single pacing lead in either right atrium or ventricle

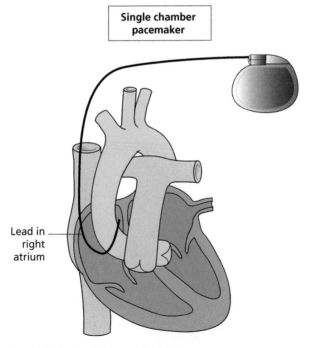

Single chamber pacemaker

Lead in right atrium

Figure 25.1 Line drawing of a single-chamber pacemaker *in situ*.

Clinical Guide to Cardiology, First Edition. Edited by Christian F. Camm and A. John Camm.
© 2016 John Wiley & Sons, Ltd. Published 2016 by John Wiley & Sons, Ltd.
Companion website: www.wiley.com/go/camm/cardiology.

Dual-chamber pacemaker
- Two leads; one in right atrium, one in right ventricle
- Coordinates contraction of the atria and the ventricles

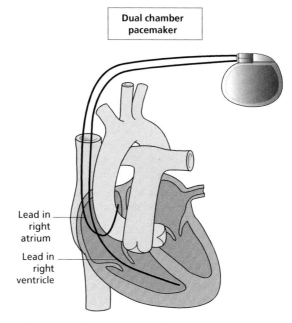

Figure 25.2 Line drawing of a dual-chamber pacemaker *in situ*.

Biventricular pacemakers
- Three leads; one in right atrium, one in right ventricle, one in left ventricle
- Increases cardiac contractility to improve heart function (cardiac resynchronization therapy)

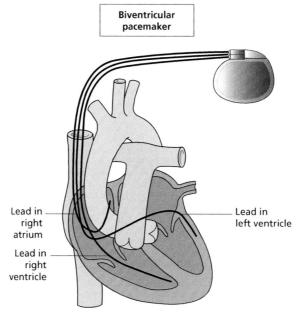

Figure 25.3 Line drawing of a bi-ventricular pacemaker *in situ*.

Implantable cardiac defibrillator
- Variable number of leads
- The lead in the right ventricle also contains a thickened coil that initiates internal defibrillation of the heart when triggered

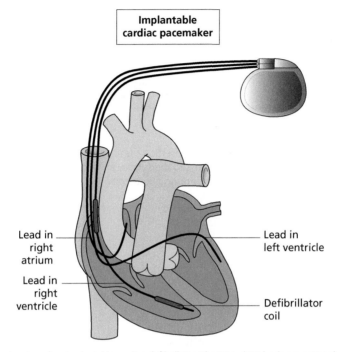

Figure 25.4 Line drawing of an implantable cardiac defibrillator. The LV and RA leads are optional.

Temporary pacing wire
- Typically a single pacing lead

Table 25.1 NASPE/BPEG pacemaker coding system consisting of three to five letters

Letter	I	II	III	IV	V
Role Coding	Chamber(s) paced O = none A = atrium V = ventricle D = dual (A+V)	Chamber(s) sensed O = none A = atrium V = ventricle D = dual (A+V)	Response to sensing O = none T = triggered I = inhibited D = dual (T+I)	Rate modulation O = none R = rate modulation – –	Multisite pacing O = none A = atrium V = ventricle D = dual (A+V)

Box 25.1   Commonly used pacemaker coding

- **AAI:** the atria are paced when the intrinsic atrial rhythm falls below threshold
- **VVI:** the ventricles are paced when the intrinsic ventricular rhythm falls below threshold
- **VDD:** able to sense both atria and ventricles, only able to pace the ventricles (coordinated with atrial activity)
- **DDD:** able to sense and pace both chambers

(See Audio Podcast 25.1 at **www.wiley.com/go/camm/cardiology**)

25.3 OUTLINE OF PROCEDURE

Table 25.2 Outline of procedure for pacemaker placement

Patient positioning	Patient on their back
Procedure length	60–90 minutes
Performing clinician	Cardiologist
Location	Cardiac catheter lab
Insertion site	Approximately 2 cm inferior to the clavicle (typically left-sided)
Medication given	Sedation given systemically
	Local anaesthetic to pacemaker insertion site
Other equipment	Fluoroscope for lead guidance and placement

Procedure
1. Local anaesthetic is administered to pacemaker insertion site
2. Leads inserted through infraclavicular incision into the subclavian vein
3. Leads guided to correct positions within heart using fluoroscopy
4. Pacemaker device inserted beneath the skin
5. Leads connected to the pacemaker using fluoroscopy
6. Pacemaker checked to ensure correct function
7. Incision closed

Box 25.2 Components of a pacemaker check

- Programmed pacing parameters
- Sensing and pacing thresholds
- Assessment of pacing capture
- Remaining battery life and estimation of time until replacement required
- Review of recorded episodes of arrhythmia detection

25.4 INDICATIONS

Indications for permanent pacemaker
1. Atrioventricular block (complete)
2. Symptomatic sinus bradycardia (see Box 25.3)
3. AF with ventricular pauses (>3 seconds) or symptomatic bradycardia
4. Cardiac resyncronization therapy (see Box 25.4)

Box 25.3 Subtypes of sinus bradycardia

- Sick sinus syndrome
- Carotid sinus syndrome
- Cardio-inhibitory vasovagal syncope

Box 25.4 Indications for cardiac resynchronization therapy

- QRS interval ≥ 120 ms
- Severe LV systolic dysfunction LVEF ($\leq 35\%$) with moderate to severe HF (NYHA III) despite optimal medical therapy

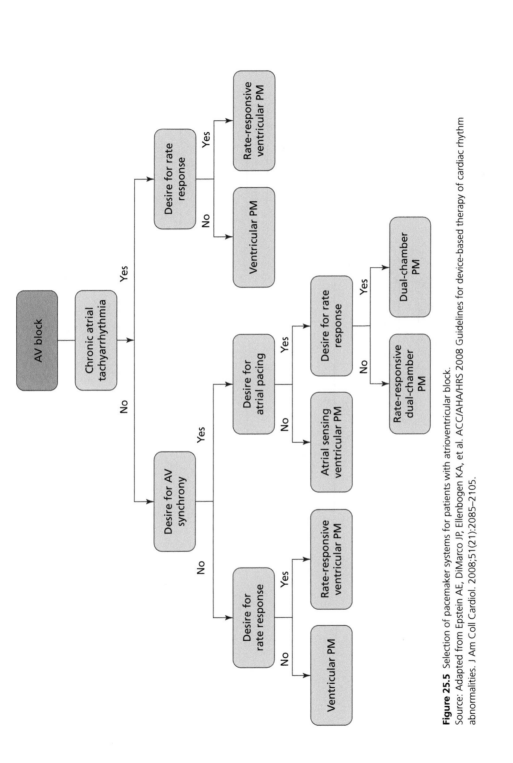

Figure 25.5 Selection of pacemaker systems for patients with atrioventricular block.

Source: Adapted from Epstein AE, DiMarco JP, Ellenbogen KA, et al. ACC/AHA/HRS 2008 Guidelines for device-based therapy of cardiac rhythm abnormalities. J Am Coll Cardiol. 2008;51(21):2085–2105.

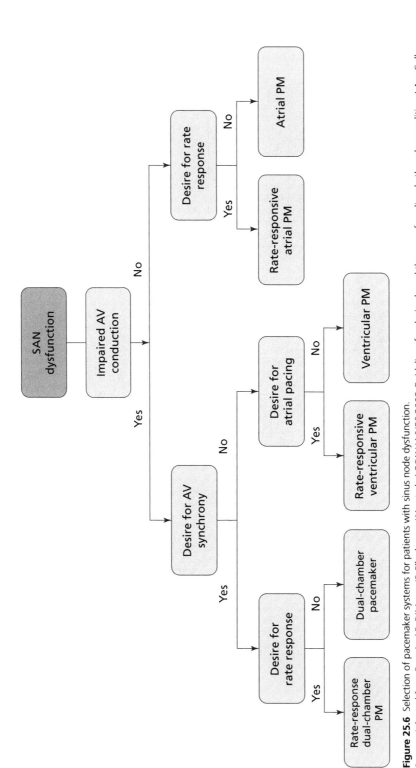

Figure 25.6 Selection of pacemaker systems for patients with sinus node dysfunction.

Source: Adapted from Epstein AE, DiMarco JP, Ellenbogen KA, et al. ACC/AHA/HRS 2008 Guidelines for device-based therapy of cardiac rhythm abnormalities. J Am Coll Cardiol. 2008;51(21):2085–2105.

Indications for temporary pacemaker
1. Symptomatic bradycardia not responding to atropine
2. Inferior MI resulting in complete heart block
3. Trifascicular block (prior to permanent pacemaker insertion)
4. Where arrhythmia requiring pacing is expected to resolve
5. Bradycardia following cardiothoracic surgery

Indications for implantable cardiac defibrillator
Primary prevention
1. LVEF ≤35% with non-sustained VT/inducible VT on electrophysiological testing
2. LVEF ≤30% and QRS ≥120 ms
3. Familial or inherited conditions with a high risk for life-threatening ventricular tachyarrhythmias

Secondary prevention
1. Cardiac arrest due to VF or VT where no reversible cause is found
2. Spontaneous sustained VT causing syncope or significant haemodynamic compromise
3. Sustained VT and with an associated reduction in ejection fraction (LVEF ≤35%)

Box 25.5   Inherited conditions with a high risk of ventricular tachyarrhythmias

- Long QT syndrome
- Brugada syndrome
- Hypertrophic cardiomyopathy
- Arrhythmogenic right ventricular dysplasia/cardiomyopathy

25.5 PERI-PROCEDURAL MANAGEMENT

Prior to procedure
- **Blood tests:** full blood count, urea and electrolytes and coagulation profile
- **Imaging:** chest X-ray (to exclude infection and structural abnormalities)
- **Fasting:** nil by mouth for 6 hours prior to the procedure
- **Cannula:** minimum 20 gauge (for IV sedation)
- **Nursing requirement:** present during procedure and throughout time spent in recovery
- **LMWH:** hold for 24 hours prior to procedure
- **Anticoagulation:** variable practice, continued with INR 2.0–2.5 or stopped 5 days prior to procedure with LMWH bridge
- **Antibiotics:** single dose of IV flucloxacillin given at insertion (unless allergies prevent) – always check local protocols

Post procedure
- **Recovery:** monitored in hospital or day-case unit – may require overnight stay
- **Cardiac monitoring:** in a cardiac-monitored bed
- **Blood tests:** not routinely needed after PM insertion
- **Imaging:** chest X-ray (to check lead positioning and to exclude pneumothorax)
- **Patient advice:** not to wash the wound site for 5–7 days. No heavy lifting for 6 weeks
- **Antibiotics:** no further doses usually required post procedure
- **Anticoagulation:** typically restarted the following day
- **Sutures:** if non-absorbable, removed after 7 days (10 days if diabetic)
- **Pacemaker check:** usually required prior to discharge

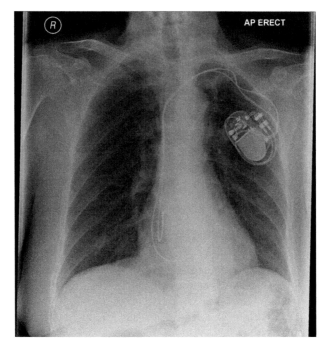

Figure 25.7 Chest radiograph of a permanent pacemaker with leads in the right atrium and right ventricle.

25.6 POTENTIAL COMPLICATIONS

1. Lead displacement (1–2%)
2. Pneumothorax (1–2%)
3. Infection (1%):
   • Localized infection of the pocket
   • Systemic infection, e.g. septicaemia
4. Cardiac tamponade

Box 25.6   Common bacteria causing infection after pacemaker insertion

• Coagulase-negative staphylococci
• *Staphylococcus aureus*
• Gram-negative enteric bacilli

(See Audio Podcast 25.2 and 25.3 at **www.wiley.com/go/camm/cardiology**)

KEY CLINICAL TRIALS

Key trial 25.1
Trial name: UKPACE.
Participants: 2000 patients >70 years of age with high-grade AV block.
Intervention: Dual-chamber pacemaker.
Control: Single-chamber pacemaker.
Outcome: Death from all causes and secondary end-points were not different between the two groups. However, procedural complications were more common in the dual-chamber group.
Reason for inclusion: Study that has been influential in pacemaker choices in the elderly.

Reference: Toff WD, Camm AJ, Skehan JD; United Kingdom Pacing: Cardiovascular Events Trial Investigators. Single-chamber versus dual-chamber pacing for high-grade atrioventricular block. N Engl J Med. 2005;353:145–155. http://www.ncbi.nlm.nih.gov/pubmed/16014884.

Key trial 25.2

Trial name: CARE-HF.

Participants: 813 patients with New York Heart Association class III or IV heart failure who are receiving standard pharmacological therapy.

Intervention: Optimal medical therapy (OMT) and CRT-D.

Control: OMT.

Outcome: CRT-D caused a 10% reduction in death rate, increased LVEF, improved symptoms and quality of life.

Reason for inclusion: One of the first studies to prove the improvement in LVF and reduction in symptoms with a CRT-D.

Reference: Cleland JGF, Daubert JC, Erdmann E, et al. The CARE-HF study (CArdiac REsynchronisation in Heart Failure study): rationale, design and end-points. Eur J Heart Fail. 2001;3:481–489. http://www .nejm.org/doi/full/10.1056/NEJMoa050496

Key trial 25.3

Trial name: CTOPP.

Participants: 2568 patients with symptomatic bradycardia.

Intervention: Dual-chamber pacemaker (atrial and ventricular pacing).

Control: Single-chamber pacemaker (ventricular pacing only).

Outcome: 9.4% relative risk reduction in stroke or death due to cardiovascular disease in dual-chamber pacing compared with single-chamber pacing. However, there were significantly more perioperative complications with dual-chamber pacing than with ventricular pacing (9.0% vs. 3.8%, $p<0.001$).

Reason for inclusion: Study that was influential in the choice of pacemaker insertion.

Reference: Connolly SJ, Kerr CR, Gent M, et al. Effects of physiologic pacing versus ventricular pacing on the risk of stroke and death due to cardiovascular causes. Canadian Trial of Physiologic Pacing Investigators. N Engl J Med. 2000;342:1385–1391. http://www.nejm.org/doi/full/10.1056/NEJM2000 05113421902

GUIDELINES

National Institute for Health and Care Excellence. Bradycardia – dual chamber pacemakers (TA88). 2005. http:// guidance.nice.org.uk/TA88.

European Society of Cardiology. 2013 ESC Guidelines on cardiac pacing and cardiac resynchronization therapy. 2013. http://www.escardio.org/guidelines-surveys/esc-guidelines/Pages/cardiac-pacing-and-cardiac-resynchronisation-therapy.aspx.

National Institute for Health and Care Excellence. Implantable cardioverter defibrillators for arrhythmias (TA095). 2006. http://www.nice.org.uk/nicemedia/live/11566/33167/33167.pdf.

American Heart Association. Guidelines for Device-Based Therapy of Cardiac Rhythm Abnormalities. 2008. http://circ.ahajournals.org/content/126/14/1784.

 For additional resources and to test your knowledge, visit the companion website at:

www.wiley.com/go/camm/cardiology

26 Percutaneous Coronary Intervention and Angioplasty

Anna Robinson

King's College Hospital NHS Foundation Trust, London, UK

26.1 DEFINITION

Coronary angiography
A method of visualizing the coronary arteries using contrast material delivered through a catheter.

Coronary angioplasty
A non-surgical method of cardiac revascularization using a catheter to dilate obstructions in the coronary artery and allow placement of a stent across an area of stenosis.

26.2 BASIC PRINCIPLES

Right coronary artery
- **Origin/Course:** arises from the right aortic sinus and descends along the right atrioventricular groove
- **Branches:** posterior descending and right marginal arteries
- **Supply:** predominantly the right atrium and ventricle, and the inferior segments of the left ventricle

---

Box 26.1   Key structures supplied by the right coronary artery

- Sinoatrial node
- Right atrium
- Right ventricle
- Atrioventricular node
- Bundle of His
- Inferior segments of the left ventricle
- +/− left atrium

Left coronary artery
- **Origin/Course:** arises from the left aortic sinus and branches early to continue down the anterior interventricular groove as the left anterior descending (LAD) artery, and the left atrioventricular groove as the left circumflex
- **Branches:** LAD, left circumflex, marginal, diagonal and septal branches
- **Supply:** the greater part of the left atrium, left ventricle and ventricular septum

---

Box 26.2   Key structures supplied by the left coronary artery

- Left atrium
- Left ventricle
- Interventricular septum
- Right and left bundle branches

Relation of ECG leads to cardiac anatomy

- **Inferior leads (II, III, aVF):** right coronary artery (RCA)
- **Anterior leads (V3, V4):** left anterior descending artery (LAD)
- **Lateral leads (I, aVL, V5, V6):** left circumflex artery (LCX)
- **Septal leads (V1, V2):** perfused by the RCA and LAD

Box 26.3   Right and left dominance

- Right dominance (70%): RCA supplies the posterior descending artery (basal interior aspect of left ventricle)
- Left dominance (20%): the left circumflex supplies the basal aspect of the left ventricle and continues as the posterior descending artery and supplies the inferior aspect of the heart
- Balanced pattern (10%): both left and right coronary arteries contribute to the supply of the posterior descending artery

---

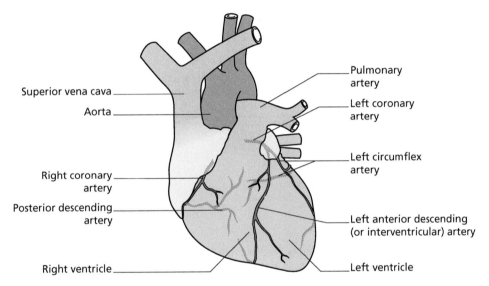

Figure 26.1 Coronary artery anatomy.

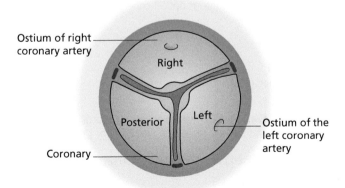

Figure 26.2 Origins of the right and left coronary artery (from above the aortic valve).

26.3 OUTLINE OF PROCEDURE

Table 26.1 Outline of procedure for PCI

Patient positioning	Supine (patient must be able to lie flat for this procedure)
Average procedure length	1–2 hours
Performing clinician	Interventional cardiologist
Other ancillary staff required	Radiographer Scrub nurse Cardiac physiologist monitoring ECG and haemodynamic data
Location	Angiography suite
Medication given	Short-acting benzodiazepine (e.g. midazolam – procedural sedation) Opiate analgesia Local anaesthetic for catheter insertion (e.g. lidocaine) Aspirin (300 mg pre-procedure) Antiplatelet agent (e.g. clopidogrel 300 mg/600 mg loading dose, 75 mg if already loaded) Heparin
Other equipment	Temporary transvenous pacemaker (if current/risk of conduction abnormality) Intra-aortic balloon pump/left ventricular assist device (if cardiogenic shock or poor LV function)

Box 26.4 Other potential antiplatelet agents used in PCI

1. Prasugrel: 60 mg loading dose (10 mg if already loaded)
2. Ticagrelor: 180 mg loading dose (90 mg if already loaded)

The procedure
1. **Arterial access:** radial (usual), femoral or brachial route
2. **Guiding catheter:** inserted and advanced around the aortic arch and into the coronary artery
3. **Contrast medium:** injected to image coronary blood flow and vessels to visualize areas of stenosis
4. **Guide wire:** inserted through the catheter and positioned across the stenosis
5. **Balloon catheter:** advanced across the stenosis and inflated – this expands the pre-mounted stent
6. **Withdrawal:** balloon and guide wire are withdrawn leaving the expanded stent *in situ*
7. **Further imaging:** intravascular ultrasound or optical coherence tomography may be required to ensure correct stent deployment

26.4 INDICATIONS

Primary (emergency) PCI
- ST-elevation myocardial Infarction (STEMI)

Urgent PCI
1. **Unstable angina/non-ST elevation ACS:** with high risk of mortality or MI within 6 months – determined using a cardiac risk stratification score (see Box 26.7) or presence of certain risk factors (see Box 26.8)
2. **Post cardiac arrest:** having sustained polymorphic VT or >30 seconds of monomorphic VT

Elective angiography +/– PCI
1. **Stable angina:** severe (class III/IV – see Table 10.1) despite optimal medical treatment
2. **High-risk CAD:** as identified on non-invasive testing

During elective angiography revascularization may be performed in the absence of complex coronary disease but often this is a diagnostic procedure and PCI is performed at a future date.

Box 26.5   Relative contraindications to PCI

- Non-amenable cardiac anatomy
- Previous (severe) contrast reaction
- Pre-existing renal failure
- Acute infection/stroke/bleeding
- Severe electrolyte abnormalities

Box 26.6   Features of stenotic lesions at high risk of PCI failure or serious complications

- Diffuse lesion
- Proximal vessels excessively tortuous
- Extremely angular segment
- Total occlusion over 3 months or bridging collateral vessels
- Bifurcated lesions – inability to protect major side branches
- Degenerated vein grafts with friable lesions in patients with previous CABG

Box 26.7   GRACE score criteria (predicts cumulative 6-month risk of mortality or myocardial infarction)

- Age
- HR
- Systolic BP
- Creatinine
- Class of heart failure
- Cardiac arrest on admission
- ST-segment deviation
- Elevated cardiac enzymes

Box 26.8   Indicators predicting high risk of thrombosis or progression to MI, requiring urgent angiography

- Ongoing or recurrent ischaemia
- Dynamic spontaneous ST changes
- Deep ST depression in anterior leads V2–V4
- Haemodynamic instability
- Major ventricular arrhythmia

 (See Audio Podcast 26.1 at **www.wiley.com/go/camm/cardiology**)

26.5 PERI-PROCEDURAL MANAGEMENT

Prior to procedure
- **Blood tests:**
  - FBC: assess for pre-existing anaemia or thrombocytopenia
  - Urea and electrolytes: renal function assessment prior to contrast
  - Clotting: INR <2 for femoral access
  - Group and save: in case a transfusion is required
- **Imaging:** baseline ECG only
- **Fasting:** 6 hours for solids, 2 hours clear liquids
- **Cannula:** minimum 20 gauge (for IV sedation)

- **Nursing requirement:** no routine nursing escort required
- **Warfarin:**
  - Typically held 2–3 days prior to procedure
  - Primary PCI: radial approach used, reversal not required
- **LMWH:**
  - Prophylactic – hold for 12 hours prior to procedure
  - Therapeutic – hold 24 hours prior to procedure
  - Fondaparinux – hold on day of procedure
- **Other considerations:** metformin held 24 hours prior to procedure

---

Box 26.9   PCI in patients with chronic renal disease

- Metformin should be stopped 48 hours prior to procedure
- Consider IV fluids and N-acetylcysteine prior to procedure (follow local guidelines)
- If previous contrast reaction, discuss this with a senior; consider giving steroids prior to procedure

---

Post procedure
- **Recovery:** transferred to recovery area for approximately 5–6 hours
- **Monitoring:**
  - Cardiac monitoring for 2 hours post procedure
  - Routine observations (heart rate, blood pressure and oxygen saturations)
- **Blood tests:**
  - Urea and electrolytes 24–48 hours post procedure if poor baseline renal function
  - Metformin can be restarted once creatinine has returned to baseline (normally a minimum period of 48 hours is observed)
  - Full blood count if concerns of significant blood loss
- **Medications:**
  - Aspirin (75 mg OD) – minimum of 12 months post stent insertion – normally life-long
  - Clopidogrel (75 mg OD) – 1–3 months (bare-metal stent), 12 months (drug-eluting stents) or alternative antiplatelets (i.e. prasugrel/ticagrelor)
  - LMWH – re-start 8 hours post procedure (often held for longer, seek senior advice if unsure)
- **Antibiotics:** none as standard

Patient advice
- **Home:** will need to be accompanied if an outpatient procedure
- **Dressings:** remove entry site dressing 1 day post procedure, keep area clean and dry
- **Showering:** not for 24 hours – increased risk of bleeding
- **Driving:** not for 1 week post angioplasty (as per DVLA guidance) – if post-MI driving restriction will depend on LVEF
- **Activity:** no heavy lifting or strenuous activity for the first 2 weeks, sexual activity can be resumed 48 hours after successful angioplasty
- **Metformin:** restart after 48 hours (unless pre-existing renal failure)

Box 26.10   Drugs eluted from stents

- Paclitaxel
- Sirolimus
- Zotarolimus
- Tacrolimus
- Biolimus
- Everolimus

26.6 INTERPRETATION

A written report should be provided by the performing physician. This will detail the following.

History
- Relevant past medical history and cardiac risk factors
- Indication for procedure

Procedure
- Entry site used
- Type/size of all equipment used – including catheter/guide wire/balloons/stent
- Medications administered
- Details of vessels imaged and any abnormalities present
- If stent inserted – details of insertion and adequacy of position
- Haemostasis – how this was achieved
- Any complications during the procedure

Management
- Summary of procedure undertaken
- Post-procedure management
- Follow-up plan

Interpretation
- **Stenosis severity:** the degree of stenosis is measured by comparing the narrowed area to an adjacent segment
- **Percentage:** stenosis reduction is given as a percentage and calculated in the most severely narrowed projection
- **Fractional flow reserve (FFR):** this is the pressure difference across an area of stenosis after induction of maximal blood flow

Angiographic indications for revascularisation
- **Significant stenosis:** defined as ≥70% diameter narrowing, or ≥50% for left main stem disease
- **Revascularization:** the American College of Cardiology recommends revascularization in significant stenosis or with a FFR ≤0.80

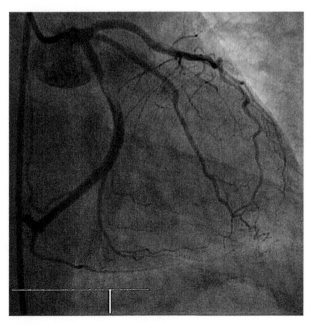

Figure 26.3 Stenosis of the proximal left circumflex artery.

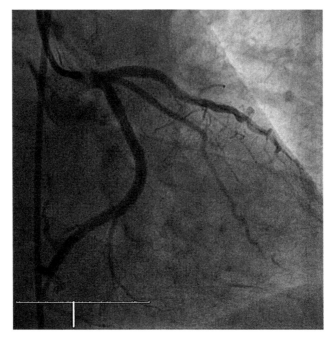

Figure 26.4 Left circumflex artery post stent insertion.

 (See Audio Podcast 26.2 at **www.wiley.com/go/camm/cardiology**)

26.7 POTENTIAL COMPLICATIONS

Most common
1. Vascular complication at access site:
- Minor bleeding (5%)
- Haematoma (2.5%)
- Pseudoaneurysm (1%)

2. Mild contrast reaction (4–6%)
3. Contrast-induced nephropathy (3%)

Dangerous
1. Major bleeding (1–2%)
2. Acute MI (1%)
3. Embolic stroke (0.5%)
4. Cardiac tamponade (0.5%)
5. Death (0.2%)
6. Infection (<0.01%)

Box 26.11   Features of a mild adverse reaction to iodinated contrast

- Scattered urticaria
- Low-grade pyrexia
- Pruritus
- Rhinorrhea
- Nausea/vomiting
- Dizziness

Box 26.12   Contrast-induced nephropathy

- Criteria: ≥25% increase in serum creatinine
- Onset: 48–72 hours after IV contrast
- High-risk patients: eGFR <45 mL/min/1.73m^2, acute illness, acute renal failure
- Risk reduction pre-procedure:
  a. Hold nephrotoxic drugs 48 hours pre-/post-procedure (or until creatinine returns to baseline)
  b. Hold metformin 48 hours pre-/post-procedure (increased risk of lactic acidosis in contrast-induced nephropathy)
  c. IV fluids at 1 mL/kg/hr for 12 hours pre-/post-procedure
  d. Consider N-acetylcysteine infusion

Box 26.13   Managing major catheter entry site bleeding post PCI

- Seek senior support early
- ABCD assessment of the patient
- Be aware: hidden retroperitoneal bleeding can occur after femoral access
- Apply firm pressure over the catheter entry site
- IV access: commence aggressive IV fluid resuscitation
- Bloods: FBC and cross-match ≥2 units
- Transfusion: if Hb <80 g/L in stable patients (<80–100 g/L for patients with ACS)
- Consider reversal of anticoagulation with senior support if life-threatening bleed or unable to achieve haemostasis

(See Audio Podcast 26.3 at **www.wiley.com/go/camm/cardiology**)

26.8 THROMBOLYSIS

Indication
Acute STEMI presenting within 12 hours of onset of symptoms when PCI cannot be delivered within 120 minutes.

Procedure
- Tissue plasminogen activators increase endogenous production of plasmin, causing degradation of the fibrin clots responsible for coronary artery occlusion
- Administered intravenously
- Followed immediately by treatment-dose subcutaneous LMWH

Drugs used
1. Alteplase
2. Reteplase
3. Tenecteplase

Complications
- Major bleeding (1.8%)
- Intracranial haemorrhage causing stroke (1.2%)
- Allergic reaction

Box 26.14   Advantages of PCI compared to thrombolysis for acute STEMI

1. Higher vessel patency rates
2. Faster ECG normalization
3. Lower rates of recurrent stenosis
4. Reduced risk of major bleeding
5. Reduced mortality
6. Angiography used – visualization of affected vessels

KEY CLINICAL TRIALS

Key trial 26.1
Trial name: RAVEL study.
Participants: 238 patients with single vessel coronary disease.
Intervention: Sirolimus drug-eluting stent.
Control: Bare-metal stent.
Outcome: Re-stenosis rates in the sirolimus-eluting stent group were significantly lower than in the control group.
Reason for inclusion: The first double-blind, randomized study performed in Europe evaluating the use of drug-eluting versus bare-metal stents.
Reference: Morice MC, Serruys PW, Barragan P, et al. Long-term clinical outcomes with sirolimus-eluting coronary stents: five-year results of the RAVEL trial. J Am Coll Cardiol. 2007;50:1299–1304. http://dx.doi.org/10.1016/j.jacc.2007.06.029.

Key trial 26.2
Trial name: SYNTAX.
Participants: 1800 patients with *de novo* three-vessel and/or left main coronary artery disease.
Intervention: PCI using paclitaxel-eluting stents.
Control: CABG.
Outcome: The incidence death, stroke, myocardial infarction or repeat revascularization were significantly higher for PCI in complex disease.
Reason for inclusion: Coronary artery bypass graft surgery is currently the revascularization method of choice in patient with proximal three-vessel disease or left main coronary artery disease.
Reference: Morice MC, Serruys PW, Kappetein AP, et al. Five-year outcomes in patients with left main disease treated with either percutaneous coronary intervention or coronary artery bypass grafting in the SYNTAX Trial. Circulation. 2014;113.006689.

Key trial 26.3
Trial name: A comparison of balloon-expandable stent implantation with balloon angioplasty.
Participants: 520 patients with stable angina and single coronary artery lesions.
Intervention: Bare-metal stent insertion.
Control: Balloon angioplasty.
Outcome: Reduced incidence of death, stroke, MI, or need for CABG in the stent insertion group (risk ratio 0.68, CI 0.50–0.92).
Reason for inclusion: Evidence for the use of stents over standard balloon angioplasty.
Reference: Serruys PW, de Jaegere P, Kiemeneij F, et al. A comparison of balloon-expandable stent implantation with balloon angioplasty in patients with coronary artery disease. N Engl J Med. 1994;331:489–495.

Key trial 26.4
Trial Name: COURAGE.
Participants: 2300 patients with objective evidence of myocardial ischaemia and significant stable coronary artery disease.
Intervention: PCI with optimal medical therapy.
Control: Optimal medical therapy alone.

Outcome: No significant difference in the incidence of death, and non-fatal MI (risk ratio 1.05, CI 0.87–1.27).

Reason for inclusion: Limited benefit of PCI over medical therapy in those with stable angina.

Reference: Boden WE, O'Rourke RA, Teo KK, et al. Optimal medical therapy with or without PCI for stable coronary disease. N Engl J Med. 2007;356:1503–1516.

GUIDELINES

National Institute for Heath and Care Excellence (NICE). CG 126 – The management of stable angina. 2011. http://www.nice.org.uk/nicemedia/live/13549/55660/55660.pdf

European Society of Cardiology (ESC) and the European Association for Cardio-Thoracic Surgery (EACTS). Guidelines on myocardial revascularization. 2010. http://www.escardio.org/guidelines-surveys/esc-guidelines/guidelinesdocuments/guidelines-revasc-ft.pdf

National Institute for Health and Care Excellence (NICE). CG 167 – The management of myocardial infarction with ST elevation. 2013. http://www.nice.org.uk/nicemedia/live/14208/64410/64410.pdf

The American College of Cardiology and The American Heart Association. Guideline for percutaneous intervention. 2011. http://content.onlinejacc.org/article.aspx?articleid=1147816

FURTHER READING

Sigwart U, Puel J, Mirkovitch V, Joffre F, Kappenberger L. Intravascular stents to prevent occlusion and restenosis after transluminal angioplasty. N Engl J Med. 1987;316:701–706.
First report of stent placement to successfully prevent re-stenosis following balloon angioplasty.

De Bruyne B, et al. Fractional flow reserved-guided PCI versus medical therapy in stable coronary disease. N Engl J Med. 2012;367:991–1001. Fame II
Study stopped early due to significantly increased risk of death, myocardial infarction, or urgent revascularization in those undergoing PCI with a fractional flow reserve 0.80.

 For additional resources and to test your knowledge, visit the companion website at:

www.wiley.com/go/camm/cardiology

27 Valvuloplasty

Akshay Garg

King's College Hospital NHS Foundation Trust, London, UK

27.1 DEFINITION

A procedure in which a stenotic valve is expanded using a balloon catheter.

27.2 OUTLINE OF PROCEDURE AND DEVICES

Table 27.1 Outline of balloon aortic valvuloplasty (BAV) procedure

Patient positioning	Supine
Procedure length	30–60 minutes
Performing clinician	Interventional cardiologist
Location	Coronary catheter lab
Catheter insertion	Femoral artery
Medication given	Local anaesthetic, sedatives
Other equipment	Image intensifier
	Temporary pacing wire
	Cardiac monitor

Procedure
- **Preparation:** local anaesthetic and sedative administered. Temporary pacing wire inserted via femoral vein, and femoral artery sheath into femoral artery. Balloon size selected
- **Insertion:** balloon catheter inserted via femoral sheath and guided across the aortic valve
- **Pacing:** the ventricle is rapidly paced to reduce movement of balloon
- **Inflation:** under fluoroscopic guidance, the balloon is correctly positioned and inflated
- **If pre-TAVI:** if undertaken to ascertain annulus size, contrast then injected upstream of the balloon. If there is contrast leaking into the left ventricle then the balloon is too small
- **Completion:** the balloon is deflated and can be inflated/deflated a number of times prior to removal

Clinical Guide to Cardiology, First Edition. Edited by Christian F. Camm and A. John Camm.
© 2016 John Wiley & Sons, Ltd. Published 2016 by John Wiley & Sons, Ltd.
Companion website: www.wiley.com/go/camm/cardiology.

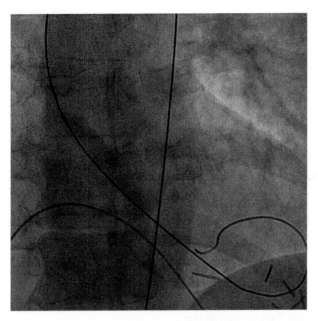

Figure 27.1 Fluoroscopy image of guide wire inserted across the aortic valve.

Device

The balloon is attached to the end of a catheter. The balloon comes in various sizes and brands.

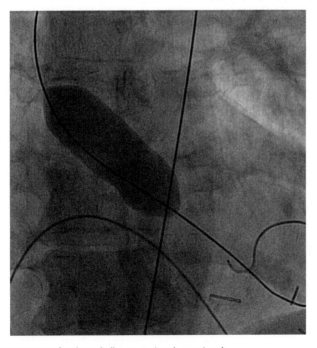

Figure 27.2 Fluoroscopy image of catheter balloon opening the aortic valve.

27.3 INDICATIONS

Valvuloplasty is most commonly used in the treatment of aortic stenosis in the following situations:

1. **Bridging therapy:** to TAVI or valve replacement
2. **Palliative:** to reduce symptoms in patients unsuitable for more definitive management
3. **Elective:** prior to other major non-cardiac operations, for example knee replacements etc.

Valvuloplasty is contraindicated in patients that have mixed aortic valve disease with predominant aortic regurgitation.

27.4 PERI-PROCEDURAL MANAGEMENT

Prior to procedure
- **Blood tests:**
  - FBC – check platelets and Hb
  - Urea and electrolytes – ensure renal function adequate
  - Clotting – to ensure INR within range
- **Imaging:** echocardiogram
- **Fasting:**
  - 6 hours for solid foods
  - 4 hours for clear fluids
- **Cannula:** minimum 20 gauge cannula
- **Nursing requirement:** standard nursing care
- **Anticoagulation:**
  - Needs to be stopped, however the cover depends on the indication
  - AF – no need for LMWH cover
  - Metallic valve – will need unfractionated heparin (UFH) in the days leading up to the procedure
  - UFH stopped 4–6 hours pre-procedure
- **Other considerations:** insulin-dependent diabetic patients should have a sliding scale

Post procedure
- **Recovery:** ward-based care, overnight observation
- **Cardiac monitoring:** not required
- **Blood tests:** urea and electrolytes – check renal function
- **Anticoagulation:** can be restarted the day following procedure if no bleeding complications

Patient advice
- **Immediate:**
  - Keep leg straight and head down on the pillow for 1 hour
  - 2 hours bed rest sitting up 45°
- **Analgesia:** not likely to be required, but can take paracetamol
- **Wound:** keep the site clean and dry for 1 week (no baths only quick shower)
- **Exercise:** no heavy lifting, pushing, pulling for 1 week
- **Driving:** no driving for 48 hours
- **Follow-up:** depends on indication for BAV

27.5 POTENTIAL COMPLICATIONS

Most common
1. Bleeding from puncture site
2. Infection
3. Vascular injury

Dangerous

1. New or worsening aortic regurgitation
2. Stroke
3. Cardiac tamponade
4. Dysrhythmias/arrhythmias

Box 27.1   Management of puncture-site bleeding

1. Assess the patient in an ABCDE manner
2. Ascertain whether bleeding is superficial or arterial:
   - Apply manual pressure to femoral artery
   - If stops, likely arterial bleed, continue to apply pressure and get help
3. Ascertain if retroperitoneal bleed:
   - Severe back pain, hypotension and bruising around puncture site
   - If suspected, get senior help immediately
4. Check peripheral pulses and other symptoms of clot forming in arterial system
5. If manual pressure does not control bleeding, get senior help:
   - Likely to suggest using Femstop temporarily. Dome-shaped object placed directly over femoral artery, strapped around patient and dome inflated to apply pressure

---

(See Audio Podcast 27.1 at **www.wiley.com/go/camm/cardiology**)

GUIDELINES

National Institute of Health and Clinical Excellence (NICE). Balloon valvuloplasty for aortic valve stenosis in adults and children. 2004. http://www.nice.org.uk/nicemedia/live/11091/30980/30980.pdf

European Society of Cardiology (ESC). Guidelines on the management of valvular heart disease. 2012. http://www.escardio.org/guidelines-surveys/esc-guidelines/GuidelinesDocuments/Guidelines_Valvular_Heart_Dis_FT.pdf

 For additional resources and to test your knowledge, visit the companion website at:

www.wiley.com/go/camm/cardiology

28 Transcatheter Aortic Valve Implantation

Akshay Garg

King's College Hospital NHS Foundation Trust, London, UK

28.1 DEFINITION

A minimally invasive alternative to conventional aortic valve replacement where an artificial valve is delivered by catheter and implanted over the native valve.

28.2 OUTLINE OF PROCEDURE AND DEVICES

Table 28.1 Outline of TAVI procedure

Patient positioning	Supine
Procedure length	2–4 hours
Performing clinician	Interventional cardiologist +/- cardiothoracic surgeon
Location	Coronary catheter laboratory
Access sites	Transfemoral (TF) approach – femoral artery
	Transapical (TA) approach – small incision in chest wall to expose apex
Medication given	General anaesthetic
Other equipment	Image intensifier – to guide valve placement
	Transoesophageal echocardiography – accurate positioning of valve
	Temporary pacing wire – to allow rapid pacing of the heart
	Cardiac monitor

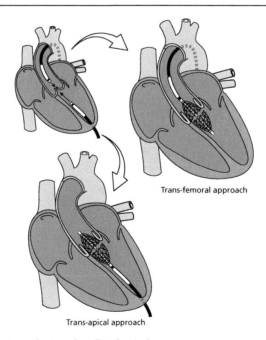

Trans-femoral approach

Trans-apical approach

Figure 28.1 Insertion of a TAVI valve into place (line drawing).

Clinical Guide to Cardiology, First Edition. Edited by Christian F. Camm and A. John Camm.
© 2016 John Wiley & Sons, Ltd. Published 2016 by John Wiley & Sons, Ltd.
Companion website: www.wiley.com/go/camm/cardiology.

Devices

There are two main devices, the Edwards Sapien® device and the Medtronic CoreValve® device.

- **Sapien®:** tri-leaflet valve of porcine pericardium inside a balloon-expandable nickel–titanium frame (for either TF or TA approach)
- **CoreValve®:** tri-leaflet valve constructed from bovine pericardium inside a self-expanding tubular metal stent (TF approach only)

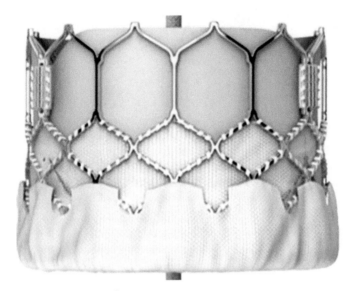

Figure 28.2 A TAVI valve (Edwards Sapien®).
Source: Image kindly provided by Edwards Lifesciences LLC, Irvine, CA. Edwards SAPIEN is a trademark of Edwards Lifesciences Corporation.

Procedure

Preparation

- Local or general anaesthetic administered
- Temporary pacing wire inserted via femoral vein
- Transoesophageal echocardiogram probe inserted
- Valve crimped on to the delivery balloon

Transfemoral approach

- Femoral sheath inserted
- BAV performed to improve valve size selection (see Chapter 27)
- Valve inserted via femoral sheath and positioned in the aortic annulus
- Under fluoroscopic guidance and rapid ventricular pacing, balloon inflated to deploy the valve
- Multiple checks to ensure correct anatomical placement and intended performance of the valve

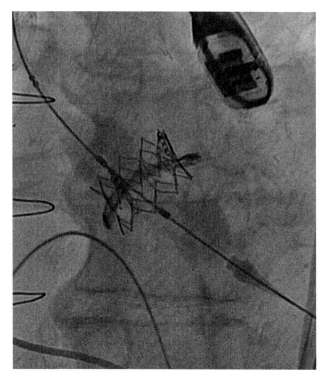

Figure 28.3 TAVI valve being inserted and expanded using a transfemoral approach.

Transapical approach
- Similar to the transfemoral approach, except the valve is delivered directly via the apex of the heart
- This procedure is performed jointly with a cardiothoracic surgeon

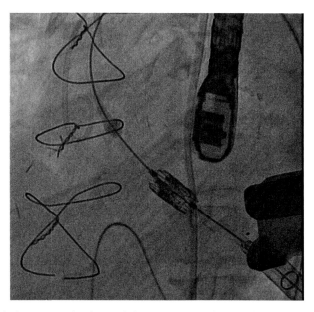

Figure 28.4 TAVI valve being inserted and expanded using a transapical approach.

28.3 INDICATIONS

Severe symptomatic aortic stenosis carries a poor prognosis if managed medically, with a predicted mortality of 25% at 1 year and 50% at 2 years. The indications for this procedure are rapidly developing.

TAVI should be considered in patients with a high predicted operative mortality with conventional aortic valve replacement. Prerequisites for TAVI usage include:

1. **Multidisciplinary team:** consisting of cardiologists, cardiac surgeons, experts in cardiac imaging, cardiac anaesthetists and other specialists as required
2. **Location:** TAVI should only be performed in locations with on-site cardiac and vascular surgery

Patients must fulfill the following criteria to be suitable for TAVI:

1. **Symptomatic AS:** not suitable for SAVR as assessed by the multidisciplinary team
2. **Improvement:** likely to gain improvement in their quality of life
3. **Life expectancy:** more than 1 year after consideration of their co-morbidities
4. **Heart failure:** symptomatic (NYHA functional class II or higher) from AS, rather than other co-morbidities

---

Box 28.1   Work up for potential TAVI candidates

1. **ECG:** ensure no conduction abnormalities pre-procedure
2. **Lung function tests:** ensure good functional reserve
3. **Chest radiograph**
4. **Carotid Doppler:** check for evidence of carotid artery stenosis
5. **Transoesophageal echocardiogram:** assess the severity, morphology and calcification of AS as well as the annular size and shape
6. **Coronary angiogram:** measure annulus to coronary ostia distance, and assess for coronary artery disease
7. **CT aorta:** determine atheroma burden in iliofemoral vessels

---

Box 28.2   Valvular requirements for consideration of TAVI

Aortic stenosis with severely calcified valve leaflets with reduced systolic motion, AND

- Mean gradient of >40 mmHg or jet velocity of >4.0 m/s; OR
- Aortic stenosis with aortic valve area of <1 cm^2 or indexed effective orifice area <0.5 cm^2/m^2

Box 28.3   Exclusion criteria for TAVI candidates

1. Bicuspid, unicuspid, or non-calcified aortic valve (not an absolute contraindication)
2. Severe aortic regurgitation
3. Native aortic valve annulus too small or too large for current available devices
4. Otherwise medically unfit for procedure – renal function, TIA/CVA within 6 months of planned procedure, intracardiac mass/thrombus, severe MR or severe incapacitating dementia
5. Estimated life expectancy <1 year

28.4 PERI-PROCEDURAL MANAGEMENT

Prior to procedure
- **Blood tests:**
  - FBC – check Hb levels, platelets and white cells
  - Urea and electrolytes – to get baseline renal function
  - Clotting – to check INR in acceptable range
  - Cross-match – 2 units of packed red cells if transapical approach

- **Imaging:** see Box 28.1
- **Fasting:**
  - Light meal – 6 hours prior to procedure
  - Clear fluids – 4 hours prior to procedure
- **Cannula:** minimum 20 gauge cannula or larger
- **Nursing requirement:** standard nursing care
- **Warfarin:**
  - Needs to be stopped, however the cover depends on the indication for warfarin
  - AF – no need for LMWH cover
  - Metallic valve (elsewhere) – will need UFH in the days leading up to the procedure
- **LMWH:** can be given the day before. UFH will need to stop 4–6 hours prior to procedure
- **Other considerations:** if insulin-dependent diabetic will require a sliding scale

Post procedure

- **Recovery:**
  - Transfemoral: cardiac HDU (1–2 days)
  - Transapical: cardiac ITU/HDU (2–3 days)
- **Cardiac monitoring:** while in high-dependency or ITU, not necessary on ward
- **Blood tests:** urea and electrolytes to check renal function
- **Antibiotics:** usually given peri-procedure, check local trust guidelines. Transapical TAVI will continue this post procedure for wound prophylaxis
- **Anticoagulation:** none needed as a tissue valve is used; if previously on warfarin, can usually be safely restarted the day after the procedure
- **Other considerations:**
  - Post-TAVI echocardiogram required
  - Transapical approach will have a drain, usually removed after 1–2 days
  - Metformin should be held for 48 hours

Patient advice

- **Analgesia:** regularly until no further discomfort
- **Wound:** TA approach – will normally have healed prior to discharge. If over 1 week and wound healthy, patient may shower
- **Sutures:** normally dissolvable
- **Follow-up:** clinic in 6 weeks, with repeat echocardiogram if required. If well, then every 6–12 months
- **Exercise:** avoid strenuous exercise for a few weeks, especially if TA approach. However important to avoid being sedentary, encourage short walks
- **Driving:** not allowed for 4 weeks post-procedure. If large goods vehicle (LGV) or passenger-carrying vehicle (PCV), will need exercise test before getting licence back

28.5 POTENTIAL COMPLICATIONS

Overall similar safety profile to surgical aortic valve replacement, however there are still significant risks associated with the procedure:

1. Acute kidney injury (common)
2. Para-valvular leaks (common)
3. Atrioventricular block – often requiring permanent pacemaker (common)
4. Vascular injury and bleeding, especially in transfemoral procedures (common)
5. Stroke (less common)
6. Annular rupture or ventricular perforation requiring emergency surgery (uncommon)
7. Coronary artery ostial occlusion (rare)

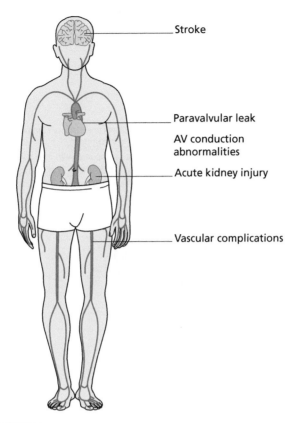

Figure 28.5 TAVI complications.

 (See Audio Podcast 28.1 at **www.wiley.com/go/camm/cardiology**)

KEY CLINICAL TRIALS

Key Trial 28.1
Trial name: PARTNER Trial.
Participants: Multicentre randomized controlled trial performed in two arms. PARTNER A (n = 699) and PARTNER B (n = 358).
Intervention: TAVI – transfemoral or transapical approach.
Control: Surgical AVR (PARTNER A) or optimal medical therapy (PARTNER B).
Outcome: Two arms of study PARTNER A (TAVI vs. SAVR) and PARTNER B (TAVI vs. OMT). PARTNER A: Mortality at 1 year is equal for TAVI and SAVR (24.2% and 26.8% respectively, p = 0.001). PARTNER B: Mortality at 1 year is better for TAVI than OMT (30.7% and 50.7% respectively, p < 0.001).
Reason for inclusion: Large RCT to demonstrate that TAVI is a viable alternative to SAVR.
Reference: Leon MB, et al. Transcatheter aortic-valve implantation for aortic stenosis in patients who cannot undergo surgery. N Engl J Med. 2010;363(17):1597–1607. http://www.ncbi.nlm.nih.gov/pubmed/20961243.

GUIDELINES

European Society of Cardiology. Guidelines on the management of valvular heart disease. 2012. http://www.escardio
.org/guidelines-surveys/esc-guidelines/Pages/valvular-heart-disease.aspx

National Institute of Health and Clinical Excellence. IPG421: Transcatheter aortic valve implantation for aortic stenosis.
2012. http://guidance.nice.org.uk/IPG421/Guidance/pdf/English

FURTHER READING

Figulla L, et al. Transcatheter aortic valve implantation: evidence on safety and efficacy compared with medical therapy.
A systematic review of current literature. Clin Res Cardiol. 2011;100:265–276.
Review discussing the relative benefits and disadvantages of TAVI compared with medical therapy.

Bagur R, Webb JG, Nietlispach F, et al. Acute kidney injury following transcatheter aortic valve implantation: predictive
factors, prognostic value, and comparison with surgical aortic valve replacement. Eur Heart J. 2010;31:865–874.
Discussion of the risks and predictive factors involved in the development of renal failure following TAVI.

 For additional resources and to test your knowledge, visit the companion website at:

www.wiley.com/go/camm/cardiology

29 Cardiac Ablation

Christian F. Camm

John Radcliffe Hospital, Oxford, UK

29.1 DEFINITION

An invasive procedure used to terminate and prevent arrhythmias by destroying arrhythmic foci or pathways using an electrode/catheter inserted into the heart.

29.2 OUTLINE OF PROCEDURE

Table 29.1 Outline of cardiac ablation procedure

Patient positioning	Supine
Procedure length	Dependent on procedure (30 minutes to 4 hours)
Performing clinician	Cardiologist (electrophysiologist)
Location	Cardiac catheter lab
Insertion site	Femoral vein (occasionally additional insertion via subclavian vein)
Medication given	Sedation given systemically (intraoperatively) or orally (preoperatively)
	Local anaesthetic to catheter insertion site
	Long/painful procedures often require light general anaesthetic
Other equipment	Fluoroscope for lead guidance and placement
	Mapping software and hardware
Procedural process	Local anaesthetic is administered to insertion site
	Leads inserted into the femoral vein
	Leads guided to correct positions within heart using fluoroscopy and mapping
	Ablation undertaken
	Leads removed

Pulmonary vein isolation (PVI)
- Used to block aberrant foci that trigger atrial fibrillation from interacting with the left atrium
- Most patients have four pulmonary veins, all of which may generate potential triggers and should be isolated
- Prior to the procedure, imaging of the left atrium (often TOE) may be required
- Catheters are inserted through the femoral vein and advanced into the right atrium
- A trans-septal catheter is then advanced across the septum into the left atrium
- Ablation is then conducted around the orifices of the pulmonary veins

AV nodal/His bundle ablation
- Used to establish ventricular rate control in atrial fibrillation
- An electrode catheter is inserted into the right heart adjacent to the AV node/His bundle
- The AV node/His bundle is ablated creating complete heart (AV) block
- Permanent ventricular pacing, usually biventricular, is then instituted

Clinical Guide to Cardiology, First Edition. Edited by Christian F. Camm and A. John Camm.
© 2016 John Wiley & Sons, Ltd. Published 2016 by John Wiley & Sons, Ltd.
Companion website: www.wiley.com/go/camm/cardiology.

AV nodal (slow-pathway) ablation
- Used to prevent AV nodal re-entrant tachycardia
- The AV node often consists of a fast and slow pathway, both of which are necessary to develop the re-entrant circuit which supports AVNRT
- An electrode catheter is inserted into the right heart and positioned between the coronary sinus and AV node/His bundle
- Energy is applied to destroy one of the AV nodal pathways (normally the slow pathway) to eliminate the re-entrant circuit

Accessory pathway ablation
- Used to ablate accessory pathways (both Wolff–Parkinson–White syndrome and concealed pathways) which can lead to AVRT
- Catheter inserted through the femoral vein and advanced into the right/left atrium
- The accessory pathway is localized by recording potentials from the region around the tricuspid and mitral valves
- Once located, the accessory pathway is ablated

Cavo-tricuspid isthmus ablation
- The tissue between the inferior vena cava and tricuspid valve is the common site for atrial flutter circuits, ablation prevents the circuit forming
- Catheter inserted through the femoral vein and advanced into the right atrium and the isthmus is ablated

RVOT ablation
- The right ventricle outflow tract is a major site for the formation of ectopic ventricular beats/sustained ventricular tachycardia
- Catheter inserted through the femoral vein and passed via the right atrium into the right ventricle
- The focus of ventricular depolarization is located by mapping the origin of induced ventricular tachycardia or artificially stimulating the myocardium and comparing traces with those found during the original arrhythmia
- Once located, the focus is ablated

Other ventricular tachycardias
- These may arise from any area of ventricular tissue (both left and right ventricles)
- Catheter is introduced into the appropriate chamber or inserted into the pericardial space (if an epicardial approach is needed)
- Origin of the arrhythmia is mapped (as for RVOT ablation)
- Once located, the focus is ablated

Box 29.1 Different energy forms for ablation

1. Radiofrequency
2. Cryothermy
3. Microwave
4. Laser

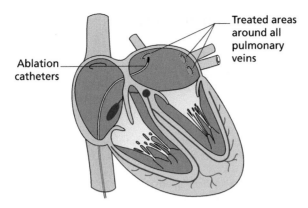

Figure 29.1 Pulmonary vein isolation.

29.3 INDICATIONS

Each form of ablation has specific indications as follows:

1. **Atrial fibrillation:** PVI, AV nodal/His bundle ablation
2. **Atrial flutter:** cavo-tricuspid isthmus ablation
3. **AV nodal re-entrant tachycardia:** AV nodal (slow pathway) ablation
4. **Ventricular tachycardia:** RVOT ablation or ablation of other ventricular sites
5. **Wolff–Parkinson–White/AVRT:** accessory pathway ablation

---

Box 29.2   Indications for PVI in atrial fibrillation

1. Symptomatic
2. Failed previous trial of anti-arrhythmic medication
3. Centre and operator with adequate expertise

Box 29.3   Features that suggest successful likelihood of PVI ablation

1. Small left atrial size (not dilated)
2. Paroxysmal > persistent > long-standing persistent
3. Good left ventricular function

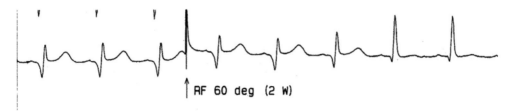

Figure 29.2 Ablation of accessory pathway conduction ECG; note disappearance of δ-wave (last two beats).

29.4 PERI-PROCEDURAL MANAGEMENT

Prior to procedure
- **Blood tests:**
  - INR: if on concomitant vitamin K antagonist (VKA)
  - Urea and electrolytes: to confirm renal function as contrast used
- **Imaging:**
  - Trans-thoracic echo – imaging of the cardiac chambers to identify/exclude underlying structural heart disease
  - Transoesophageal echo – to exclude thrombus in left atrial appendage (PVI)
  - ECG/Holter: to assess the nature of the arrhythmias experienced and confirm the type of ablation required
- **Fasting:** 6 hours for solids, 2 hours for clear liquids
- **Cannula:** minimum 20 gauge (for sedation/anaesthesia)
- **Anticoagulation:**
  - Warfarin normally continued through ablation (INR target 2.0–2.5), if stopped LMWH bridging should be used
  - Novel oral anticoagulants (NOACs) normally stopped 12–24 hours prior to procedure (but may need to be continued)
- **LMWH:** omitted the night before, can be restarted after procedure
- **Other considerations:** some centres require detailed pre-procedural anatomical imaging (CT or MRI) to allow for electro-anatomical mapping

Post procedure
- **Recovery:** held overnight
- **Monitoring:** cardiac monitoring for first 6 hours
- **Blood tests:** urea and electrolytes to confirm post-procedural renal function
- **Medications:** warfarin should be continued for minimum of 3 months, LMWH should be used to bridge if necessary (PVI ablation)
- **Imaging:** trans-thoracic echo – monitor cardiac function and exclude potential complications (e.g. pericardial effusion)
- **Antibiotics:** none as standard

Patient advice
- **Home:** normally discharged the following day
- **Showering:** as normal
- **Driving:** may resume on the following day
- **Activity:** heavy exertion and competitive sports should be avoided for at least 1 week
- **Follow-up:** normally at 3 months (but dependent on clinician preference)

29.5 POTENTIAL COMPLICATIONS

Most common
1. Peripheral vascular complications (e.g. haematoma, pseudoaneurysm)
2. Bleeding (including pericardial bleeding)
3. TIA/stroke (left-sided ablations only)
4. Recurrence of arrhythmia
5. Development of additional arrhythmias (e.g. atrial tachycardia/atrial flutter)

Dangerous
1. Pericardial tamponade (1.0%)
2. Atrial–oesophageal fistula (< 0.05%)
3. Pulmonary vein stenosis
4. Perforation of the aortic root (when making a trans-septal puncture)
5. Embolization (air/charred tissue/left atrial thrombus)

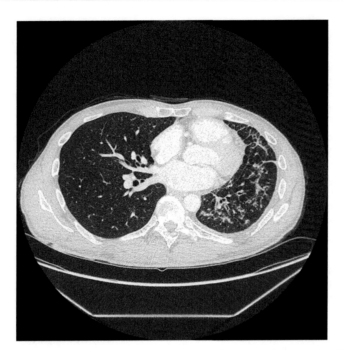

Figure 29.3 Chest CT showing left-sided pulmonary vein obliteration following pulmonary vein isolation ablation.

Box 29.4   Features of oesophageal perforation

- A rare side effect of pulmonary vein isolation
- Occurs 3–40 days after ablation
- Mortality >50%
- Symptoms relate to air embolism and infection
- Common features:
  a. Fever (75%)
  b. Neurological symptoms (69%)
  c. Chest pain (28%)

KEY CLINICAL TRIALS

Key trial 29.1

Trial name: ThermoCool.

Participants: 160 patients with three or more AF episodes who did not respond to one or more anti-arrhythmic drug.

Intervention: Pulmonary vein isolation ablation.

Control: Anti-arrhythmic drug therapy.

Outcome: 66% of catheter arm remained free from treatment failure compared with 16% of the anti-arrhythmic drug arm (p < 0.001).

Reason for inclusion: Large-scale RCT highlighting the benefit of pulmonary vein isolation in those who have failed previous ant-arrhythmic drug therapy.

Reference: Wilber DJ, et al. Comparison of antiarrhythmic drug therapy and radiofrequency catheter ablation in patients with paroxysmal atrial fibrillation: a randomized controlled trial. JAMA. 2010;303(4):333–340. http://www.ncbi.nlm.nih.gov/pubmed/20103757

Key trial 29.2

Participants: 43 patients with recurrent paroxysmal AF not controlled with three or more anti-arrhythmic drugs.

Intervention: AV nodal ablation and DDDR PPM insertion.

Control: Anti-arrhythmic drug therapy.

Outcome: Ablation significantly improved reported quality of life scores ($p < 0.001$), palpations ($p < 0.001$), effort dyspnoea ($p = 0.04$) and exercise intolerance scores ($p = 0.02$) over anti-arrhythmic drug therapy.

Reason for inclusion: Supports the use of AV nodal ablation in AF patients when AF continues despite multiple anti-arrhythmic drugs.

Reference: Brignole M, et al. Assessment of atrioventricular junction ablation and DDDR mode-switching pacemaker versus pharmacological treatment in patients with severely symptomatic paroxysmal atrial fibrillation: a randomized controlled study. Circulation. 1997;96(8):2617–2624. http://www.ncbi.nlm.nih.gov/pubmed/9355902

GUIDELINES

European Society of Cardiology. Guidelines for the management of atrial fibrillation. 2010. http://eurheartj .oxfordjournals.org/content/31/19/2369.full.pdf

American College of Cardiology, American Heart Association, European Society of Cardiology. Guidelines for the management of patients with supraventricular arrhythmias. 2003. http://www.escardio.org/guidelines-surveys/esc-guidelines/GuidelinesDocuments/guidelines-SVA-FT.pdf

America College of Cardiology, American heart Association, Heart Rhythm Society. 2015 ACC/AHA/HRS guideline for the management of adult patients with supraventricular tachycardia http://content.onlinejacc.org/article.aspx?articleid=2443667

FURTHER READING

Haïssaguerre M, Jaïs P, Shah DC, et al. Spontaneous initiation of atrial fibrillation by ectopic beats originating in the pulmonary veins. N Engl J Med. 1998;339(10):659–666. http://www.ncbi.nlm.nih.gov/pubmed/9725923
First paper highlighting the importance of pulmonary veins in the arrhythmogenesis of AF.

 For additional resources and to test your knowledge, visit the companion website at:

www.wiley.com/go/camm/cardiology

PART 6
Pharmacology

30 Anti-Arrhythmic Agents

George Davies
Oxford University Hospitals NHS Trust, Oxford, UK

30.1 ADENOSINE

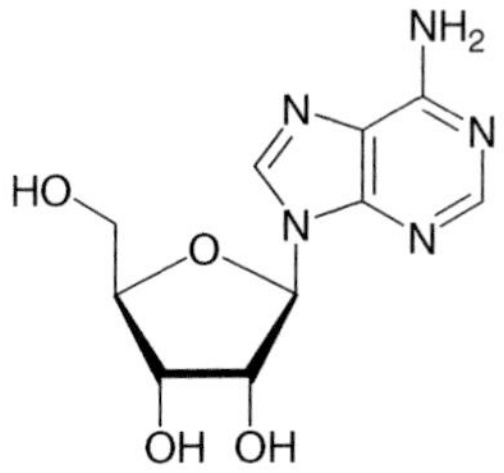

Figure 30.1 Structure of adenosine.

Drug class
• Purine nucleoside

Pharmacology
• **Agonist to A1 receptors:** activated in the AV node, triggering K$^+$ channels
• **Hyperpolarization:** increased conduction of K$^+$ hyperpolarizes the conduction tissue thus increasing the AV node refractory period

Indications
Termination of narrow-complex regular tachycardia involving the AV node:

1. AV nodal re-entrant tachycardia
2. Atrioventricular re-entrant tachycardia

Contraindications
1. Asthma (caution COPD)
2. Second-/third-degree AV block
3. Sick-sinus syndrome

Interactions
1. Dipyridamole: mutually increase each other's effects
2. Digoxin: may increase risk of VF
3. Anti-arrhythmics: increased myocardial depression
4. Theophylline: adenosine effect antagonized by theophylline

Side effects
A transient period of asystole is likely to occur on giving adenosine.

Dangerous
1. Bronchospasm
2. Severe hypotension
3. Angina

Clinical Guide to Cardiology, First Edition. Edited by Christian F. Camm and A. John Camm.
© 2016 John Wiley & Sons, Ltd. Published 2016 by John Wiley & Sons, Ltd.
Companion website: www.wiley.com/go/camm/cardiology.

Common
1. Metallic taste
2. Apprehension
3. Flushing
4. Dizziness
5. Nausea

Excretion/metabolism
Half-life
- 10 seconds

Metabolism
- Metabolized on luminal surface of vascular endothelium

Route
- IV only

Starting dose
- 3–6 mg IV bolus through proximal vein followed by flush
- If unsuccessful, up to 12 mg can be given
- Repeat every 1–2 minutes if necessary

Monitoring/equipment
- Cardiac monitoring is required
- If Wolff–Parkinson–White syndrome is suspected, external pacing equipment must be available

30.2 AMIODARONE

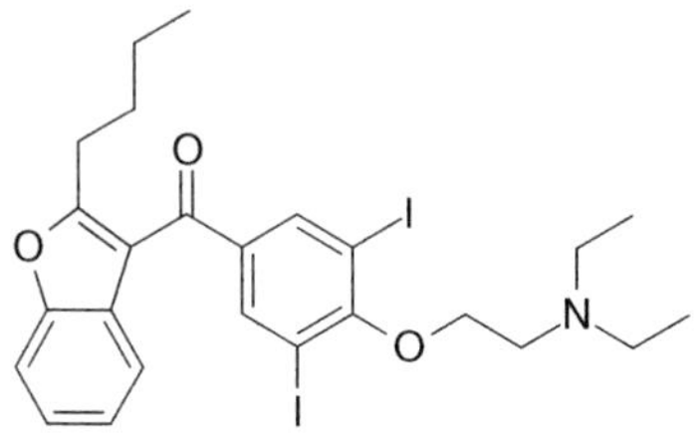

Figure 30.2 Structure of amiodarone.

Drug class
- Group III anti-arrhythmic

Pharmacology
- **K⁺ channels:** blockage is responsible for delay in repolarization
- **Action potential:** prolongation of duration throughout the myocardium
- **Refractory period:** this is prolonged causing suppression of ectopic related and re-entrant circuit related tachycardias
- **QT interval:** increased by the same mechanism as the refractory period

Indications
Highly effective in controlling/terminating many tachyarrhythmias:

1. Regular broad-complex ventricular tachycardia: first-line, alone or in conjunction with DC cardioversion
2. Cardiac arrest: after third shock for pulseless shockable rhythm

Due to adverse effects second- or third-line drug for other tachyarrhythmias.

Contraindications
1. **SAN disease:** risk of bradycardia
2. **AVN block without pacemaker:** risk of bradycardia
3. **Pregnancy:** excreted in breast milk

Cautions
1. **Hypotension/respiratory failure (non-arrhythmia related):** hypotensive effect can worsen
2. **Pre-existent QT prolongation:** can prolong the QT interval further, risking torsades de pointes
3. **History of thyroid disease:** increased risk of hyper-/hypothyroidism
4. **Hypokalaemia:** increased risk of torsades de pointes
5. Moderate to severe renal/hepatic impairment

Interactions
1. **Digoxin, phenytoin:** amiodarone reduces clearance
2. **Class I/III anti-arrhythmics:** increase risk of arrhythmia
3. **Antipsychotics, tricyclics, lithium:** increase risk of arrhythmia
4. **Cytochrome inhibitors:** reduce clearance and increased risk of arrhythmia
5. **Verapamil, diltiazem, beta-blockers:** increased risk of bradycardia and conduction block

Side effects
Dangerous
1. Torsades de pointes – particularly if long QT or in electrolyte abnormalities (low K^+, high Ca^{2+})
2. Interstitial lung disease
3. Hepatotoxicity
4. Hypotension if IV (related to solvent and rate of delivery)
5. Conduction block

Common
1. Fatigue
2. Photosensitivity: warn to avoid sun/use sunscreen even several months after halting
3. Hyper-/hypothyroidism
4. Nausea and vomiting

Excretion/metabolism
Half-life
- 58 days, highly variable from 15–142 days

Metabolism
- Hepatic via CYP2C8 and CYP3A3/4
- Note that amiodarone itself inhibits CYP2C9, CYP2D6, CYP3A3/4

Route
- Oral
- Intravenous

Starting dose
- **Oral:** 200 mg TDS 1st week, BD 2nd week, OD 3rd week
- **IV (emergency termination of arrhythmia):** 150–300 mg in 10–20 mL 5% dextrose/3 min (bolus in cardiac arrest)
- **Infusion:** 5 mg/kg over 20–120 mins (1.2 g maximum daily)

Monitoring/equipment
- IV doses should ideally be given through central or large, proximal peripheral line
- ECG and blood pressure monitoring required if used to terminate acute tachyarrhythmia
- Should be started under supervision (hospital or specialist clinic)
- If starting in a non-acute situation, liver and thyroid function should be checked prior to and a week following starting therapy

30.3 FLECAINIDE

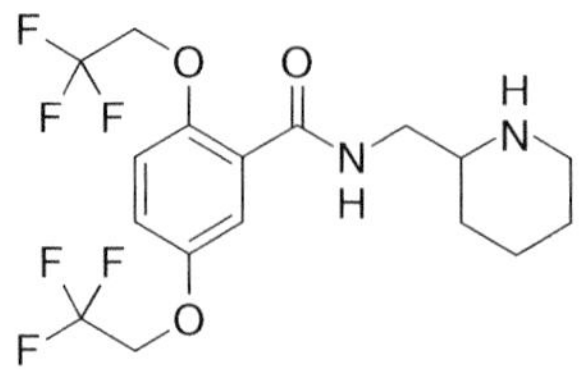

Figure 30.3   Structure of flecainide.

Drug class
• Group IC anti-arrhythmic

Pharmacology
• **Blockade:** causes a use-dependent block of voltage-gated Na^+ channels (Nav1.5)
• **Action potential:** prolonged due to delayed repolarization
• **Effective refractory period:** increased within the myocardium
• **Slowed conduction:** a use-dependent slowing of action potential conduction is effective at disrupting re-entrant tachycardia circuits
• **Myocardial excitability:** causes a general reduction throughout the action potential

Indications
1. Paroxysmal atrial fibrillation in structurally normal hearts (e.g. pill in pocket therapy)
2. Paroxysmal SVT termination and prophylaxis
3. Ventricular tachycardia termination and prophylaxis

Contraindications
1. **IHD:** increased incidence of sudden death due to VF in patients who have had an MI
2. **Second-degree AV block:** increased risk of conversion to complete heart block
3. **Third-degree AV block:** increased risk of loss of escape rhythm
4. **Bifascicular block:** increased risk of conversion to complete heart block
5. **AF following cardiac surgery:** increased risk of developing VT/VF
6. **Permanent AF:** increased risk of VF without benefit on AF
7. **Haemodynamic compromise:** negative inotropic effect of flecainide

Cautions
1. **Electrolyte abnormalities:** must be normalized prior to use
2. **Non-programmable pacemakers/poor thresholds:** interference with pacing spike conduction in the endocardium
3. **Moderate to severe renal impairment:** renal clearance of flecainide metabolites
4. **Left ventricular dysfunction:** reduced initial dosage, risk of exacerbating pre-existing CCF

Interactions
1. **Amiodarone:** increases levels of flecainide through CP450 inhibition
2. **Antipsychotics:** increased risk of arrhythmias
3. **Tricyclic antidepressants:** increased risk of arrhythmias
4. **Beta-blockers/verapamil:** synergistic effect on myocardial depression
5. **Digoxin:** flecainide causes slightly increased levels

Side effects
Dangerous
1. Arrhythmia: VT, torsades de pointes
2. Negatively inotropic

Common
1. Visual disturbance
2. Dizziness
3. Dyspnoea
4. Nausea
5. Headache
6. Peripheral oedema

Excretion/metabolism
Half-life
- 12–27 hours – increased by renal impairment

Metabolism
- Extensive hepatic metabolism – including via CYP2D6
- 80% of metabolites are renally cleared

Routes
- Oral
- Intravenous

Starting dose
- **Pill-in-pocket therapy:** 200–300 mg PO (taken when symptoms occurs)
- **SVT prevention:** 50 mg PO BD (maximum 300 mg daily)
- **VT prevention:** 100 mg PO BD (can be increased 50 mg every 4 days, maximum 400 mg daily)
- **Acute termination:** 2 mg/kg IV over 10–30 mins (maximum 150 mg). If necessary, a further 1.5 mg/kg IV over 1 hour followed by 100–250 µg/kg/hr for 24 hours
- **Total flecainide:** should not exceed 600 mg in the initial 24 hours
- Considerations should be made for both hepatic and renal impairment

Monitoring/equipment
- **Acute scenario:** ECG and blood pressure monitoring are essential
- **Plasma levels (pre-dose):** should be monitored if hepatic or renal impairment. Target 0.2–1.0 mg/L

30.4 DIGOXIN

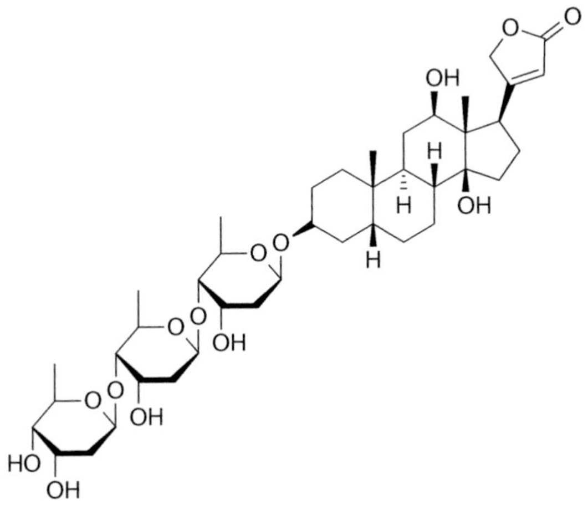

Figure 30.4 Structure of digoxin.

Drug class
- Cardiac glycoside

Pharmacology
- **Inhibition of Na$^+$/K$^+$ pump:** resultant reduction of inward Na$^+$ gradient, thus reducing cellular Ca^{2+} extrusion via Na$^+$/Ca^{2+} exchange transporter
- **Increased Ca^{2+} storage:** reduced Ca^{2+} extrusion causes more intracellular storage and greater intra-cellular release of calcium, increasing the force of myocardial contraction
- **Anti-arrhythmic:** less Ca^{2+} extrusion increases the refractory period of the AV node thus reducing its maximal rate of conduction

Indications
1. Supraventricular tachycardia: particularly for control of fast AF when hypotension is a risk
2. Heart failure: evidence of symptomatic (fewer hospital admissions) benefit in patients with EF <45% (if already taking ACEi + diuretic)

Contraindications
1. Second-/third-degree heart block: reduced conduction through the AV node
2. Wolff–Parkinson–White: increased antegrade conduction through the accessory pathway due to increased refractory period of AV node

Interactions
1. Furosemide, thiazide diuretics: agents lower K$^+$, increasing digoxin effect on myocardium and risk of toxicity
2. ACEi, spironolactone: decrease excretion
3. Calcium antagonists, amiodarone: increased toxicity

Side effects
Dangerous (mostly only during toxicity)
1. Arrhythmias: bradyarrhythmias
2. Conduction: development of heart block

Common
1. Nausea
2. Diarrhoea and vomiting
3. Anorexia
4. Visual blurring/yellow halo

Excretion/metabolism
Half-life
- 36–48 hours (normal renal function)

Metabolism
- Hepatic metabolism (16%) and renal excretion
- **Hepatic:** p-glycoprotein
- **Renal:** dose should be reduced in renal impairment and the elderly

Routes
- Oral
- Intravenous

Starting dose
- **Acute SVT:** 500 μg PO repeated 12 hours later
- **Emergency loading:** 0.75–1 mg IV over 2 hours
- **Maintenance for AF/flutter:** 125–250 μg PO OD
- **Heart failure:** 62.5–125 μg PO OD

Monitoring/equipment
- ECG monitoring and blood pressure if used for acute SVT
- ST depression on ECG may signify development of toxicity
- Blood levels: not routinely required; if required, take sample 6 hours post dose

30.5 ATROPINE

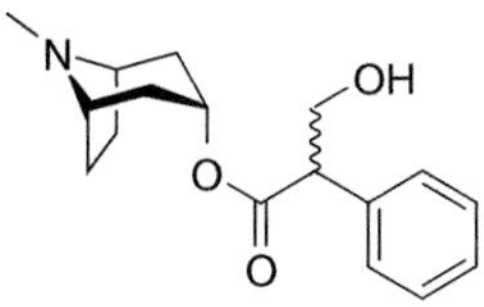

Figure 30.5 Structure of atropine.

Drug class
- Endogenous alkaloid

Pharmacology
- **Antagonist:** blocks parasympathetic muscarinic receptors (M2) on SAN and AVN
- **Reduced parasympathetic:** blockade of vagus-mediated limitation of heart rate at SAN and AVN
- **Positive chronotropism:** this increases the rate at the SAN and conduction through the AVN

Indications
1. Bradycardia: sinus, atrial, nodal or AV-block related bradycardia with haemodynamic/cardiac instability or recent asystole/pauses >3 seconds
2. No evidence for use in cardiac arrest

Contraindications
1. Myasthenia gravis: blockade of acetylcholine receptors increasing symptoms
2. Paralytic ileus: decreased gut stimulation
3. Toxic megacolon: decreases gut stimulation increasing risk of perforation
4. Prostatic enlargement: increased risk of urinary retention

Interactions
1. Antimuscarinic agents (e.g. tricyclics): potentiate antimuscarinic adverse effects
2. Metaclopramide: atropine antagonizes effect on gastrointestinal activity
3. Digoxin: increased levels of digoxin, mechanism unknown

Side effects
Dangerous
1. Acute confusion/hallucinations: particularly in the elderly, atropine is able to cross the blood–brain barrier
2. Cardiac hyperstimulation: VF, VT, SVT

Common
Anticholinergic symptoms are the primary adverse effects:

1. Blurred vision
2. Dry mouth
3. Urinary retention
4. Palpitations
5. Constipation

Excretion/metabolism
Half-life
- 2 hours

Metabolism
- **Hepatic (50%):** metabolized by hydroxylation
- **Renal (50%):** excreted unchanged

Routes

- Intravenous
- Intramuscular

Starting dose

- **Bradycardia:** 500 µg IV, repeated to a maximum of 3 mg

Monitoring/equipment

- ECG monitoring and blood pressure essential

KEY CLINICAL TRIALS

Key trial 30.1

Trial name: CAST I trial.

Participants: 2300 patients with asymptomatic/mildly symptomatic ventricular arrhythmia who had an MI >6 days but <2 years previously.

Intervention: Encainide, flecainide, moricizine.

Control: Placebo group.

Outcome: Encainide and flecainide had a mortality rate at 10 months of 4.5% compared with 1.2% for placebo.

Reason for inclusion: Flecainide should not be used in patients who have had an MI – translated to those with any structural heart disease.

Reference: The Cardiac Arrhythmia Suppression Trial (CAST) Investigators. Preliminary Report: Effect of encainide and flecainide on mortality in a randomized trial of arrhythmia suppression after myocardial infarction. N Engl J Med. 1989;321(6),406–412. http://www.nejm.org/doi/full/10.1056/NEJM198908103210629

Key trial 30.2

Trial name: DIG.

Participants: 6800 patients with symptomatic heart failure (LVEF ≤ 45%) in sinus rhythm.

Intervention: Digoxin + diuretics and ACEi.

Control: Placebo + diuretics and ACEi.

Outcome: No effect on mortality (34.8% digoxin, 35.1% control) – 37-month mean follow-up. Fewer patients admitted to hospital for worsening heart failure (26.8% digoxin, 34.7% placebo, $p < 0.001$).

Reason for inclusion: This trial underlies the use of digoxin in heart failure for symptomatic benefit.

Reference: Digitalis Investigation Group. The effect of digoxin on mortality and morbidity in patients with heart failure. N Engl J Med. 1997;336 (8):525–533. http://www.nejm.org/doi/full/10.1056/NEJM199702203360801

 For additional resources and to test your knowledge, visit the companion website at:

www.wiley.com/go/camm/cardiology

31 Beta-Blockers

George Davies

Oxford University Hospitals NHS Trust, Oxford, UK

31.1 GENERAL NOTES

These agents are competitive antagonists to the beta (β)-adrenoceptor, present on many tissues.

Box 31.1   Sites of clinically significant beta-adrenoceptors

- Myocardium
- Bronchial smooth muscle
- Vascular smooth muscle
- Juxtaglomerular renin-releasing tissue
- Presynaptic receptors on sympathetic neurons
- Liver

Myocardial effect
- Decreases the action of cathecholamines released by the sympathetic nervous system on the β1-adrenoceptor
- **β1-receptors:** stimulation in the myocardium increases the rate and force of myocyte contraction:
    1. **Negative chronotropic:** beta-blockade reduces the rate of myocyte contraction and can terminate or prevent tachyarrhythmias
    2. **Negative inotropic:** beta-blockade reduces the force of myocyte contraction thus reducing myocardial oxygen consumption, making these agents of use in ischaemic heart disease

Effect on smooth muscle
β2-receptors are present in vascular smooth muscle cause vasodilatation, thus β2-blockade causes relative vasoconstriction:

1. IHD: the reduction in myocardial oxygen consumption is sufficiently greater than the effect of coronary artery constriction with beta-blockade

2. Airway disease: β2-receptors on bronchial smooth muscle cause relaxation and dilatation of the airways, therefore beta-blockade can cause bronchospasm (comparatively selective β1-antagonists are not free from this effect)

Hypertension
Beta-blockers are also useful for hypertension. This is most likely to be multifactorial:

1. Reduction of cardiac output: negative chronotropic and inotropic effect
2. Reduction of renin release: from renal juxtaglomerular apparatus
3. Reduced catecholamine release: from sympathetic neurons by blockade of presynaptic receptors
4. Block α1-receptors: some agents (e.g. carvedilol) have this effect on vascular smooth muscle causing vasodilatation

---

Clinical Guide to Cardiology, First Edition. Edited by Christian F. Camm and A. John Camm.
© 2016 John Wiley & Sons, Ltd. Published 2016 by John Wiley & Sons, Ltd.
Companion website: www.wiley.com/go/camm/cardiology.

Heart failure

Beta-blockers have been shown to reduce mortality in heart failure.

1. Mechanism: most likely through the same mechanism useful in their benefit in angina and post MI
2. Haemodynamic instability: beta-blockers are negatively inotropic so they should not be used in acute heart failure

Liver

Blockade of liver adrenoceptors reduces glucose release by the liver. In diabetic subjects this may delay the recovery of blood glucose following administration of insulin and can increase the risk of exercise-induced hypoglycaemia.

31.2 NON-SELECTIVE

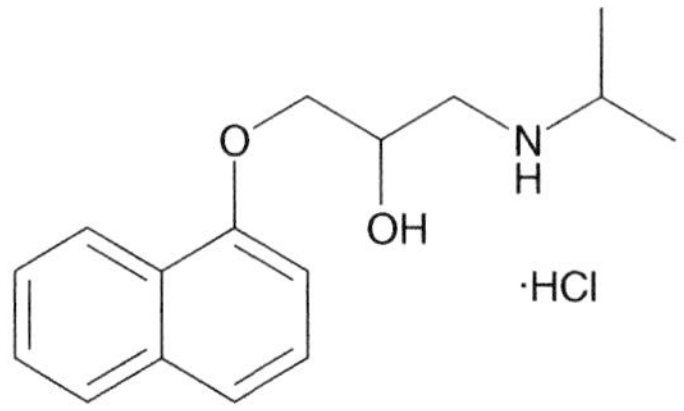

Figure 31.1 Chemical structure of propranolol.

Drug examples
• Propranolol

Pharmacology
• No preference for $\beta 1/2$

Indications (cardiac)
1. Hypertension
2. Portal hypertension
3. Ischaemic heart disease
4. Tachyarrhythmias (particularly symptomatic for palpitations)

Box 31.2   Non-cardiac indications for non-selective beta-blockers

• Anxiety
• Essential tremor
• Migraine

Contraindications
1. Asthma/bronchospasm
2. Severe peripheral arterial disease
3. Bradycardia/sick sinus syndrome
4. Second-/third-degree heart block
5. Cardiogenic shock/hypotension
6. Acute heart failure

Cautions
1. COPD
2. First-degree heart block
3. Diabetes mellitus

Interactions
1. Calcium-channel blockers: serious risk of bradycardia and heart block (especially verapamil/diltiazem)
2. Anti-arrhythmics: there is increased risk of bradycardia and AV block

Side effects
Dangerous
1. Bradycardia
2. Hypotension
3. Bronchospasm

Common
1. Peripheral vasoconstriction
2. Fatigue
3. Depression
4. Sleep disturbances
5. Raynaud phenomenon

Excretion/metabolism
Half-life
- 4–6 hours

Metabolism
- Majority hepatic metabolism: CYP2D6, CYP1A2
- Renal excretion of metabolites

Route
- Oral
- Intravenous

Starting dose
- **Hypertension:** 40 mg PO BD (maximum 240 mg BD)
- **Portal hypertension:** 10 mg PO TDS – titrated to heart rate (maximum 60 mg QDS)
- **Ischaemic heart disease:** 40 mg PO BD (maximum 80 mg QDS)
- **Arrhythmia:**
  - 10 mg PO TDS (maximum 30 mg QDS)
  - 1 mg IV/min repeated every 2 minutes as required to a maximum of 5 mg
- **Anxiety**: 40 mg PO OD
- **Migraine:** 20 mg PO QDS (maximum 60 mg QDS)
- **Essential tremor**: 40 mg PO BD (maximum 80 mg TDS)

31.3 CARDIOSELECTIVE

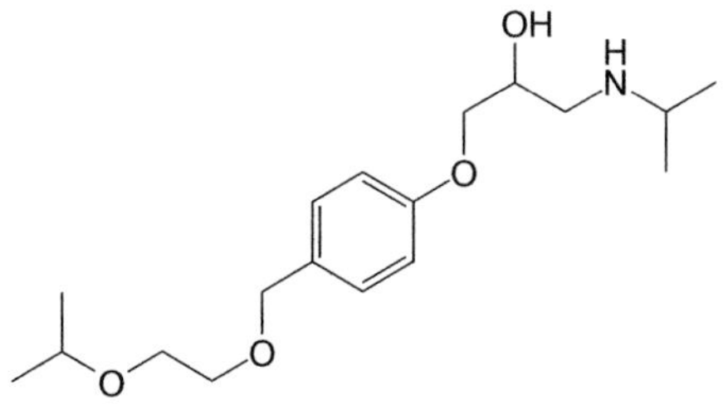

Figure 31.2 Chemical structure of bisoprolol.

Drug example
- Bisoprolol
- Atenolol
- Metoprolol

Pharmacology
- Relative selectivity β1 > β2

Indications
1. Hypertension
2. Ischaemic heart disease
3. Arrhythmia (treatment and prophylaxis of SVT, particularly AF)
4. Heart failure (bisoprolol and metoprolol have shown benefit)

Box 31.3 Indications for metoprolol

- Metoprolol is primarily used IV for acute SVTs
- Short-acting beta-blocker preparation to terminate SVTs
- Minimizes bradycardia and bronchospasm

Contraindications
Largely as for propranolol

Cautions
- **Psoriasis:** increased risk of exacerbation with bisoprolol
- Otherwise as for propranolol

Interactions
As for propranolol

Side effects
As for propranolol

Excretion/metabolism
Half life
- Metoprolol: 3–7 hours
- Bisoprolol: 10–12 hours

Metabolism
- Hepatic: primarily CYP2D6
- Excretion: faeces (50%), urine (50%)

Route
- Oral
- Intravenous (metoprolol only)

Starting dose
Oral starting dose
- Start small and build up for hypertension, angina and HF
- **Bisoprolol:** 1.25 mg PO OD (maximum 10 mg OD; for hypertension/angina 5–20 mg OD)
- **Atenolol:** 25 mg PO OD (maximum 100 mg PO OD)
- **Metoprolol:** 50 mg PO BD (maximum 100 mg PO TDS)

Termination of arrhythmia
- **Bisoprolol:** 5 mg PO (repeat as necessary, generally to maximum of 10 mg)
- **Atenolol:** 50–100 mg PO
- **Metoprolol:** 2–5 mg IV at a rate of 1–2 mg/min (repeat as necessary to maximum of 10–15 mg)

KEY CLINICAL TRIALS

Key trial 31.1

Trial name: ISIS-1.

Participants: 16 000 patients with suspected MI within 12 hours of onset of symptoms.

Intervention: Atenolol 5–10 mg IV STAT with 100 mg/day PO OD for 7 days.

Control: Equivalent medical therapy but no beta-blockers.

Outcome: Significant reduction in vascular cause of mortality in the week of treatment and at 1 year in the intervention group. Much of the benefit occurred within the first 24 hours.

Reason for inclusion: Seminal demonstration of benefit of beta-blockers in acute myocardial infarction.

Reference: ISIS-1 (First International Study of Infarct Survival) Collaborative Group. Randomised trial of intravenous atenolol among 16027 cases of suspected acute myocardial infarction: ISIS-1. Lancet. 1986;328(8498):57–66. http://www.thelancet.com/journals/lancet/article/PIIS0140-6736(86)91607-7/abstract.

Key trial 31.2

Trial name: CIBIS-II.

Participants: 2600 patients with NYHA III or IV with LVEF ≤35% who were receiving standard therapy with diuretics and ACE inhibitors.

Intervention: Bisoprolol 1.25 mg OD increasing to 10 mg.

Control: Placebo.

Outcome: Significant mortality benefit compared with placebo (11.8% compared with 17.3%). In the intervention group there was also a significantly lower number of sudden deaths.

Reason for inclusion: Significant survival benefit in heart failure with bisoprolol.

Reference: CIBIS-II Investigators and Committees. The Cardiac Insufficiency Bisoprolol Study II (CIBIS-II): a randomised trial. Lancet. 1999;353(9486):9–13. http://www.thelancet.com/journals/lancet/article/PIIS0140-6736(98)11181-9/fulltext.

 For additional resources and to test your knowledge, visit the companion website at:

www.wiley.com/go/camm/cardiology

32 Calcium-Channel Blockers

George Davies

Oxford University Hospitals NHS Trust, Oxford, UK

32.1 GENERAL NOTES

- **Voltage-gated calcium channel:** all agents of this group bind to the L-type voltage-gated Ca^{2+} channel
- **Open state:** agents bind more strongly when the channel is in a depolarized (i.e. open) state
- **Selectivity:** agents are selective for either cardiac or smooth-muscle myocytes
- **Blockade:** reduces the inward Ca^{2+} current into the cell
- Three broad agent classes:
  a. **Dihydropyridines:** nifedipine, amlodipine
  b. **Phenylalkylamines:** verapamil
  c. **Benzothiazepines:** diltiazem
- **Inward Ca^{2+} current:** is key to propagation of the action potential in SAN and AV node
- **Depolarization:** Ca^{2+} current blockade reduces the rate of depolarization through the AV node
- **Negative inotropism:** reduced Ca^{2+} entry during depolarization reduces both the force of contraction and the chance of spontaneous depolarizations
- **Afterload:** smooth muscle relaxation dilates coronary and systemic vessels reducing afterload
- **Reflex tachycardia:** results from vasodilatation with some agents in response to blood pressure reduction

32.2 CARDIAC SELECTIVE

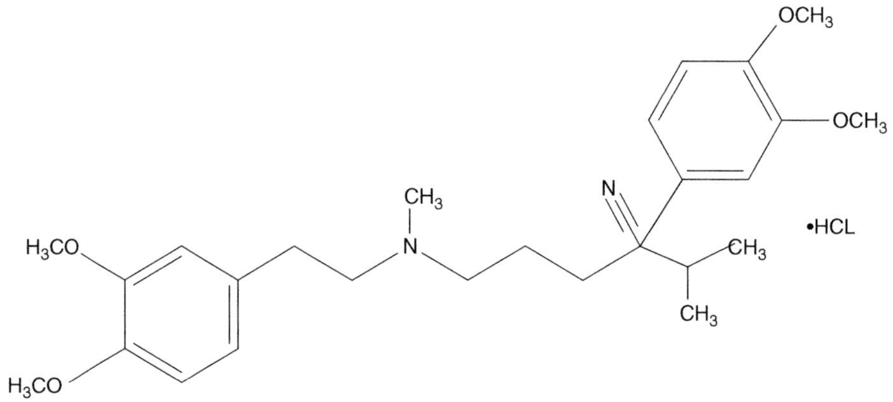

Figure 32.1 Chemical structure of verapamil.

Drug examples
- Diltiazem
- Verapamil

Clinical Guide to Cardiology, First Edition. Edited by Christian F. Camm and A. John Camm.
© 2016 John Wiley & Sons, Ltd. Published 2016 by John Wiley & Sons, Ltd.
Companion website: www.wiley.com/go/camm/cardiology.

Pharmacology
- Greater action on cardiac L-type calcium channels than on smooth-muscle channels
- Verapamil is the more cardioselective of the two and has increased effect on the AV node (decreased chronotropic effect)

Indications
1. **Arrhythmias:** in particular SVT prevention – verapamil is the agent most often used
2. **Angina:** diltiazem is the agent of choice
3. **Hypertension:** diltiazem is the agent of choice

Contraindications
1. **Heart failure:** negatively inotropic
2. **Hypotension:** can exacerbate this condition
3. **Bradycardia:** can exacerbate this condition
4. **Second-degree heart block:** can lead to complete AV nodal block
5. **Third-degree heart block:** can reduce the aberrant ventricular depolarization required in complete heart block
6. **Atrial flutter/fibrillation with associated accessory pathway:** risk of accessory pathway dominance and resultant VF
7. **Acute porphyria:** reports of inducing acute exacerbation

Cautions
1. Post myocardial infarction
2. First-degree heart block
3. Aortic stenosis
4. H(O)CM

Interactions (selected)
1. **Beta-blockers:** risk of asystole, complete heart block, serious bradycardia and heart failure if combined
2. **Dantrolene:** absolute contraindication as risk of VF
3. **CYP3A4 inducers:** (e.g. carbamazepine/phenytoin) decrease the effects of verapamil
4. **Digoxin:** increases the level by decreasing renal clearance
5. **Statin:** verapamil increases risk of statin-induced myopathy

Side effects
Dangerous
1. Conduction block
2. Arrhythmias
3. Hypotension
4. Hepatotoxicity (diltiazem)

Common
1. Headache
2. Gingival hyperplasia
3. Flushes
4. Peripheral oedema
5. Reflex tachycardia
6. Rash (verapamil)
7. Constipation (verapamil)
8. Fatigue

Excretion/metabolism
Half-life
- **Diltiazem:** 3–4.5 hours (extended release: 4–10 hours)
- **Verapamil:** 3–7 hours

Metabolism
- Primarily hepatic: CYP3A4

Route
- Oral
- Intravenous

Starting dose
Diltiazem
- **Angina:** 60 mg TDS PO (maximum 360 mg daily)
- **Hypertension:** 180 mg daily OD/BD PO (maximum 480 mg) – modified-release preparations are used in this context

Verapamil
- **Angina/hypertension**: 80 mg TDS PO (maximum 160 mg TDS)
- **Arrhythmias (chronic):** 40 mg TDS PO (maximum 120 mg TDS)
- **Arrhythmias (acute):** 5–10 mg IV over 2–3 minutes + ECG monitoring +/– additional 5 mg after 5–10 minutes

32.3 ACTION PRIMARILY ON VASCULAR SMOOTH MUSCLE

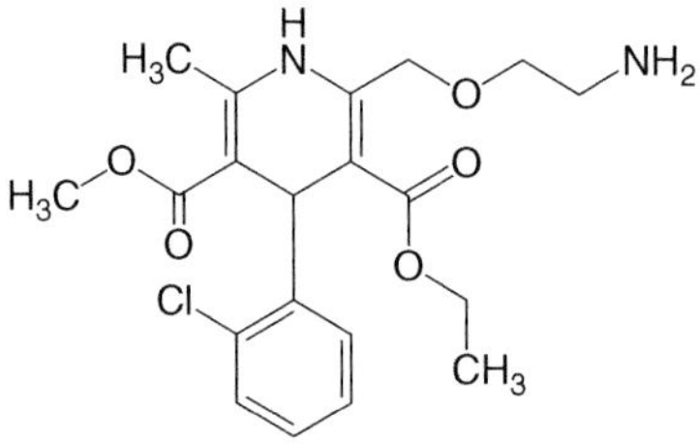

Figure 32.2 Chemical structure of amlodipine.

Drug examples
- Amlodipine
- Felodipine
- Nifedipine

Pharmacology
- Long-acting dihydropyridines
- Action on smooth-muscle L-type calcium channels predominates
- Felodipine is similar to amlodipine but is less negatively ionotropic
- Nifedipine is short acting, causing reflex tachycardia; it may be used as long-acting preparations

---

Box 32.1   Particulars of nifedipine

- Nifedipine is short acting and is also the oldest of the three agents
- It causes a reflex sympathetic response – tachycardia and contractility
- For these reason nifedipine can cause erratic BP control and worsen IHD
- These effects can be overcome when nifedipine is used in long-acting preparations

---

Indications
1. Angina
2. Hypertension

Contraindications
1. **Cardiogenic shock:** due to negative inotropic effect and hypotension
2. **Acute coronary syndrome:** due to hypotensive effects
3. **Aortic stenosis (clinically significant):** risk of hypotension

Caution
1. **Acute porphyria:** also reported to cause acute exacerbations, less data
2. **Chronic liver disease:** primarily hepatic metabolism

Interactions
1. Less than other class, amlodipine may increase levels of theophylline
2. Metabolism is affected by enzyme inhibitors and inducers

Side effects
Dangerous
1. Hypotension
2. Symptoms of worsening heart failure
3. Worsening angina

Common
1. Ankle swelling (particularly amlodipine, related to angioedema)
2. Headache
3. Flushing
4. Dizziness (particularly nifedipine)

Excretion/metabolism
Half-life
- **Amlodipine:** 30–50 hours
- **Felodipine:** 10–15 hours
- **Nifedipine:** 2–5 hours

Metabolism
- Primarily hepatic: CYP3A4

Route
- Oral

Starting dose
Amlodipine
- **Hypertension:** 5 mg OD PO (maximum 10 mg OD)

Felodipine
- **Hypertension:** 5 mg OD PO (maximum 20 mg OD)

Nifedipine
- **Hypertension:** 30 mg PO OD – extended-release preparations (maximum 90 mg OD)
- **Angina:** 30 mg PO OD – extended-release preparations (maximum 120 mg OD)

Box 32.2 Dosing of nifedipine

- Due to short half-life, long-acting preparations should be used for hypertension and angina
- Normal preparations are only really useful to acutely lower blood pressure (e.g. subarachnoid haemorrhage, aortic dissection)
- Different long-acting preparations may have different doses – if in doubt, look up the specific preparation

KEY CLINICAL TRIALS

Key trial 32.1

Trial name: VALUE.

Participants: 12 570 patients with cardiovascular disease or three or more risk factors for cardiovascular disease (male, >50 years, diabetes, smoker etc.).

Intervention: Amlodipine 5 mg OD (doubled to 10 mg after 1 month).

Control: Valsartan 80 mg OD (doubled up to 160 mg after 1 month).

Outcome: Amlodipine had better BP control than valsartan particularly in first month. No significant difference in cardiovascular morbidity.

Reason for inclusion: Demonstration of amlodipine as effective in control of hypertension and at least as effective as ACEi at reducing cardiovascular morbidity, however there is no comparison to control in this trial.

Reference: Julius S, *et al*. Outcomes in hypertensive patients at high cardiovascular risk treated with regimens based on valsartan or amlodipine: the VALUE randomised trial. Lancet. 2004;363(9426):2022–2031. http://www.thelancet.com/journals/lancet/article/PIIS0140-6736(04)16451-9/fulltext

Key trial 32.2

Trial name: PREVENT.

Participants: 825 patients with angiographically documented coronary artery disease.

Intervention: Amlodipine.

Control: Placebo.

Outcome: No difference in angiographic progression or the risk of major cardiovascular events. The amlodipine group had significantly fewer hospitalizations with non-fatal unstable angina and congestive cardiac failure and received less revascularization.

Reason for inclusion: When given to individuals with IHD, amlodipine resulted in significantly fewer admissions with unstable angina, supporting its role in management of angina symptoms.

Reference: Pitt B, et al. Effect of amlodipine on the progression of atherosclerosis and the occurrence of clinical events. Circulation. 2000;102(13):1503–1510. http://www.ncbi.nlm.nih.gov/pubmed/11004140.

 For additional resources and to test your knowledge, visit the companion website at:

www.wiley.com/go/camm/cardiology

33 Nitrates

George Davies
Oxford University Hospitals NHS Trust, Oxford, UK

33.1 GENERAL NOTES

- Nitrate agents are converted to nitric oxide (NO) at the vascular endothelium
- NO is an endogenous signalling molecule which causes local relaxation of vascular smooth muscle
- NO plays a key role both in physiological maintenance of tissue perfusion and in pathological states (e.g. septic shock)
- NO activation and release is induced by shear wall stress and other signalling molecules (acetylcholine, bradykinin, substance P)
- Produced in the endothelium, NO diffuses into smooth muscle cells and activates guanylate cyclase
- Guanylate cyclase activation increases production of cyclic guanosine monophosphate (cyclic-GMP)
- Cyclic-GMP causes activation of protein kinase G, eventually resulting in the dephosphorylation and deactivation of the contractile apparatus and a reduction of intracellular calcium
- The summative effects are vascular smooth muscle relaxation

33.2 ORAL NITRATES

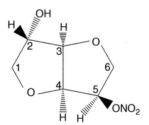

Figure 33.1 Chemical structure of isosorbide mononitrate.

Drug examples
- Glyceryl trinitrate (GTN)
- Isosorbide mononitrate (ISMN)

Pharmacology
- A systemic increase in nitric oxide causes vascular dilatation
- In angina, coronary blood flow is limited by vessel stenosis. Either the stenosis or oxygen demand is such that endogenous dilatation of downstream arterioles is insufficient
- Nitrates dilate coronary arteries, opposing coronary spasm and globally increasing coronary blood flow
- Dilatation of collaterals may be central to their action, as vessels in ischaemic areas are already maximally relaxed
- Relaxation of systemic arteries decreases systemic resistance, afterload and oxygen demand

Clinical Guide to Cardiology, First Edition. Edited by Christian F. Camm and A. John Camm.
© 2016 John Wiley & Sons, Ltd. Published 2016 by John Wiley & Sons, Ltd.
Companion website: www.wiley.com/go/camm/cardiology.

Indications
1. Stable angina
2. Acute coronary syndrome

Contraindications
1. Hypotension
2. Severe anaemia
3. Closed-angle glaucoma

Caution
Primarily in situations in which hypotension is a risk:

1. Hypovolaemia
2. Severe aortic stenosis/mitral stenosis
3. Constrictive pericarditis
4. Tamponade
5. HOCM
6. Raised intracranial pressure (high BP essential for perfusion)

Interactions
- **Phosphodiesterase inhibitors:** (e.g. sildenafil) cause significant hypotension

Side effects
Dangerous
1. Hypotension
2. Nitrate withdrawal

Box 33.1   Nitrate withdrawal

- Occurs if long-term therapy stopped too rapidly
- Symptoms include:
  a. Headache
  b. Hypertension
  c. Angina

Common
1. Headache
2. Dizziness
3. Flushing

Excretion/metabolism
Half-life
- GTN: 1–4 minutes
- ISMN: 4–6 hours

Metabolism
- Primarily hepatic

Route
- Oral

Starting dose
- **GTN:** two sprays/tablets PRN sublingual
- **ISMN:** 30 mg BD PO standard starting dose (maximum 40 mg BD)

1. Can occur with long-acting preparations (IMDUR/ISMN, slow-release GTN patches, continuous IV infusions)
2. Twice daily preparations should be given 8 hours apart
3. This allows for a nitrate-free period overnight

33.3 NITRATES USED AS AN INFUSION

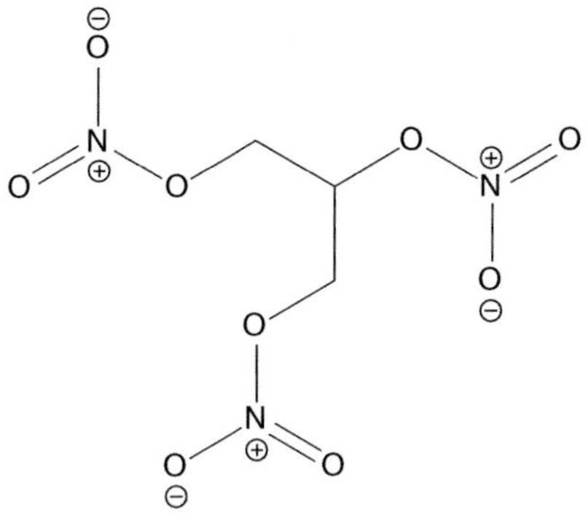

Figure 33.2 Chemical structure of glyceryl trinitrate.

Drug examples
- GTN infusion

Pharmacology
- As discussed in Section 33.2, nitrates increase coronary blood oxygenation
- In pulmonary oedema, their primary benefit is reduction of preload and afterload
- In acute pulmonary oedema, the heart is compromised by volume of venous return (preload) or the tension required to eject fluid in systole (afterload)
- Reduction in preload and afterload reduces cardiac workload and pulmonary oedema
- The two effects combined make nitrates very effective but with the significant side effect of hypotension

Indications
1. ACS with ongoing chest pain despite initial management
2. Acute heart failure

Contraindications
As for oral nitrates

Interactions
As for oral nitrates

Side-effects
As for oral preparations – tolerance and caution in withdrawal are more prevalent

Excretion/metabolism
Half-life
- 1–4 minutes

Metabolism
- Primarily hepatic

Starting dose

- In most situations, prescribe GTN 50 mg in 50 mL IV (is usually pre-prepared)
- Usual starting rate 0.5–1.0 ml/hr
- Rate is titrated (up to 10 mL/hr) to clinical response and blood pressure (keep systolic BP >90 mmHg)

KEY CLINICAL TRIALS

Key trial 33.1

Trial name: GISSI-3.

Participants: 19 394 patients admitted to CCU within 24 hours of onset of acute MI.

Intervention: Either lisinopril (5 mg initial then 10 mg OD) or GTN (IV for first 24 hours then 10 mg patch daily) or both.

Control: Standard medical therapy but neither of the above agents.

Outcome: Lisinopril alone or both agents group had significantly reduced overall mortality. GTN alone did not show any significant reduction in these outcomes.

Reason for inclusion: Supports ACEi inclusion in ACS protocol. Suggestive that, although GTN may be symptomatically beneficial, it may not have any concrete benefit to outcome.

Reference: GISSI group. GISSI-3: effects of lisinopril and transdermal glyceryl trinitrate singly and together on 6-week mortality and ventricular function after acute myocardial infarction. Lancet. 1994;343(8906):1115–1122. http://www.ncbi.nlm.nih.gov/pubmed/7910229.

Key trial 33.2

Participants: 110 patients admitted with severe pulmonary oedema and SaO_2 <90%.

Intervention: Isosorbide dinitrate 3 mg bolus IV every 5 minutes + oxygen 10 L/min, furosemide 40 mg IV, morphine 3 mg IV.

Control: Furosemide 80 mg IV bolus every 15 minutes + isosorbide dinitrate 1 mg/hr increasing by 1 mg/hr every 10 min + oxygen 10 L/min, morphine 3 mg IV.

Outcome: Decreased need for mechanical ventilation with nitrate boluses (13% vs. 40%, p = 0.004). Decreased MI with nitrate boluses (17% vs. 37%, p = 0.047).

Reason for inclusion: Although very small, one of the few randomized trials to assess nitrates in acute pulmonary oedema and their combination with furosemide. This trial would support bolus administration of nitrates with low-dose furosemide over the nitrate infusion method.

Reference: Cotter G, et al. Randomized trial of high-dose isosorbide dinitrate plus low-dose furosemide versus high-dose furosemide plus low-dose isosorbide dinitrate in severe pulmonary oedema. Lancet. 1998;351(9100):389–393. http://www.ncbi.nlm.nih.gov/pubmed/9482291.

 For additional resources and to test your knowledge, visit the companion website at:

www.wiley.com/go/camm/cardiology

34 Drugs Targeting the Angiotensin Axis

George Davies
Oxford University Hospitals NHS Trust, Oxford, UK

34.1 GENERAL NOTES

- **Renin–angiotensin axis:** global function in the maintenance of circulating volume and sodium balance
- **Renin:** secreted in response to a range of factors including renal perfusion pressure, glomerular filtration and the control of other control systems (e.g. sympathetic nervous system)
- **Angiotensin I (AI):** production is caused by renin, neither have any end-organ effects in themselves
- **Angiotensin-converting enzyme (ACE):** present on vascular endothelium (particularly lung), catalyses the cleavage of two amino acid residues from angiotensin I to produce angiotensin II
- **Angiotensin II (AII):** acts on AT1 receptors to cause vasoconstriction, increased release of noradrenaline, increased reabsorption of sodium by the kidney and release of aldosterone from the renal cortex
- **Aldosterone:** causes increased sodium and water absorption in the kidney
- **Key target:** the effect of this axis on circulating volume, salt and water balance makes it important in the management of hypertension and heart failure

34.2 ACE INHIBITORS (ACEi)

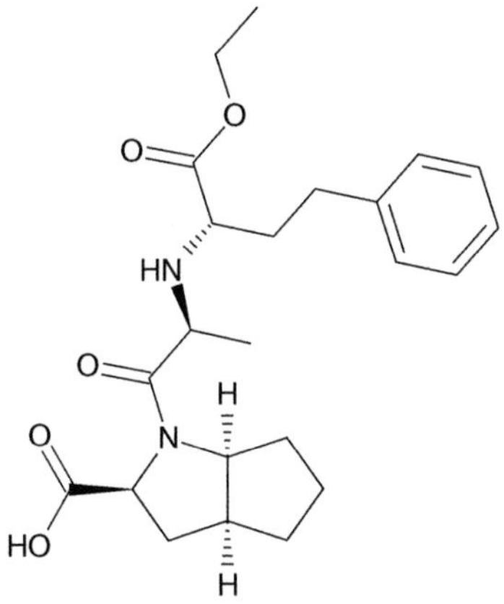

Figure 34.1 Structure of ramipril.

Drug examples
- Captopril
- Lisinopril
- Ramipril

Clinical Guide to Cardiology, First Edition. Edited by Christian F. Camm and A. John Camm.
© 2016 John Wiley & Sons, Ltd. Published 2016 by John Wiley & Sons, Ltd.
Companion website: www.wiley.com/go/camm/cardiology.

Pharmacology
- **Competitive antagonist:** ACEi block the site of the enzyme to which angiotensin I binds, thereby inhibiting its conversion
- **Vasodilatation:** results from decreased amount of AII, and affects the small arteries and arterioles reducing peripheral vascular resistance (decreased afterload, increased cardiac output)
- **Aldosterone:** decreased AII reduces aldosterone release and thus reduces salt and water reabsorption
- The effect is marked in hypertensives and marked for those in high-renin states (e.g. already on diuretic)
- **Bradykinin:** ACE also catalyses the degradation of bradykinin; the dry cough common as a side effect of ACEi is caused by bradykinin elevation

Indications
1. Hypertension
2. Heart failure
3. Cardioprotection post MI

Contraindications
1. **Bilateral renal artery stenosis:** prerenal failure will result, AII constricts the efferent arteriole
2. **Acute renal failure:** decreased renal blood flow will exacerbate the condition
3. **Hyperkalaemia:** exacerbated by ACEi
4. **Pregnancy:** risk of birth defects
5. **Breast feeding:** can cause profound neonatal hypotension

Cautions
1. Clinically significant aortic stenosis
2. Those at risk of falls or postural hypotension
3. Chronic renal disease: increased risk of hyperkalaemia

Interactions
1. NSAIDs: prostaglandins dilate afferent arteriole, synergistic effect to reduce GFR
2. Other agents that cause rise in K^+ (potassium-sparing diuretics, K^+ supplements)
3. Other angiotensin agents (e.g. angiotensin-receptor blockers)
4. Lithium: increased risk of lithium toxicity

Side effects
Dangerous
1. Renal failure
2. Hyperkalaemia
3. Hypotension (particularly first dose)
4. Hypersensitivity/angioedema

Common
1. Dry cough
2. Photosensitivity
3. Pharyngitis/sinusitis

Excretion/metabolism
- Primarily renal excretion – prolonged in heart failure and greatly increased if creatinine clearance <20 mL/min

Half-life
- **Captopril:** 1.9 hours
- **Lisinopril:** 12 hours
- **Ramipril:** 13–17 hours

Metabolism
- Metabolism: hepatic (50%)
- Excretion: renal (50–60%)

Starting dose
Captopril
- **Hypertension:** 12.5 mg BD PO (maximum 50 mg BD)
- **Heart failure:** 6.25 mg BD (maximum 50 mg TDS)

Lisinopril
- **Cardioprotection/heart failure:** 2.5 mg OD PO (maximum 20 mg OD)
- **Hypertension:** 10 mg OD PO (maximum 20 mg OD)

Ramipril
- All: 1.25 mg OD PO (maximum 10 mg OD)

Monitoring
- Renal function and electrolytes at baseline and after 1 week: $\leq 50\%$ increase in creatinine and K^+ <5.5 mmol/L are acceptable

34.3 ANGIOTENSIN-RECEPTOR BLOCKERS

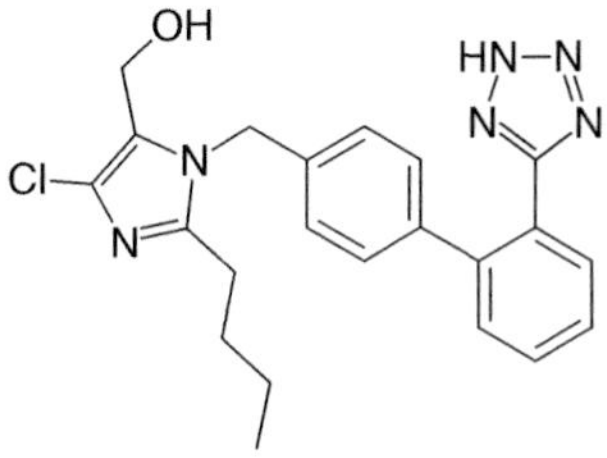

Figure 34.2 Structure of losartan.

Drug examples
- Losartan
- Irbesartan

Pharmacology
- Blockade of AT1 receptors has the same effect on vasoconstriction and fluid status as ACEi
- AT1 blockers do not increase bradykinin and thus can be better tolerated

Indications
1. Hypertension
2. Heart failure
3. Cardioprotection post MI

Contraindications
As with ACEi

Caution
As with ACEi

Interactions
As with ACEi

Side effects
Dangerous
1. Renal failure
2. Hyperkalaemia
3. Hypotension (particularly first dose)
4. Hypersensitivity/angioedema

Common
1. Photosensitivity
2. Pharyngitis/sinusitis

Excretion/metabolism
Half-life
- **Losartan:** 1.5–2 hours
- **Irbesartan:** 11–15 hours

Metabolism
- Primarily hepatic P450 enzyme CYP2C9
- Dose should be reduced in both renal and hepatic impairment

Starting dose
Losartan
- 25 mg PO OD (maximum 100 mg)

Irbesartan
- 150 mg PO OD (maximum 300 mg)

Monitoring
- Renal function and electrolytes at baseline and after 1 week: ≤50% increase in creatinine and K$^+$ <5.5 mmol/L are acceptable

For additional resources and to test your knowledge, visit the companion website at:

www.wiley.com/go/camm/cardiology

35 Diuretics

George Davies

Oxford University Hospitals NHS Trust, Oxford, UK

35.1 LOOP DIURETICS

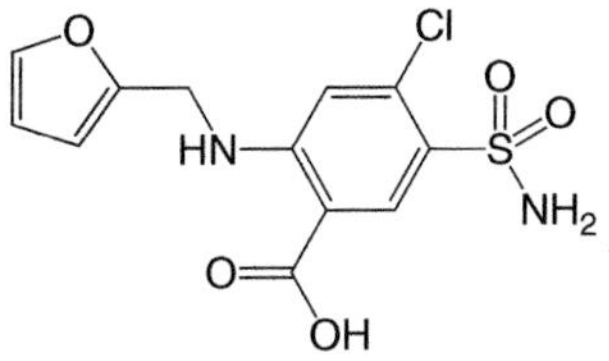

Figure 35.1 Structure of furosemide.

Drug examples
- Furosemide
- Bumetanide

Pharmacology
- **$Na^+/K^+/2Cl^-$:** loop diuretics bind to the chloride site of the $Na^+/K^+/2Cl^-$ co-transporter on the thick ascending limb of the loop of Henle
- **Osmolality gradient:** reduced between glomerular filtrate and renal parenchyma due to inhibition of solute absorption which in turn disrupts free water absorption
- **Salt depletion:** prevention of reabsorption of K^+ and Na^+ can lead to a depletion of these salts
- **Vasodilatation:** secondary effect of IV furosemide which precedes diuresis and is not fully understood; it may include actions via angiotensin, sympathetic and prostaglandin signalling cascades
- **Reducing demand:** cardiac demand is reduced by the overall effect of diuresis and vasodilatation thus reducing circulating volume, preload and afterload

Indications
1. Heart failure (both acute and chronic)
2. Hypertension

Contraindications
1. Severe hypotension
2. Hypokalaemia
3. Hyponatraemia
4. Anuric renal failure
5. Advanced cirrhosis

Caution
1. Those at risk of renal impairment
2. Those at risk of hypotension, particularly postural and in the elderly

Interactions

1. **Digoxin, sotalol and flecainide:** disturbances of K^+ and Mg^{2+} increase toxicity
2. **Gentamicin, lithium:** increases toxicity
3. **Hypoglycaemic agents:** decreases effects of oral hypoglycaemics
4. **Any drug which reduces GFR:** has worse toxicity with furosemide (e.g. ACEi, NSAIDs)

Side effects

Dangerous

1. Hypotension
2. Hypokalaemia
3. Hyponatraemia
4. Hypomagnesaemia

Common

1. Hypocalcaemia
2. Gout (increased urate)
3. Alkalosis (increased loss of H^+ from distal tubule)
4. Tinnitus (dose related, recovers)

Excretion/metabolism

Note GI absorption is impaired in CCF due to poor intestinal perfusion and mesenteric oedema (furosemide > bumetanide).

Half-life

- **Furosemide:** 30–120 minutes (normal renal function), 9 hours (severe CKD)
- **Bumetanide:** 1–1.5 hours

Metabolism

- **Conjugation:** hepatic (10% furosemide, limited in bumetanide)
- **Excretion:** urine (50% furosemide, 80% bumetanide)

Routes

- Oral
- Intravenous

Starting dose

Furosemide

- **Acute pulmonary oedema:** 40–120 mg IV slow bolus. Infusion 120–240 mg/24 hours (less initial vasodilatory effect)
- **Heart failure, hypertension:** 40 mg OD PO (maximum 80 mg BD, second dose at noon)

Bumetanide

- **Heart failure, hypertension:** 1 mg OD PO (maximum 2 mg BD, second dose at noon)

35.2 THIAZIDES AND THIAZIDE-LIKE DIURETICS

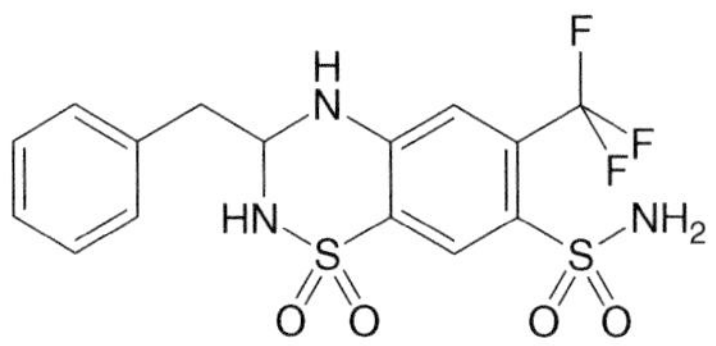

Figure 35.2 Structure of bendroflumethiazide.

Drug examples
- Bendroflumethaizde (thiazide)
- Indapamide (thiazide-like)
- Metolazone (thiazide-like)

Pharmacology
- **Na$^+$/Cl$^-$ co-transporter:** thiazide diuretics act via this co-transporter in the distal convoluted tubule
- **Chloride site:** binding to this site prevents reabsorption of sodium and chloride
- **Circulation volume:** reduced due to loss of these salts and water
- **Electrolyte loss:** disturbance at the distal nephron also causes loss of K$^+$ and Mg^{2+}
- **Thiazide-like diuretics:** also act via the same co-transporter but differ significantly in structure from thiazides and cause less electrolyte disturbance
- **Renin–angiotensin axis:** a reduction in circulating volume is mitigated by a corresponding increase in angiotensin II and thus increased total peripheral resistance
- **Off-target actions:** poorly understood in both classes; they are known to cause a degree of vasodilatation and hyperglycaemia

Indications
1. Congestive cardiac failure
2. Hypertension

Contraindications
1. Hypokalaemia
2. Hyponatraemia
3. Addison's disease: will increase electrolyte abnormalities
4. Severe liver disease
5. Not effective if GFR <30 mL/min/1.73 m^2

Caution
1. **Gout:** increases uric acid level
2. **Diabetes:** increased glucose intolerance
3. **Hypercalcaemia:** increased imbalance
4. **Mild/moderate liver disease:** if loop diuretics are already prescribed, synergistic effect

Interactions
1. **Digoxin, lithium, amiodarone, flecanide, sotalol:** toxicity increased by hypokalaemia
2. **Allopurinol:** increases hypersensitivity
3. **Hypoglycaemic agents:** decreases effects of oral hypoglycaemics
4. Synergistic effect of hypotension/nephrotoxicity when combined with other antihypertensive agents (especially loop diuretics)

Side effects
Dangerous
1. Hypotension
2. Hyponatraemia
3. Hypokalaemia
4. Hypomagnesaemia
5. Haematological: agranulocytosis, leucopenia, thrombocytopenia
6. Pancreatitis

Common
1. GI upset
2. Hyperuricaemia: competes with uric acid for excretion
3. Hyperglycaemia
4. Erectile dysfunction (reversible)
5. Deranged lipid metabolism

Excretion/metabolism
Half-life
- **Bendroflumethiazide:** 3–3.9 hours
- **Indapamide:** 14–25 hours
- **Metolazone:** 20 hours

Metabolism
- **Metabolism:** indapamide is extensively metabolized (CYP3A4)
- **Excretion:** renal excretion predominates for bendroflumethiazide and metolazone

Routes
- Oral

Starting dose
Bendroflumethiazide
- **Heart failure:** 5–10 mg OD PO
- **Hypertension:** 2.5 mg OD PO

Indapamide
- **All:** 2.5 mg OD PO

Metolazone
- **All:** 5 mg OD PO (maximum 20 mg OD)

35.3 POTASSIUM-SPARING DIURETICS

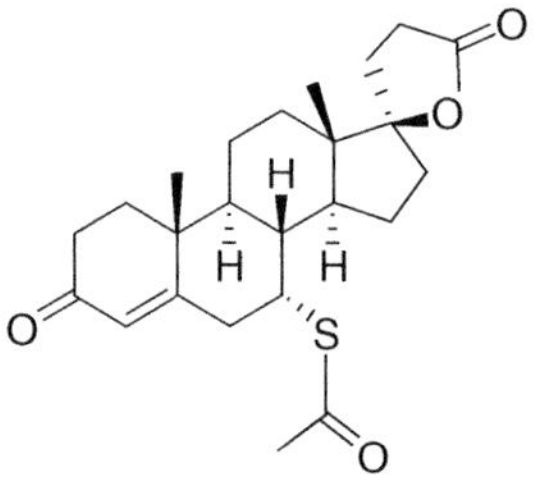

Figure 35.3 Structure of spironolactone.

Drug examples
- Spironolactone
- Eplerenone
- Amiloride

Pharmacology
- Distinguished from other diuretics by the fact that they do not cause hypokalaemia
- **Distal tubule:** reabsorption of sodium at this site is an active process driven by a basal Na^+/K^+ ATPase
- **Aldosterone:** causes transcription changes, upregulating Na^+ reabsorption (Na/K ATPase plus mitochondrial upregulation, upregulation of luminal sodium channels)
- **Blockade:** of this axis causes loss of Na^+ (and thus free water and circulating volume) and retention of K^+
- **Amiloride:** blocks Na^+ channels on the luminal surface of cells in the distal nephrons
- **Spironolactone/eplerenone:** antagonists to intracellular receptors for aldosterone within the epithelium of the distal nephron
- **Poorly antihypertensive:** these agents have a reduced antihypertensive effect compared to other diuretics
- **Survival benefit:** seen with spironolactone/eplerenone in heart failure

Indications
1. **Heart failure:** spironolactone/eplerenone
2. **Hypertension:** essential and secondary
3. **Potassium conservation:** when used with other diuretics

Contraindications
1. Hyperkalaemia
2. Significant risk of hyperkalaemia (e.g. CKD, ACEi)
3. Addison's disease
4. Significant hypotension

Caution
1. Individuals predisposed to hypotension and at risk of falls
2. Cirrhotic liver disease: metabolic acidosis with spironolactone

Interactions
1. **Diuretics:** synergistic effect
2. **Lithium:** increased risk of toxicity
3. **Ciclosporin and tacrolimus:** increase risk of hyperkalaemia
4. **Enzyme inhibitors:** risk of hyperkalaemia increased for spironolactone/eplerenone
5. **Potassium replacements:** should not be co-prescribed due to risk of hyperkalaemia

Side effects
Dangerous
1. Hyperkalaemia
2. Hyponatraemia
3. Metabolic acidosis: spironolactone + cirrhosis

Common
1. Gynaecomastia (off-target effects on sex steroid receptors – less prevalent with eplerenone)
2. Hypotension
3. Abdominal pain

Excretion/metabolism
Half-life
- **Spironolactone:** 1.4 hours
- **Eplerenone:** 3.5–6 hours
- **Amiloride:** 6–9 hours

Metabolism
- **Metabolism:** hepatic (spironolactone/eplerenone)
- **Excretion:** amiloride is not metabolized, only excreted – 50% urine, 50% faeces

Starting dose
Spironolactone
- **Heart failure:** 25 mg OD PO (maximum 50 mg OD)
- **Hypertension:** 100 mg OD PO (maximum 400 mg OD PO)

Eplerenone
- **All:** 25 mg OD PO (maximum 50 mg OD)

Amiloride
- **All:** 10 mg OD PO (maximum 20 mg OD)

KEY TRIALS

Key trial 35.1

Trial Name: RALES.

Participants: 1663 patients with NYHA grade ≥3 receiving an ACE-i and loop diuretic.

Intervention: Spironolactone 25 mg OD with the option to increase to 50 mg after 8 weeks.

Control: Placebo.

Outcome: Spironolactone group had a significantly lower all-cause mortality and frequency of hospitalization (p<0.001 for both).

Reason for inclusion: Key demonstration of the prognostic benefit of spironolactone in heart failure. Emphasizes the role of renin–angiotensin–aldosterone in the pathogenesis of heart failure.

Reference: Pitt B, et al. The effect of spironolactone on morbidity and mortality in patients with severe heart failure. Randomized Aldactone Evaluation Study Investigators. N Engl J Med. 1999;341(10):709–717. http://www.nejm.org/doi/full/10.1056/NEJM199909023411001.

   For additional resources and to test your knowledge, visit the companion website at:

www.wiley.com/go/camm/cardiology

36 Anticoagulants

George Davies

Oxford University Hospitals NHS Trust, Oxford, UK

36.1 HEPARIN

Pharmacology
- Heparin is an endogenous anticoagulant originally extracted from liver
- It is a large glycosaminoglycan of varying lengths
- Binds to antithrombin III and facilitates its binding to thrombin (direct interaction between heparin and thrombin)
- Binding of Factor Xa is also facilitated by heparin but not by direct interaction
- Due to its structure it cannot be absorbed orally, given IV or SC
- When given SC, action is delayed by approximately 60 minutes
- Heparin is generally preferred over more convenient LMWH in three scenarios:
  a. **Severe renal impairment:** heparin has a greater hepatic component to its metabolism
  b. **Accurate monitoring is required:** activated partial thromboplastin time (aPTT) can be used
  c. **Very high bleeding risk:** quicker reversal due to short half-life

Indications
1. Prophylaxis and treatment of VTE
2. May be part of ACS protocol
3. Bridging anticoagulant

Contraindications
1. Active bleeding
2. Thrombocytopenia/history of heparin-induced thrombocytopenia

Caution
1. Bleeding risk: this has to be based on clinical scenario
2. Hyperkalaemia: especially if diabetic, CKD or taking drugs predisposing to hyperkalaemia
3. Chronic liver disease: especially alcoholic liver disease (ALD) + varices

---

Box 36.1   Bleeding risks to consider with anticoagulants

1. Bleeding disorder, e.g. haemophilia
2. GI ulcer
3. Severe uncontrolled hypertension
4. Recent ICH or major infarct
5. Acute/subacute bacterial endocarditis
6. Purpuric events
7. Recent surgery or trauma to CNS structures, including eye
8. Spinal/epidural anaesthesia

Clinical Guide to Cardiology, First Edition. Edited by Christian F. Camm and A. John Camm.
© 2016 John Wiley & Sons, Ltd. Published 2016 by John Wiley & Sons, Ltd.
Companion website: www.wiley.com/go/camm/cardiology.

Interactions

1. Increased bleeding risk with other anticoagulants, antiplatelets and NSAIDs
2. IV GTN may decrease effectiveness

Side effects

Dangerous

1. Haemorrhage
2. Heparin-induced thrombocytopenia (HIT): see Box 36.2
3. Hyperkalaemia: particularly problematic with longer-term use – due to decreased production of aldosterone

---

Box 36.2 Heparin-induced thrombocytopenia (HIT)

1. Mechanism: serious immune-mediated reaction – IgM/G
2. Timing: 5–10 days after initiation of heparin
3. Definition: 50% reduction in platelets +/- skin reaction
4. Thrombosis: may paradoxically accompany HIT
5. Management: stop heparin and obtain specialist advice
6. Alternative: danaparoid can be used a substitute for heparin in HIT

Common

1. Osteoporosis: associated with prolonged therapy
2. Alopecia: associated with prolonged therapy
3. Platelet fall: early transient fall in platelets can occur and is not necessarily clinically important

Excretion/metabolism

Half-life

- 60–90 minutes

Metabolism

- Metabolism: partial hepatic metabolism (non-cytochrome)
- Excretion: urinary

Starting dose

- **VTE prophylaxis/ACS:** 5000 units SC BD
- **VTE treatment:** 5000 units IV bolus, then 15–25 units/kg/hr IV (adjustment following should be based on aPTT ratio and local guidelines)

Monitoring

- aPTT can be used reliably
- Check FBC if use continues >5 days
- Check U&E if use continues >7 days

Box 36.3 Reversal of heparins

- Protamine sulphate
- Inactivates heparin by forming complex
- Only partially effective with LMWH, not effective with fondaparinux
- Dose is based on heparin dose that has already been given
- Seek specialist advice

36.2 LOW MOLECULAR WEIGHT HEPARINS (LMWHs)

Drug examples
- Dalteparin
- Enoxaparin
- Tinzaparin

Pharmacology
- **Fragments:** LMWHs are fragments of heparin (hence lower molecular weight)
- **Antithrombin III:** LMWHs still bind to antithrombin III, however, they have limited activity on thrombin and are targeted towards factor X
- **Predictable kinetics:** for this reason they can be given once daily and do not require routine monitoring (note they may not prolong aPTT, anti-Xa assay should be used instead)

Table 36.1 Molecular weight and anticoagulant activities of LMWHs

LMWH	Average molecular weight	Ratio anti-Xa/anti-IIa activity
Dalteparin	6000	2.5
Enoxaparin	4500	3.9
Tinzaparin	6500	1.6

Indications
1. Prophylaxis and treatment of VTE
2. May be part of ACS protocol
3. As bridging anticoagulant

Contraindications
1. Active bleeding
2. Moderate to severe renal impairment (heparin is preferred)

Caution
1. Bleeding risk: see Box 36.1
2. Hyperkalaemia
3. Moderate to severe renal impairment

Interactions
1. Increased bleeding risk with other anticoagulants, antiplatelets and NSAIDs

Side effects
Dangerous
1. Haemorrhage
2. HIT (much less common with LMWHs than unfractionated heparin)
3. Hyperkalaemia: particularly problematic with longer-term use due to decreased production of aldosterone

Common
1. **Osteoporosis:** associated with prolonged therapy (less common for LMWHs)
2. **Alopecia:** associated with prolonged therapy (less common for LMWHs)

Excretion/metabolism
Half-life
1. **Dalteparin:** 3–5 hours
2. **Enoxaparin:** 4.5 hours
3. **Tinzaparin:** 3–4 hours

Metabolism
- Metabolism: minimal hepatic component
- Excretion: primarily renal

Starting dose
Dosing should be based on local guidelines and patient's weight as different formulations may have markedly different doses.

Monitoring
- aPTT cannot be used with LMWH, anti-Xa assay is the test of choice

36.3 FONDAPARINUX

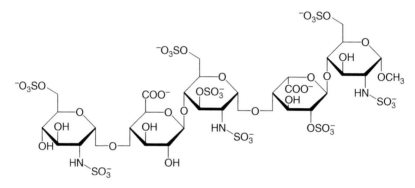

Figure 36.1 Structure of fondaparinux.

Pharmacology
- **Pentasaccharide:** fondaparinux is a synthetic pentasaccharide LMWH analogue
- **Factor Xa:** fondaparinux directs antithrombin to inhibit factor Xa in a similar way to LMWHs
- **Long half-life:** can be administered once daily similarly to LMWHs

Indications
- Similar to unfractionated heparin and LMWH
- There is an evidence base to specifically support fondaparinux usage in ACS

Contraindications
1. Active bleeding
2. Creatinine clearance <30 mL/min
3. Bacterial endocarditis
4. History of serious hypersensitivity reaction

Caution
1. Bleeding risk: see Box 36.1
2. Moderate to severe renal impairment
3. Platelets <100 × 10^9/L

Interactions
- Increased bleeding risk with other anticoagulants, antiplatelets and NSAIDs

Side effects
Dangerous
1. Haemorrhage
2. Hypokalaemia
3. HIT (much less common than with unfractionated heparin)

Common
1. Headache
2. Nausea/vomiting
3. Anaemia
4. Rash
5. Constipation/diarrhoea

Excretion/metabolism
Half-life
- 17–21 hours

Metabolism
- Metabolism: minimal hepatic component
- Excretion: primarily renal

Starting dose
- **ACS:** 2.5 mg SC STAT then OD following
- **VTE prophylaxis:** 2.5 mg SC OD
- **VTE treatment:** <50 kg – 5 mg SC OD; 50–100 kg – 7.5 mg SC OD; >100 kg – 10 mg SC OD

Monitoring
- Not routinely required
- If an individual has high bleeding risk or risk of accumulation, unfractionated heparin should be considered as an alternative

36.4 WARFARIN

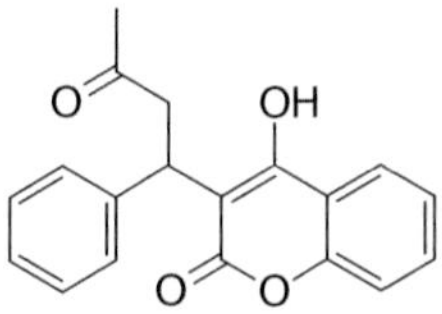

Figure 36.2 Structure of warfarin.

Pharmacology
- **Clotting factors:** warfarin has effects on factors II, VII, IX and X
- **Synthesis:** these clotting factors require conversion of glutamic acid residues to carboxyglutamic residues
- **Vitamin K:** a key co-factor for the enzyme which catalyses this process, during which it converted to its epoxide form
- **Vitamin K reductase:** catalyses the conversion of vitamin K back to the reduced form
- **Inhibition:** warfarin inhibits vitamin K reductase thereby depleting reduced vitamin K available
- **Route:** warfarin is readily absorbed enterally
- **Timing:** effect on prothrombin time (PT) is detectable after approximately 14 hours, peak effect takes 48 hours to develop due to the half-lives of factors II, VII, IX and X
- **Supplementation:** warfarin binds to vitamin K reductase competitively, additional vitamin K can not only reverse but also impair warfarin's effect
- **Anticoagulant factors:** proteins C and S are anticoagulant factors also dependent on vitamin K for production, their short half-lives mean warfarin can initially be pro-coagulant

Table **36.2** Half-lives of clotting
factors dependent on vitamin K

Clotting factor	Half-life (hours)
Factor II	60
Factor VII	6
Factor IX	24
Factor X	48
Protein C	8
Protein S	30

Indications
1. Atrial fibrillation
2. Metallic heart valves
3. Thromboembolic disease (PE, DVT, ventricular thrombus)
4. Pulmonary hypertension
5. Dilated cardiomyopathy

Contraindications
1. Active bleeding
2. Pregnancy (teratogenic in first trimester, risk of intracerebral haemorrhage (ICH) in later stages)
3. Severe hepatic dysfunction

Caution
1. **Bleeding risk:** see Box 36.1
2. **Sepsis:** high states of basal metabolic rate, increase degradation of clotting factors
3. **Thyrotoxicosis:** will increase degradation of clotting factors and increase warfarin's effect

Interactions
Many and various interactions, check with every new agent. Those listed here are a limited selection.

1. Increased bleeding risk with other anticoagulants, antiplatelets and NSAIDs
2. Alcohol and cranberry juice increase effect
3. Vitamin K-containing foods reduce effect (e.g. green vegetables)
4. Cephalosporins inhibit reduction of vitamin K. Other broad-spectrum antibiotics can reduce availability of vitamin K through suppression of gut flora

Box 36.4 Key agents increasing warfarin's effect

1. Alcohol (binge)
2. Amiodarone
3. Ciprofloxacin
4. Co-trimoxazole
5. Erythromycin
6. Metronidazole
7. Simvastatin

Box 36.5 Key agents to decrease warfarin's effect

1. Rifampicin
2. Carbemezapine
3. Phenytoin
4. Vitamin K

Side effects

Dangerous
1. Haemorrhage (especially intracranial)
2. Hepatoxicity
3. Skin necrosis

Common
1. Bruising
2. Rash/pruritus
3. Headache
4. Alopecia

Excretion/metabolism

Half-life
- Highly variable – aproximately 40 hours

Metabolism
- Hepatic cytochromes – CYP2C90

Starting dose
Loading – refer to local recommendations for loading.

Generally
- Load with 5 mg PO OD for 2 days then check INR and adjust
- **Acute thrombo-embolic disease:** cover with LMWH or heparin for at least 5 days and/or the INR is >2 for 24 hours
- **For other indications (e.g. AF):** LMWH cover is not necessary

Monitoring
- INR – based on laboratory PT ratio compared against international sensitivity index for laboratory's thromboplastin

---

Box 36.6   INR targets with warfarin use

1. Thromboembolic disease: 2–3
2. AF +/- valvular disease: 2–3
3. Mitral bioprosthetic heart valve: 2–3 for at least 3 months
4. Mechanical heart valve: normally 3–4

Reversal
- Dependent on the INR and nature of bleeding event (see Box 36.7)

Box 36.7   Reversal of warfarin

1. **If major bleeding, falling Hb, haemodynamically unstable:**
   - Vitamin K 5–10 mg IV
   - Prothrombin complex concentrate (PCC) 25–50 units/kg (not exceeding 3000 units)
   - Fresh frozen plasma (FFP) is suboptimal (give if PPC not available)
2. **Non major bleeding:**
   - Give vitamin K 1–3 mg IV
3. **Not bleeding, INR >5.0**
   - Hold two doses
   - Reduce maintenance dose
   - Look for cause
   - INR >8.0 give 1–5 mg oral vitamin K

Note: PCC will reverse INR in approximately 10 minutes, however its factors have a half-life (shortest = 6 hours). IV vitamin K will have effect in 6–8 hours.

- In all scenarios stop warfarin and restart when INR <5.0 with adjusted dose

36.5 NOVEL ORAL ANTICOAGULANTS

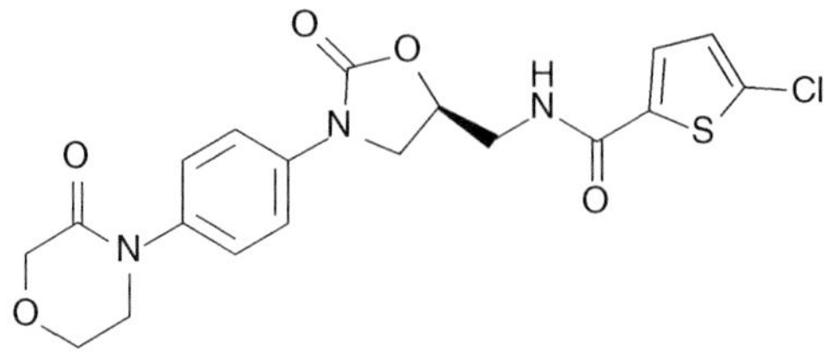

Figure 36.3 Structure of rivaroxaban.

Drug examples
- Dabigatran
- Rivaroxaban

Pharmacology
- **Dabigatran:** a direct thrombin inhibitor with good oral absorption and rapid onset
- **Rivaroxaban:** a factor Xa inhibitor, also with good oral absorption and rapid onset
- **Monitoring:** not required owing to more reliable pharmokinetics between patients and less effect by diet, alcohol, other medications
- **Shorter half-lives:** anticoagulant effect wears off quicker as a result

Indications
1. Established role for anticoagulation in AF
2. VTE treatment (rivaroxaban)
3. VTE prophylaxis following hip surgery (rivaroxaban)

Contraindications
1. Active bleeding
2. Severe renal impairment (creatinine clearance <15 mL/min)
3. Mechanical heart valves – significant increase in thrombotic events c.f. warfarin

Caution
1. **Bleeding risk**
2. **Dabigatran:** caution/dose adjustment necessary in renal impairment (contraindicated if creatinine clearance <30 mL/min)
3. **Rivaroxaban:** caution/dose adjustment necessary in both renal and hepatic impairment

Interactions
1. Increased bleeding risk with other anticoagulants, antiplatelets and NSAIDs
2. **Rivaroxaban:** potent hepatic cytochrome inhibitors, e.g ketoconazole, ritonavir, clarithromycin, increase levels and should not be co-prescribed
3. **Dabigatran:** interaction with potent hepatic enzyme inducers (e.g. St. John's wort, rifampin) which may decrease levels
4. **Amiodarone:** increases levels of both

Side effects
Dangerous
1. Haemorrhage

Common
1. **Dabigatran:** gastritis/dyspepsia
2. **Rivaroxaban:** nausea/vomiting, pruritis

Excretion/metabolism
Half-life
- **Dabigatran:** 12–14 hours
- **Rivaroxaban:** 5–9 hours (>75 years 11–13 hours)

Metabolism
- **Rivaroxaban:** mixed renal/hepatic (CYP3A4)
- **Dabigatran:** 80% renal excretion

Starting dose
- **Dabigatran:** AF – 150 mg PO BD (110 mg PO BD if age >80 years)
- **Rivaroxaban:** AF – 20 mg PO OD (15 mg if creatinine clearance <50 mL/min)

Monitoring
- Not routinely required
- **Rivaroxaban** – anti-Xa assay can be used
- **Dabigatran** – specific thrombin inhibitor assay is available

Box 36.8   Use of coagulation tests with novel oral anticoagulants

- Both drugs will often affect the PT or aPTT
- However, there is a non-linear relationship between effect on aPTT/PT and effect on clotting
- Thus PT and aPTT cannot reliably be used for monitoring
- aPTT is moderately sensitive for dabigatran at lower levels of the drug
- If aPTT is normal, can be inferred that there is minimal drug circulating and likely to be normal clotting

Reversal
- Activated factor VII/PCC may be considered in life-threatening overdose
- Limited benefit compared with FFP/PCC on warfarin
- However reversal is often not required if renal function is acceptable

KEY TRIALS

Key trial 36.1
Trial name: OASIS 5.
Participants: 20 000 patients ≥60 years admitted with biochemical or electrocardiographic evidence of cardiac ischaemia.
Intervention: Fondaparinux 2.5 mg OD.
Control: Enoxaparin 1 mg/kg.
Outcome: The fondaparinux group had significantly lower 30-day mortality (p = 0.02) mainly due to the lower incidence of major bleeding (hazard ratio 0.52, p < 0.001).
Reason for inclusion: Part of the evidence body underlying the preference for fondaparinux in ACS.
Reference: Yusuf S, et al. Comparison of fondaparinux and enoxaparin in acute coronary syndromes. N Engl J Med. 2006;354(14):1464–1476. http://www.nejm.org/doi/full/10.1056/NEJMoa055443.

Key trial 36.2
Trial name: OASIS 6.
Participants: 12 000 patients admitted with STEMI.
Intervention: Fondaparinux 2.5 mg OD for up to 8 days.
Control: Unfractionated heparin for 48 hours followed by placebo for up to 8 days or placebo throughout if UFH not indicated.
Outcome: Reduced death/re-infarction at 30 days in fondaparinux group (p = 0.008).
Reason for inclusion: With Key trial 36.1, these two studies underlie the choice for fondaparinux in ACS as it, in general, has comparable if not better effect and reduced major bleeding events.
Reference: Yusuf S, et al. Effects of fondaparinux on mortality and reinfarction in patients with acute ST-segment elevation myocardial infarction: the OASIS-6 randomized trial. JAMA. 2006;295(13);1519–1530. http://jama.jamanetwork.com/article.aspx?articleid= 202628.

Key trial 36.3

Trial name: RE-LY.

Participants: 18 000 patients with atrial fibrillation + $CHA_2DS_2VASc > 2$.

Intervention: Dabigatran 110 mg or 150 mg BD.

Control: Warfarin.

Outcome: Dabigatran group (150 mg) had a significantly lower incidence of stroke or systemic embolism (1.69% vs. 1.11%, $p < 0.001$). Risk of a major bleeding event was significantly reduced (110 mg group) (2.71% v 3.36%, $p = 0.003$).

Reason for inclusion: Major trial detailing the first novel oral anticoagulant released. Dabigatran 110 mg has comparable protection with reduced rate of major bleeding events, whereas dabigatran 150 mg has significantly better protection but with not significantly reduced rate of major bleeding events.

Reference: Connolly SJ, et al. Dabigatran versus warfarin in patients with atrial fibrillation. N Engl J Med. 2009;361(12):1139–1151. http://www.nejm.org/doi/full/10.1056/NEJMoa0905561.

For additional resources and to test your knowledge, visit the companion website at:

www.wiley.com/go/camm/cardiology

37 Antiplatelets

George Davies
Oxford University Hospitals NHS Trust, Oxford, UK

37.1 ASPIRIN

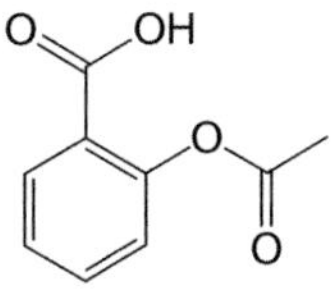

Figure 37.1 Structure of aspirin.

Pharmacology
- **Cyclo-oxygenase (COX) inhibitor:** aspirin primarily inhibits COX-1 (this is the only isoform found inside platelets)
- **Thomboxane A2 (TXA2):** COX-1 inhibition decreases production of TXA2 in platelets and prostaglandin I2 (PGI2) in the vascular endothelium
- **Aggregation:** TXA2 promotes platelet aggregation, PGI2 inhibits it
- **Vascular endothelial cells:** counter PGI2 production reduction by increasing production of COX-1 and by utilizing COX-2 (platelets cannot)
- **Irreversible:** the binding of aspirin to COX-1 is irreversible, platelet function does not recover until affected platelets are replaced (7–10 days)

Indications
1. Acute coronary syndrome
2. Prophylaxis of stable IHD
3. Post coronary stenting
4. Peripheral vascular disease

Contraindications
1. Active bleeding
2. Severe renal impairment (GFR <10 mL/min/1.73 m^2)
3. Severe liver failure
4. Haemophilia
5. Hypersensitivity to any NSAID
6. Avoid in children <16 years (Reye's syndrome)
7. Avoid if known GI ulcer (or give GI protection: proton-pump inhibitor)

Caution
1. Bleeding risk (see Box 36.1)
2. Asthma
3. Gout
4. Glucose-6-phosphate dehydrogenase (G6PD) deficiency
5. Uncontrolled hypertension
6. Surgical procedures (in general stop 7 days before)

Clinical Guide to Cardiology, First Edition. Edited by Christian F. Camm and A. John Camm.
© 2016 John Wiley & Sons, Ltd. Published 2016 by John Wiley & Sons, Ltd.
Companion website: www.wiley.com/go/camm/cardiology.

Interactions

1. Increased bleeding risk with other anticoagulants, antiplatelets and NSAIDs
2. Selective serotonin reuptake inhibitors (SSRIs) + venlafaxine: serotonin reuptake transport is also present on platelets, down- and upregulation can lead to anti- and pro-thrombotic states

Side effects

Dangerous

1. Haemorrhage
2. Acute kidney injury
3. Hepatoxicity
4. If overdosed may cause ototoxicity
5. Angioedema
6. Bronchospasm (in asthmatic patients)
7. GI ulceration

Common

1. Gastritis
2. Nausea

Excretion/metabolism

Half-life

- Low dose 2–3 hours, higher dose 15–30 hours

Metabolism

- Metabolism: hepatic – microsomal enzyme system
- Excretion: renal (80–100%)

Starting dose

- **ACS:** 300 mg PO/PR STAT, then 75 mg OD
- **Other indications:** 75 mg PO OD

37.2 CLOPIDOGREL

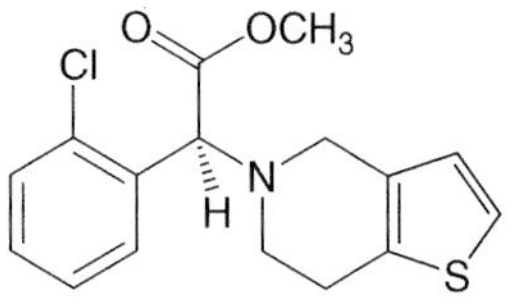

Figure 37.2 Structure of clopidogrel.

Pharmacology

- **ADP receptor:** clopidogrel is converted into an active metabolite which binds irreversibly to the ADP receptor on platelets (P2Y12)
- **ADP:** platelets respond to ADP and initiate activation and aggregation
- **Peak concentration:** occurs in approximately 60 minutes

Box 37.1   The metabolism of clopidogrel

- Clopidogrel is metabolized by CYP2C19 to its active form
- >50% of Asians have a genetic variant of CYP2C19 which inhibits clopidogrel metabolism
- PPIs can act to inhibit CYP2C19, decreasing formation of the active metabolite

Indications (cardiac)
1. Acute coronary syndrome
2. Prophylaxis of stable IHD
3. Post coronary stenting

Contraindications
1. Active bleeding
2. Severe hepatic impairment

Caution
1. Bleeding risk (see Box 36.1)
2. Surgical procedures (in general stop 7 days before)
3. Hepatic or renal impairment

Interactions
1. Increased bleeding risk with other anticoagulants, antiplatelets and NSAIDs
2. SSRIs + venlafaxine: serotonin reuptake transport is also present on platelets, down- and upregulation can lead to anti- and pro-thrombotic states
3. PPIs can reduce the efficacy of clopidogrel (minimal evidence)

Side effects
Dangerous
1. Haemorrhage
2. Bradycardia/dyspnoea
3. Pancreatitis
4. Neutropenia/aplastic anaemia
5. Thrombotic thrombocytopenic purpura
6. Acute liver failure/hepatitis

Common
1. Upper respiratory tract infection
2. Chest pain
3. Headache
4. Arthralgia
5. Diarrhoea
6. Dizziness
7. Fatigue
8. Rash

Excretion/metabolism
Half-life
- Parent drug: 6 hours
- Active metabolite: 30 minutes

Metabolism
- Metabolism: hepatic (CYP2C19 generates active metabolite)
- Excretion: urine (50%), faeces (45%)

Starting dose
- **ACS:** 300 mg (or 600 mg) PO STAT then 75 mg OD
- **Other indications:** 75 mg PO OD

37.3 NOVEL ANTIPLATELETS

Drug examples
- Ticagrelor
- Prasugrel

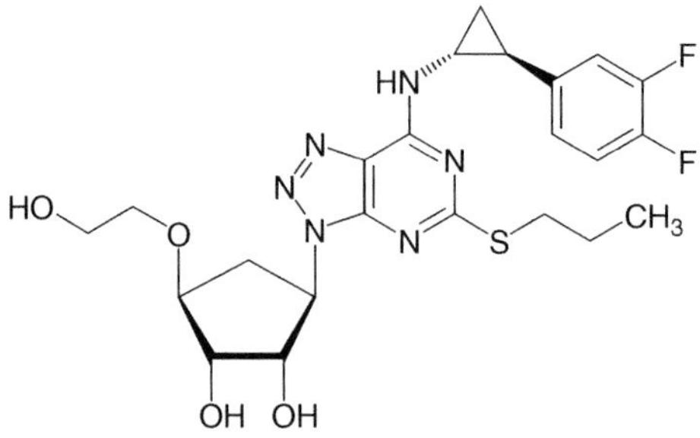

Figure 37.3 Structure of ticagrelor.

Pharmacology
- These agents are starting to replace clopidogrel for use in acute coronary syndromes
- **Prasugrel:** acts via an active metabolite which binds irreversibly to the same receptor as clopidogrel (P2Y12)
- **Faster onset:** prasugrel acts with faster onset (peak concentration, 30 minutes)
- **Ticagrelor:** acts directly as a reversible inhibitor of P2Y12
- **Mortality:** both agents significantly reduce mortality from cardiovascular causes at the expense of a significant increase in the risk of some bleeding events
- **Newer agents:** evolving opinion that these agents should be used preferentially in ACS and primary PCI
- **Clopidogrel:** used in those with cautionary factors for the newer agents and/or are at increased risk of bleeding events
- **P2Y12 inhibitors:** all have off-target effects causing dyspnoea and bradycardia, a significant issue with ticagrelor

Indications
1. Acute coronary syndrome
2. Primary coronary intervention

Contraindications
Prasugrel
1. Active bleeding
2. Prior stroke or TIA
3. Severe hepatic impairment
4. End-stage renal disease
5. Weight <60 kg

Ticagrelor
1. Active bleeding
2. History of intracranial haemorrhage
3. Severe hepatic impairment
4. Surgery: consider discontinuing 5 days prior
5. CABG: do not start if urgent CABG planned

Caution
- Bleeding risk (see Box 36.1)

Prasugrel
1. Age >75 years (increased risk of fatal bleeding)
2. Moderate hepatic impairment
3. End-stage renal disease

Ticagrelor
1. Asthma/COPD

Interactions
- Increased bleeding risk with other anticoagulants, antiplatelets and NSAIDs

Prasugrel
1. Potent inhibitors of CYP3A4/5 (e.g. ritonavir/indinavir) are contraindicated – they reduce drug effect (requires hepatic conversion to active metabolite)
2. Other liver enzyme inhibitors have not been shown to have an interaction

Ticagrelor
1. Cytochrome inhibitors (ketoconazole, clarithromycin, ciprofloxacin, verapamil, diltiazem) increase exposure
2. Cytochrome inducers may decrease effect
3. Statins: ticagrelor is a weak inhibitor of CYP3A (reduce dose of statin)
4. Digoxin, ciclosporin: ticagrelor is a weak inhibitor of p-glycoprotien (use with extreme caution)

Side effects
Dangerous
- Haemorrhage
- **Prasugrel:** rarely thrombotic thrombocytopenic purpura, liver dysfunction, haemolysis, bradycardia, dyspnoea
- **Ticagrelor:** dyspnoea, atrial fibrillation

Common
1. **Prasugrel:** rash/hypersensitivity, anaemia, headache
2. **Ticagrelor:** headache, cough, dizziness, chest pain

Excretion/metabolism
Half-life
- **Prasugrel:** 7 hours (range 2–15 hours)
- **Ticagrelor:** 7 hours (major metabolite 9 hours)

Metabolism
- **Prasugrel:** hydrolysed to active metabolite by CYP3A4 and CYP2B6
- **Ticagrelor:** CYP3A4 forms active metabolite, elimination of both via cytochrome and p-glycoprotein

Starting dose
- **Prasugrel:** 60 mg PO STAT, then 10 mg PO OD
- **Ticagrelor:** 180 mg PO STAT, then 90 mg PO BD

 For additional resources and to test your knowledge, visit the companion website at:

www.wiley.com/go/camm/cardiology

38 Lipid Regulation

George Davies

Oxford University Hospitals NHS Trust, Oxford, UK

The drug class of main relevance to cardiology in this section is HMG-CoA reductase inhibitors (statins). Drugs such as fibrates and bile acid sequestrants are used to lower blood lipid profiles but are reserved for specialist treatment of hyperlipidaemia.

38.1 STATINS

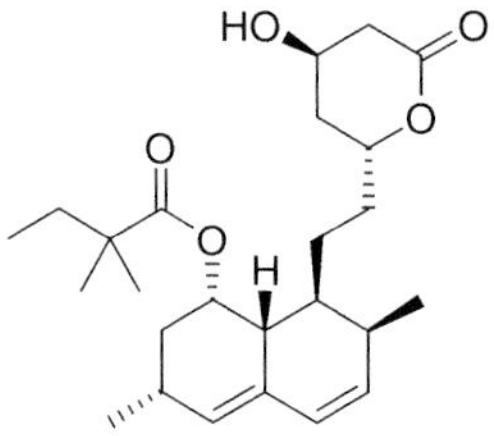

Figure 38.1 Structure of simvastatin.

Drug examples
- Simvastatin
- Atorvastatin
- Pravastatin

Pharmacology
- **Endogenous:** most plasma cholesterol is endogenously made; the rate limiter in synthesis is 3-hydroxy-3-methylglutaryl-coenzyme A (HMG-CoA)
- **Statins:** inhibit HMG-CoA and decrease cholesterol synthesis by the liver
- **LDL receptor:** reduction in cholesterol synthesis upregulates LDL receptor synthesis, increasing plasma LDL clearance
- **LDL reduction:** overall there is a reduction in LDL-C, a small increase in HDL-C and reduction in plasma triglyceride
- **IHD prevention:** the effect of lowering LDL-C is beneficial in both primary and secondary prevention
- **Off-target effects:** the subject of ongoing research and may lie behind some of their therapeutic benefits and adverse effects

Indications
1. Treatment of hypercholesterolaemia
2. Primary prevention of IHD
3. Secondary prevention of IHD
4. Familial hypercholesterolaemia

Contraindications
1. Liver failure (acute, chronic, deranged LFTs, caution in alcohol excess)
2. Acute porphyria
3. Pregnancy: evidence of neurological malformations (contraception 1 month before and after)
4. Concomitant use of strong CYP3A4 inhibitors

Clinical Guide to Cardiology, First Edition. Edited by Christian F. Camm and A. John Camm.
© 2016 John Wiley & Sons, Ltd. Published 2016 by John Wiley & Sons, Ltd.
Companion website: www.wiley.com/go/camm/cardiology.

Cautions
1. Hypothyroidism
2. Severe renal impairment (dose may need reduction)
3. Heavy alcohol use
4. History of liver disease
5. Age >65 years (increased risk of myopathy)

Interactions
1. **Fibrates, macrolides (erythro-/clarithromycin), ketoconazole, ciclosporin:** all increase statin levels and risk of myositis (should be stopped)
2. **Colchicine, amiodarone, verapamil, diltiazem and furanocoumarins:** caution for the same reasons

Side effects
Dangerous
1. Myositis (rhabomyolysis)
2. Hepatitis
3. Rarely pancreatitis
4. Angioedema

Common
1. Nausea
2. Headache
3. Rash
4. Myalgia
5. Abdominal pain
6. Constipation

Excretion/metabolism
Half-life
- **Simvastatin:** 2 hours
- **Atorvastatin:** 14 hours
- **Pravastatin:** 2.5–3 hours

Metabolism
- Metabolism: hepatic (CYP3A4)
- Excretion: faeces (60%), urine (15%)

Starting dose
- **Simvastatin:** 20 mg PO nocte (maximum 80 mg PO nocte)
- **Atorvastatin:** 10 mg PO nocte (maximum 80 mg PO nocte)
- **Pravastatin:** 10 mg PO nocte (maximum 40 mg PO nocte)

 For additional resources and to test your knowledge, visit the companion website at:

www.wiley.com/go/camm/cardiology

Index

Note: Page numbers in *italic* refer to figures, those in **bold** to tables.

Printed and bound by CPI Group (UK) Ltd, Croydon, CR0 4YY

27/10/2024

14580195-0003

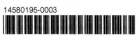